PSYCHIATRIC ASPECTS OF EPILEPSY

Contributors

David Bear, M.D.
Assistant Professor of Psychiatry, Harvard Medical School, Boston; and Staff Psychiatrist, New England Deaconess Hospital, Boston

Dietrich Blumer, M.D.
Chairman, Department of Psychiatry, Henry Ford Hospital, Detroit; and Clinical Professor of Psychiatry, University of Michigan School of Medicine

Shirley M. Ferguson, M.D., F.A.P.A.
Associate Professor of Psychiatry and Director, Section of Neuropsychiatry, Department of Psychiatry; and Associate Professor of Neuropsychiatry in Neurosciences and Director, Division of Behavioral Neurology, Department of Neurosciences, Medical College of Ohio, Toledo

Roy Freeman, M.D.
Instructor in Neurology, Harvard Medical School, Boston; Staff Neurologist, Beth Israel Hospital, Boston; and Fellow, Neuropsychiatry, New England Deaconess Hospital, Boston

Norman Geschwind, M.D.
James Jackson Putnam Professor of Neurology, Harvard Medical School, Boston; Professor of Psychology, Massachusetts Institute of Technology, Cambridge; and Director, Neurological Unit, Beth Israel Hospital, Boston

Mark Greenberg, Ph.D.
Instructor of Psychology in Psychiatry, Harvard Medical School, Boston; and Staff Psychologist, New England Deaconess Hospital, Boston

Jonathan M. Himmelhoch, M.D.
Professor of Psychiatry, University of Pittsburgh School of Medicine, Western Psychiatric Institute and Clinic, Pittsburgh

Ernst Niedermeyer, M.D.
Director of EEG and Adult Seizure Clinic, Johns Hopkins Hospital, Baltimore; and Associate Professor of Neurology and Neurological Surgery, Johns Hopkins University School of Medicine

Mark Rayport, M.D. C.M., Ph.D., F.A.C.S.
Professor of Neurological Surgery; Director, Division of Neurological Surgery; and Co-Chairman, Department of Neurosciences, Medical College of Ohio, Toledo

Ernst Rodin, M.D.
Medical Director, Epilepsy Center of Michigan, Detroit; and Professor of Neurology, Wayne State University, Detroit

A. Earl Walker, M.D.
Adjunct Professor, Department of Neurology and Neurosurgery, University of New Mexico School of Medicine, Albuquerque

Janusz J. Zielinski, M.D., D.Sci.
Director, Clinical Studies, Epilepsy Center of Michigan, Detroit

PSYCHIATRIC ASPECTS OF EPILEPSY

Edited by

Dietrich Blumer, M.D.

Chairman, Department of Psychiatry,
Henry Ford Hospital, Detroit; and
Clinical Professor of Psychiatry,
University of Michigan School of Medicine

American Psychiatric Press, Inc.

1400 K Street, N.W.
Washington, D.C. 20005

Note: The authors have worked to ensure that all information in this book concerning drug dosages, schedules, and routes of administration is accurate as of the time of publication and consistent with standards set by the U.S. Food and Drug Administration and the general medical community. As medical research and practice advance, however, therapeutic standards may change. For this reason and because human and mechanical errors sometimes occur, we recommend that readers follow the advice of a physician who is directly involved in their care or the care of a member of their family.

Cover design by Cindy Grooms
Text design by Tim Clancy and Richard E. Farkas
Typeset by VIP Systems, Inc.
Printed by R. R. Donnelley & Sons Co.

Library of Congress Cataloging in Publication Data
Main entry under title:
Psychiatric aspects of epilepsy.

Includes index.
1. Epilepsy—Psychological aspects. 2. Epilepsy—Patients—Mental health. 3. Psychiatry. I. Blumer, Dietrich.
[DNLM: 1. Epilepsy—Psychology. WL 385 P974]
RC372.P75 1984 616.8′53′0019 84-6236
ISBN 0-88048-024-6

Contents

Dedicated
to
Leopold Szondi

Introduction

If I wished to show a student the difficulties of getting at truth from medical experience, I would give him the history of epilepsy to read.

——Oliver Wendell Holmes (1891)

As we stand at the threshold of understanding the interface of behavior and its neural substrates, we are ignoring what is perhaps the most dramatic expression of that relationship. Together with the schizophrenic and manic-depressive disorders, epilepsy formed the triad of major psychiatric disorders referred to as "insanity" in the leading textbooks of the earlier part of this century. Our understanding of the cerebral substrate of the major psychoses has developed very slowly. In the case of epilepsy, with its obvious physical aspects, the psychiatric aspects have been largely forgotten and overlooked.

Epilepsy came to be part of neurology following the splendid early progress in the understanding of the neurologic aspects of epilepsy, pioneered by Hughlings Jackson and Hans Berger, and the subsequent success in the medical treatment of the most striking paroxysmal manifestations, the seizures. Moreover, with much improved seizure control, the previously most troublesome psychiatric disturbance, referred to as "postepileptic insanity" or "twilight state," which had so often required institutionalization, almost became a rarity. However, the wealth of more or less subtle mental changes associated with major forms of epilepsy is still present and can be identified.

Although a number of neurologists have made major contributions to our knowledge of the behavioral aspects of epilepsy, most, by nature of their interests and training, do not focus on the psychiatric aspects of their patients. Psychiatrists, on the other hand, have favored purely psychologic theories and treatment approaches for a long time, while ignoring the brain and anything labeled a "brain disease." Even modern, biologically oriented psychiatrists seem to be content to consider epilepsy outside their fields of expertise and interest. The neglect of the psychiatric aspects of epilepsy has been most marked in the United States with its high degree of medical specialization. Our modern textbooks of psychiatry still tend to show a singular lack of coverage of the psychiatric aspects of epilepsy compared with British and other European textbooks.

Three points need to be emphasized. First, no psychiatric disorder has ever been discovered through statistical methods. The reason for this is obvious: What clinicians recognize as a disorder distinct from all others known to them is invariably a complex entity that presents in many variations, with linkage to and overlap with other disorders, and defies mathematical formulations. Genetic and other biologic factors, psychodynamic scrutiny, and treatment response all need to be considered along with the premorbid findings, the clinical presentation, and the course of the illness. Once a homogeneous group is defined, then sufficiently large samples can be compared with other groups and statistically analyzed for similarities or differences in specific areas. The thorough understanding of the individual case represents the necessary basis for any meaningful group analysis, and in the field of psychiatry individual patients are usually not understood unless we can relate to them and elicit sufficient information from them. Thus, a skilled, sympathetic interview of a patient with temporal lobe epilepsy can reveal findings otherwise inaccessible.

Second, if we discuss epilepsy we must be aware that we are dealing with a variety of disorders. As much as 6–10 percent of the population suffers a seizure at one time or another, and the occurrence of seizures may simply point to the presence of one of many brain diseases or metabolic disorders. Then there are forms of epilepsy that do not involve the limbic system, are not associated with any emotional changes, and tend to have a benign course with early remission. Although there appear to be many mild forms of temporal lobe epilepsy, this seizure disorder tends to be chronic and, as a rule, is complicated by various degrees of psychic peculiarities; it corresponds to the disorder previously termed "genuine epilepsy." One is tempted to differentiate an "epileptiform reaction" from an "epileptiform process." However, the line between the benign epileptic reaction and the less benign temporal lobe epileptic process is not easily drawn.

Finally, those devoted to the well-being of epileptic patients are well justified in being concerned with removing the stigma of insanity and violence from epilepsy. A majority of patients with epilepsy suffer from few if any psychiatric problems. The previously common "postepileptic insanity," feared for its association with the "epileptic furor," has been nearly abolished. However, there remain highly significant mental changes that can be particularly related to temporal lobe seizure disorders. The bias against any relationship between epilepsy and psychiatry presupposes that psychiatric disorders must be considered shameful and more or less intractable. Nobody refrains from mentioning the fact that there are malignant forms of hypertension because this would give benign hypertension a bad name and blemish those who suffer from the disease. In fact, by concentrating on malignant hypertension, so much progress has been made that the number of sufferers from the more critical form of the disease has been significantly reduced.

We are convinced that substantial progress can likewise be made in the field of epilepsy by concentrating on its psychic aspects. The often-debated proportion of epileptics who require psychiatric intervention is of interest, but is irrelevant as far as the needs to understand the role of epilepsy in their psychiatric problems and to render better treatment are concerned.

This volume is clinically oriented and includes many illustrative cases. It is a book for neurologists and all health professionals dealing with epileptic patients. In particular, it is a book for every psychiatrist and clinical psychologist, because it describes disorders that tend to go undetected, and because it addresses a dimension of the mind that is still poorly understood.

The history of epilepsy, reviewed in the first chapter, presents a fascinating record of the human understanding and prejudices about one illness. The view of epilepsy as a supernatural possession, so popular in the Middle Ages, is still encountered (see Chapter 6), but may be safely rated a superstition. The current official bias is that of considering solely the physical at the expense of the psychic aspects of the disease. Chapter 1 relates what Taylor and Marsh were able to reveal about a pivotal historic case, Hughlings Jackson's Dr. Z; it sets forth Kraepelin's observations on epilepsy prior to the era of modern anticonvulsants; and then it delineates the efforts of Gastaut and Szondi toward an integration of the mental, neural, and genetic factors in epilepsy. It includes a discussion of the sometimes very potent psychotropic effects of the anticonvulsant carbamazepine.

The epidemiologic chapter by Janusz Zielinski, which had to be based on much data that did not qualify the different forms of epilepsy, conveys knowledge of the scope of the disorder. The reports of a high incidence of suicide among epileptics and his own finding that temporal lobe epilepsy frequently eludes diagnosis are of particular significance to us.

Ernst Niedermeyer's chapter on the neurologic aspects of epilepsy details the various forms of seizure disorders, their etiologies, the role of age, the focal aspects, and the diagnostic procedures. Ernst Rodin has contributed one chapter on differential diagnosis and another on anticonvulsants and the medical treatment of epilepsy.

David Bear, Roy Freeman, and Mark Greenberg discuss the behavioral alterations in patients with temporal lobe epilepsy and have included a section on the pitfalls in the assessment of these alterations, a neuropsychologic section, and a discussion of therapeutic approaches. Shirley Ferguson and Mark Rayport describe psychosis in epilepsy, which has been termed "schizophrenia-like" but is very different from schizophrenia proper; the chapter includes rich case material.

Jonathan Himmelhoch's chapter breaks new ground. His observation that as much as 10 percent of the population of an affective disorder clinic suffers from mood disorders related to epileptic changes is of importance to every psychiatrist. My own experience confirms the soundness of Himmelhoch's findings. It has to be clearly recognized that some of these patients will show only very subtle neurologic signs of epilepsy and that the major diagnostic criteria presently are those of highly labile moods ("rapid cycling") and other mental changes characteristic for temporal lobe epilepsy. The importance of Himmelhoch's findings is highlighted by the fact that these formerly intractable patients tend to respond, often remarkably well, to anticonvulsant treatment.

The long-term study by A. Earl Walker and myself of a series of temporal lobe epileptic patients surgically treated attempts to relate what are often dramatic behavioral changes to the changes in the neural substrate. The findings tend to confirm Gastaut's concept of a specific temporal lobe syndrome.

As Szondi has pointed out, the characteristic mental changes associated with epilepsy are but extraordinary variants of basic human needs and conflicts. The heightened and labile emotionality of temporal lobe epileptics, with its extremes of intense anger at one pole and hyperethical and hyperreligious fervor at the other, is brilliantly depicted in the world of characters brought to life for everybody by the genius of Dostoievsky. Norman Geschwind's chapter, the final one of this book, relates Dostoievsky's epilepsy to his biography and to his writings.

I must acknowledge a great debt of gratitude to the editorial assistance rendered by Diana Maslanka. Barbara Ahlberg also assisted very competently with the editing of portions of this volume. Barbara Klinger gave untiring assistance in the typing, correction, and assembling of parts of the manuscript.

This volume is dedicated to Leopold Szondi, to whom I owe much for his concepts and his inspiration.

Dietrich Blumer, M.D.

1

The Psychiatric Dimension of Epilepsy: Historical Perspective and Current Significance

Dietrich Blumer, M.D.

THE HISTORY OF EPILEPSY THROUGH THE NINETEENTH CENTURY (SYNOPSIS OF *THE FALLING SICKNESS* BY OWSEI TEMKIN)

> *Showing both physical and psychic symptoms, epilepsy more than any other disease was open to interpretation both as a physiological process and as the effect of spiritual influences.*
>
> —Owsei Temkin, *The Falling Sickness*

Temkin's masterful history of epilepsy in Western civilization (1) begins with the Hippocratic collection of medical writings, dating to about the year 400 B.C., and extends to the age of Hughlings Jackson, the beginnings of modern neurology. This synopsis is entirely indebted to Temkin's scholarly classic.

Antiquity

The Hippocratic book *On the Sacred Disease* describes epilepsy as a hereditary disease seated in the brain and represents the first record of the battle between magic beliefs and their refutation by scientific physicians (2). Wherever epilepsy is mentioned in the Hippocratic corpus, it is never viewed as a supernatural disturbance. The assumption of the divine character of the disease is attributed to the inexperience and amazement of people to whom it seemed quite different from all other diseases.

The name "sacred disease" for epilepsy has survived in some parts of the world to this day, but its origin is somewhat a mystery. The ancients themselves proffered a great variety of speculations about the meaning of the term. Plato (3) in *Timaeus* thought the name was justified because the disease disturbed the revolutions in the head, and these were the most divine. Others assumed the disease was called sacred or divine on account of its greatness, "for the crowd has called great things sacred" (4). The Hippocratic corpus already used the name "great disease" for epilepsy, a term that over the Latin "morbus maior" found its way into medieval French as "grand mal." Temkin lists the beliefs that a deity had sent the disease, that a demon had been thought to enter the patient, and that it attacked those who had sinned against the goddess of the moon as more authentic explanations, and then states: "At the bottom of these alleged reasons lies the basic belief that the disease is an infliction or possession by a higher power and that its cure must be supernatural. . . . What is seized by gods or demons may also be 'sacred' in the sense of inspiring fear. It may be abhorred and fled from, just as the epileptic was. The 'sacred disease' would then be an 'awesome disease' and the epileptic an untouchable person, 'taboo' particularly during his attacks."

The physicians of antiquity equated epilepsy with the sacred disease, and differentiated this disease from hysterical attacks as well as from madness. To the ancients the epileptic was an object of horror and disgust rather than a saint or a prophet as has sometimes been contended. Thus, Pliny (5) wrote, "In cases of epilepsy we spit, that is, we throw back contagion." The warped notion that epilepsy was a contagious disease and the interpretation of the disease as a sign of sin made the sight of a paroxysm even more repulsive, thus rendering epilepsy a disgraceful disease.

> The epileptic who felt an attack coming on rushed home or to a deserted place . . . and covered his head. And whether he did it from shame for the disease, as the author of *On the Sacred Disease* thinks, or from fear of the deity, as the crowd believed, his behavior was the same as that of the murderer who fled, his head covered (1, p 9).

In Euripides' *Madness of Hercules* (6) the hero is confused and has illusions during which he kills his wife and children. Then he falls to the ground and sleeps. Finally, he awakens cured, but with no memory of the whole episode. Similar actions of epileptics during twilight states were related in the psychiatric literature from the nineteenth century on. Interpretation of the ancient term "Herculean Disease" as epilepsy, however, is not securely founded.

The term "epilepsy" is of Greek origin, from the verb "epilambanein"—to seize or to attack. With the magical concept of epilepsy as the demoniac disease par excellence, the term may have come to signify epileptic seizure specifically. Early rational explanations stated that epilepsy earned its name because it "attacks" both the senses and mind of the victim. The term "epileptic" referred to the attacks and the afflicted, but the term "epilepsy" meaning the underlying disease was not used by the Hippocratic physicians.

Aretaeus (7) recognized epilepsy as an illness of varying form and horror. Epilepsy was defined by Galen (8) as "a seizure of the mind and the senses together with a sudden fall, in some with convulsions, in others, however, without convulsions." To some of the ancient physicians, the convulsions seemed entirely incidental. Vertigo had been called "a little epilepsy" by very early sources, and other minor attacks were well known to the ancient physicians.

Many types of subjective experience at the onset of an attack, tactile, sensory, motor, and psychic aura, were known in antiquity. The word "aura," meaning "a breeze," was introduced to medical terminology by a patient examined by Galen (8). A 13-year-old boy described his condition as originating in the lower leg and climbing upward through thigh, flank, and side to the neck and as far as the head; as soon as it touched his neck he was no longer able to follow it. When he was asked what exactly rose up to the head, he could not tell. But another youth said "that it was like a cold breeze." The peculiar undefinable nature of the primictal experience is thus recorded at the earliest time, and its approximation by the term "aura" became well established.

Associated with the attacks were mental changes that are familiar to the modern reader: "The mind is anxious and troubled, and they are readily roused to anger for no major reason. There is forgetfulness for what has been done shortly beforehand and a ready disposition for things causing gloom. . . . They are listless and go about accustomed tasks with sluggish movements; they have a feeling of heaviness and are sleepy and depressed" (4). With chronicity of the disease the whole personality of the patients would be affected. Because of the torpidity of their comprehension and their senses, they became languid, spiritless, unsociable, sleepless, and slow to learn (7).

It was well recognized that epilepsy tended to impair the mind. A particular kinship to melancholia is alleged in the Hippocratic saying that "most melancholics usually also become epileptics, and epileptics melancholics. One or the other [condition] prevails according to where the disease leans: if towards the body, they become epileptics, if towards reason, melancholics" (2). The differential diagnosis of epilepsy from mental diseases, however, was not detailed.

Epilepsy was viewed as an idiopathic disease of the brain, and in those cases where the patients noticed the upward movement of the aura, a sympathetic involvement of the brain originating from a primary peripheral lesion was assumed. The symptomatic nature of many seizures was not understood.

Treatment was often directed at the locus of the aura. Dietetic and pharmacologic treatments were employed; purgatives, exercises, and changes of climate were prescribed; and phlebotomy was practiced. Wrath and sexual intercourse were viewed as having deleterious effects. The best chances of treatment were offered when the attacks originated in the hands and feet and the patients were young and fond of work, not mentally impaired nor victims of apoplexy (2).

The Middle Ages

In the medieval literature of many European nations, the terms "falling evil" and "falling sickness" were used for epilepsy. Like the older names "sacred disease," "epilepsy," and "morbus comitialis," these medieval terms were of popular origin. The term "falling evil" or "morbus caducus," however, like other medieval terms ("morbus demoniacus" and "morbus lunaticus"), was less precise and referred not only to epilepsy, but to all kinds of morbid conditions characterized by a sudden fall of the victim.

From about the beginning of the Christian era, epilepsy became increasingly associated with periodic ecstasies, raptures, and prophetic trances comprehended vaguely under the name of "possession." A hitherto normal individual became possessed by a god, demon, or ghost and behaved like a willing or reluctant instrument of the intruder. Possession expressed itself from crude convulsions, by which an evil spirit seemed to torment its victim, to an exalted state of inspiration, when a deity revealed past and future through the mouth of a prophet.

Intrusive possession was not described in the writings from ancient Greece. With the extension of Oriental religions and demonologies, its occurrence became increasingly accepted in the

West, and was rarely doubted during the Middle Ages and Renaissance. The difficult question of whether a person afflicted with the falling evil was possessed or was suffering from epilepsy as a natural disease was thus posed.

The educated class of pagan society, whose notions have been transmitted to us, looked with disdain upon the display of violent emotions, including those of religious life. Aristotle (9) had compared incontinence to epilepsy. The trembling, moving, and yet paralyzed limbs of an angry man reminded some stoic philosophers of the same symptoms in epilepsy (10), and it was thought best to remain calm or, if angered, to run and hide, just as one did if he felt the approach of an epileptic attack (11). Such people, if confronted with a case of possession and cure by exorcism, would not be so easily impressed as to confound it with a natural disease like epilepsy.

The biblical story of Jesus delivering a boy from the attacks of a foul spirit became of great importance for many centuries to come (Mark 9:14–29; Matt. 17:14–20; Luke 9:37–43). The boy showed all the main symptoms of epilepsy recognized by the ancient physicians: The intruding spirit cries, but is otherwise dumb and deaf; during the attack the boy foams, grinds his teeth, is convulsed; the attacks have dated from childhood, and the boy may fall into fire or water; after the attack he falls into a state of coma. Since this miracle was performed by none other than Jesus, the naturalistic explanation of the physicians for such cases was hitherto rejected, and the popular belief that epileptics are possessed by demons formed itself into an accepted body of lay opinion.

Epilepsy was also widely associated with the moon, and an epileptic was sometimes defined as one seized by "the disease of the moon." The term "lunatic," however, referred to all abnormal states that manifested themselves at more or less regular intervals, especially those affecting the mind. The association of epilepsy, possession, madness, and similar states with the moon and other stars can be seen in the astrologic literature of the time. The confusion of epilepsy with possession and mental disorders prevailed into the later centuries of the Middle Ages.

St. Hildegard of Bingen (12) distinguished two kinds of epilepsy, depending on the moral character of the sufferers. The first kind would occur in people with an angry look and wrathful movements. When they were angered by some worldly troubles, the devil would notice it and frighten them with his suggestions, whence their soul would succumb and as a result the body would fall down and remain thus until the soul restored its strength. The second kind of epilepsy was more easily cured. It would affect people of attractive look and gentle gestures but with unstable and easy morals.

The account of Abulqasim, an Arabic physician (c. 1000 A.D.), of how he came to believe in a demoniac form of epilepsy is interesting (13). He had long doubted the symptoms that pointed to such a cause, until the matter was demonstrated to him. Among the many forms of the disease he had seen was that of people who fell down, whose appearance changed, who talked in a tongue formerly unknown to them, and read books, wrote, and talked about scientific matters of which they had hitherto been ignorant. The similarity to modern descriptions of the mental changes peculiar to some temporal lobe epileptics is striking.

Through the Middle Ages, the role of the humors and vapors was further emphasized. Magic and religious forms of treatment, however, were now more prevalent than in antiquity. On the other hand, there were clear distinctions between major and minor forms of epilepsy (i.e., with and without convulsions), and the role of inheritance was much more emphasized than it had been in the writings of the ancients.

At a time when even the educated were inclined to mistake a disease for demoniac possession, it was no small merit that the medieval physicians kept alive the tradition of epilepsy as a natural disease caused by natural factors. However, the Middle Ages added little to the physiologic understanding of epilepsy.

The Renaissance

Toward the end of the fifteenth century, physicians began to discuss the possibilities of possession, magic, and witchcraft more freely. Furthermore, during the sixteenth century physicians moved away from traditional medical views, and a large body of new facts, both clinical and anatomic, was accumulated.

In the discussions of the sphere of influence of Satan and his evil helpers on the human mind and body, epilepsy often stood in the center of the debate because of its peculiar relation to the various forms of possession. Thus, Jean Taxil, physician at Arles, maintained that it was scarcely possible to find any case in the literature of a demoniac who was not epileptic; that in the fury of their affliction, the possessed were seized by epileptic convulsions (14). Priests and physicians debated the differential diagnosis between epilepsy and possession. Natural causes, i.e., the influence of humors and vapors, were often assumed. An unusual clinical picture and the futility of rational treatment suggested a malign influence. If patients began to speak or understand foreign languages, of if they prophesied, the matter was clear beyond doubt. Many temporal lobe epileptics must have been taken for demoniacs.

Some believed the actual disease epilepsy could be brought about by witchcraft and allied powers of hell. Johann Weyer and other physicians of the sixteenth century opposed superstition and refuted the accusation of witchcraft by emphasizing the natural symptoms of epilepsy in alleged cases of possession.

Epileptic visions and raptures could be explained naturally, or as the influence of demons, or they could be accepted as divine inspirations. Some believed that the minds of epileptics might transcend to heaven and thus defended epileptic prophets against the charge of demoniac possession. Antonius Guainerius (15) cited the case of such a young epileptic prophet: "I have seen a certain choleric young man who said that during his paroxysms he always saw wondrous things which he very much wished to set down in writing, for without doubt he expected them to come to pass. For this reason the ancients called this disease divination."

Some people credited the disease with inducing dissociation, allowing the soul to develop mantic power in the ecstatic states of disease. The prophet Mohammed, with his visions and inspirational states, was considered an epileptic by Western historians, theologians, and physicians, an opinion that was branded by others as an absurd slander of Christian origin. Taxil (14) listed the Sibyls and Saul (St. Paul) among the prophesying epileptics.

Drusus, Julius Caesar, Caligula, and the emperor Charles V were statesmen listed with a degree of certainty as great epileptics, together with the poet Torquato Tasso. In an extension of the old thesis that melancholy and genius went together, there was also a belief that most epileptics were men of great intelligence (14).

Nevertheless, epilepsy in general was looked upon as a heinous disease through the centuries. The illness was considered difficult to treat, and the epileptic was considered by many a poor wretch, deserving pity, compassion, and special consideration. Some beggars, therefore, found it profitable to pose as epileptics. Others feigned epilepsy to evade punishment.

Beginning with the Renaissance, a renewed interest in individual cases kept the physicians in touch with reality. Attention was paid to head injuries preceding the onset of epilepsy. The occurrence of seizures with syphilis and other diseases was noted, and the concept of symptomatic epilepsy was formed around 1600 (16).

The affinity between vertigo and epilepsy was stressed anew. Instances of epileptic attacks were related in which the patients had neither fallen to the ground nor suffered from convulsions or vertigo. Benivenius (17) was one of the first to describe the occurrence of an epileptic automatism with amnesia in a man who later began to suffer from typical epileptic attacks. It was no longer deemed necessary for the whole body to convulse or even for the patient to fall to the ground. Slight movements of the head or the feet, or perhaps a scarcely noticeable contraction of the lips together with a short state of confusion, might be the only symptoms. The differential diagnosis between epilepsy and hysteria was further refined.

A number of observations confirmed the opinion that epilepsy was due to an irritation of the brain by some poisonous substance. The idea of irritation as the fundamental cause stood in the foreground after the beginning of the seventeenth century.

The Seventeenth and Eighteenth Centuries

Some iatrochemists of the Renaissance had already attempted to give the vague notion of poisonous vapors a more concrete chemical meaning, blaming the vitriolic vapor of mercury. A real break with tradition set in with the development of the great chemical systems of Sylvius and Willis, on the one hand, and with the iatrophysicists, on the other.

Sylvius (1614–72) assumed acid spirits or vapors to be the main factor in epilepsy, irritating the spinal cord and brain and mingling fatally with the animal spirits (18). The former action explained the convulsive motions, the latter the mental symptoms of epilepsy. Willis (1622–75) assumed the existence of a "spasmodic explosive copula" to explain paroxysms (19). Well acquainted with the experimental work of his time, he knew that irritation of the spinal nerves with a knife would bring about a response in the muscles. In epilepsy, a strong spasmodic copula being distilled from the blood in the brain, the animal spirits that lie in the middle of the brain would be affected and would explode. This would cause all the mental symptoms of the epileptic attack, and a series of similar explosions occurring along the rest of the nervous system would bring about the convulsions of the body. Willis was among the first to point out that the initial symptoms of seizures did not correspond to some lesion or corruption in the particular part of the body, but that their cause very often resided in the brain.

The epileptic attack was then viewed by the iatrochemists chiefly as a necessary result of chemical forces. The seizure was not seen as a purposeful act, but as a physical consequence. The iatrophysical school, on the other hand, with Baglivi as its most radical representative, developed a great number of mechanical explanations of epilepsy, e.g., a disturbed elastic equilibrium of fibers or pressure in blood vessels.

Toward the end of the seventeenth century, opposition to a purely mechanical physiology and pathology began to gain momentum. There was a renewed emphasis upon a teleologic principle, and the epileptic attack was viewed as a purposeful and essentially beneficial reaction of the soul or of "nature." This movement reached a climax with the animism of Stahl.

Wepfer (1620–95) had anticipated Stahl's doctrine of convulsions and epilepsy (20). This Swiss physician had investigated the action of poisons, particularly the irritative effects of hemlock. Having observed spasms and convulsions in various cases, Wepfer posed the question of whether epilepsy could be explained by irritative agents that resulted from diseases like syphilis and cancer. His answer was negative, since in reality these diseases were rarely complicated by epilepsy. Wepfer therefore assumed the existence of a higher selective principle that he referred to as "president" (archeus) of the nervous system. According to Stahl (1660–1734) it was the soul that ruled the living body (21). Mechanical stimuli may provoke epileptic convulsions as a purposeful reaction, but some idea generated by wrath or anxiety expresses itself through the disturbed motions and lies at the bottom of the disease. The causes of the epileptic seizure do not come from outside but lie inside the human organism; its true architects are sufferings of the soul brought about by anxious and terrifying "prefigurations." The fact that convulsions were seen so often in psychic disturbances was one of the main arguments for their moral rather than mechanical origin.

In England a process commonly called "Enlightenment" began in the late seventeenth century. The Enlightenment followed the intense religious excitement of the Puritan age, and slowly spread to other countries. A new type of physician began to assume a leading role in this period: a scientifically trained and scientifically interested practitioner who was an eclectic rather than a dogmatist, a classical scholar, yet progressive and inclined toward contempt for the Middle Ages.

Through the second half of the seventeenth century, most physicians did not exclude the infliction of epilepsy by the devil and witches. After all, Christ had cured the lunatic boy who was possessed by an unclean spirit and who had obviously been an epileptic. The scholar of the Enlightenment now allowed only biblical exceptions, and the final step in the progress of enlightened medicine was the denial of demoniac influence even in the biblical cases. The miracle consisted in Christ's curing natural diseases immediately by the mere command of his voice and thus superseding the laws of nature.

Thus, persons deemed possessed were again seen as suffering from a nervous disease—an answer as old as the book *On the Sacred Disease*. However, there were no consistent or clear definitions of hysterical or hypochondriacal, of ecstatic or convulsive disorders. The practical distinction between hysteria and epilepsy was often very difficult. Individuals with temporal lobe epilepsy were diagnosed as hysterical cases (22), whereas epidemics of ecstatic convulsive states were mistaken as epileptic in nature. On the other hand, writings as early as the middle of the eighteenth century document the diagnosis of hysterical paroxysms based on the astute observation of the preserved responses of the pupils to light and darkness (23).

The confirmation by Newtonian physics of the physical influence of celestial bodies upon the earth seemed to offer a new mechanical basis for the assumed relationship between the moon and epilepsy. Tissot (1728–97) rejected the chimeric influences of the moon but established a new superstition (24, 25): For more than a century and a half, masturbation figured as one of the main causes of epilepsy in medical literature. Sexual excesses as well as, in some individuals, excessive continence were again alleged to bring about epilepsy, as had been variously assumed since antiquity. In spite of his major misconceptions, Tissot was apparently the first to describe petit mal (24).

Continuing with ancient traditions, the medieval physician ordered diet, drugs, cauterization (application of a hot iron, usually to several places on the head), and trephining. These methods remained in use. From the sixteenth century on, but particularly in the seventeenth, the number of old and medieval specifics had been largely supplemented by chemical preparations, very often of an equally doubtful character. The change in therapeutics in the eighteenth century manifested itself most strikingly in the rejection of occult "specifics" (mistletoe, elk's foot, and peony root, among many others, had been considered antiepileptics) in favor of drugs.

The Nineteenth Century

1800–1860. Once the former prisons for the insane began to assume the character of asylums or hospitals, around the time of

Pinel (1745–1826), confined epileptics became the object of systematic medical attention. Epileptics who were insane, or not tolerated by society for other reasons, had been confined with the insane, and it was only around the middle of the nineteenth century that their segregation in separate wards of lunatic asylums became the established procedure. Slowly thereafter special institutions for epileptics were established in various places.

Maisonneuve had been stimulated by his teacher, Pinel, to study epilepsy at the Salpêtrière, under the new and more favorable conditions. In his book published in the year 12 of the French Revolution (1804), he gave programmatic expression to this principle of investigation: "And first of all, epilepsy, like all chronic diseases, can be studied well only in the hospitals; there alone is it possible to find all its varieties together, to see it in all its nuances, and to acquire in short time more experience of this disease than in the whole course of ordinary practice" (26). Most of the studies of epilepsy that appeared in France and England during the following years were conducted by physicians who were closely connected with hospitals for the insane, asylums for epileptics, or epileptic wards of general hospitals. A new terminology was established, statistics were increasingly used, and the psychiatric side of epilepsy received much more attention.

The fully developed seizure was referred to as "grand mal." Passing mental confusions with no definite physical symptoms were characterized as "absences." "Epileptic vertigo" tended to include mental aspects of epilepsy, whereas "petit mal" remained a convenient term for the great variety of attacks that did not have the character of grand mal. Calmeil (27), who had introduced the term "absence," seems to have been the first author to differentiate between severe seizures and "état de mal" (status). Galen's old concept of the aura as an ascending cold breeze was discredited when the rarity of this initial seizure event was noted. Physicians began to list sensory, sensitive, psychic, and motor auras.

Statistical methods were employed to study the influence on epilepsy of heredity, the age at onset, the role of menstruation, and various other "determining causes." Violent passions such as fear, wrath, and sadness were listed as causes of epilepsy. These early studies are solely of historic interest.

Esquirol and Calmeil, attempting to determine the frequency of mental disturbances, studied the case histories of 385 women located in a ward for epileptics. From this number 46 had to be deducted as suffering from hysteria. Of the remaining 339 epileptic women, 12 suffered from monomania, 30 from mania (some with tendency to suicide), 34 from fury, 145 were demented, 8 idiots, 50 showed periodic loss of memory, exalted ideas, etc., and the remaining 60 were marked only by peculiarities of character (28). Esquirol claimed that minor attacks (epileptic vertigo) had a much stronger influence upon the brain (i.e., the mind) than grand mal, a thesis upheld by many later authorities.

Among the psychiatric complications mentioned by Esquirol, none was studied so carefully and assumed such far-reaching importance as the furor epilepticus ("epileptic mania," "epileptic delirium"). The "raving fits" of lunatics had been found associated with epileptic symptoms by some writers since the latter part of the seventeenth century (29). This aspect had been neglected formerly for two reasons: The existence of epileptic attacks was overlooked and the case considered one of "furor," "delirium," or "mania" without reference to epilepsy; and epileptics had been believed possessed, in which case they were cited before the spiritual rather than the civil powers. The furor epilepticus was generally observed following the seizures, but was also noticed preceding them or in the absence of any classic seizure. Furor epilepticus was dangerous; patients in this condition might even commit murder, and the forensic significance was very important.

The concept of what was later termed "psychic equivalents" was anticipated by Prichard (30) in his discussion of somnambulic and ecstatic states: "Where they do not coexist with epilepsy, they often seem to stand in the place of it, and to depend on those particular circumstances of the constitution which are the fundamental causes of epilepsy." Not much later Meyer (31) observed that maniacal states might increasingly and vicariously become the chief manifestation upon cessation of the convulsions. The same author considered transitory states of heightened vivacity and rhetorical prowess as possible epileptic equivalents.

In 1825 Bouchet and Cazauvieilh (32) found hardening of the brain in 11 cases among 18 autopsies performed on mentally ill epileptics, documenting for the first time the presence of Ammon's horn sclerosis (medial temporal sclerosis) in such patients. Induration of the Ammon's horn was noted in four cases, softening in one. This finding would continue to be of crucial importance in the debate over the localization of higher nervous functions.

During the second third of the century, it was realized that observations made in hospitals did not necessarily give a true picture of the disease. In 1852 Theodore Herpin (1799–1865) reported his observations of private patients, arriving at a much more optimistic view than had prevailed (33). Physiologic theories focused on the roles of reflex action, cerebral angiospasm, and changes in the molecular state of the brain through malnutrition or poisoning. Reynolds (34) proposed a more restricted use of the term "epilepsy," implying only those cases that, in the present state of medical science, were irreducible. Only idiopathic epilepsy was to be called "epilepsy." Localized seizures and attacks with preserved consciousness were excluded. This explains why Hughlings Jackson called such attacks "epileptiform."

Herpin had shown great faith in the antiepileptic effects of zinc oxide. Shortly thereafter, bromide of potassium was introduced and became the first true antiepileptic drug.

Jackson's Forerunners. The chain of those who noted partial seizures goes as far back as the Hippocratic corpus and Aretaeus. In the nineteenth century, several authors preceded Hughlings Jackson with important observations of Jacksonian fits and temporal lobe epilepsy.

Bravais in 1827 published a thesis under the title of *Investigations on the Symptoms and the Treatment of Hemiplegic Epilepsy* (35). However, he did not venture an explanation of the causes of the unilateral seizures he had described. Only a few years later, Bright (36, 37) combined the clinical and anatomic approaches and reached conclusions that made him one of the closest forerunners of Jackson. Bright studied cases of "Jacksonian epilepsy," observed their connection with impaired sight, paresthesia, and weakness of the convulsed parts, noticed the presence of consciousness, and associated these symptoms with local lesions affecting the surface of the brain (membranes and cortex) on the side opposite to the one convulsed.

Two French psychiatrists and directors of asylums, Benedict Augustin Morel (1809–1879) and Jules Falret (1824–1902), were particularly concerned with the epileptic who had committed acts of violence. Of Morel, his friend Lasègue said, "One must do justice to him and admit that he was the first, or one of the first, to discern the epileptic within epilepsy; and instead of limiting himself to the description of the attacks, he has recounted the biography of the patient" (38).

Morel (39) found irritability and anger to be salient features of the epileptic character. Any trifle could provide "epileptic anger," which might last 1–2 hrs and repeat itself again and again during the day. But there also existed epileptic fury, which appeared in two forms: either in continuity with an epileptic attack, i.e., preceding or following it, or without such continuity, bursting forth "like lightning and being condensed in terrible deeds." According to Morel, suffering played a role in the pathogenesis of epileptic mental disturbance: "It is an incessant suffering whose fateful periodicity accumulates an even greater amount of irritability in their nervous system. The latter phenomenon expresses itself not only in the form of perversion in their ideas and feelings, it also manifests itself by the most serious lesion in the physiologic realm" (40). In 1860 Morel described "larval" or "masked" epilepsy (épilepsie larvée). This masked form was diagnosed by the main symptoms of epileptic insanity. Morel's list of these symptoms was taken largely from his picture of the epileptic character. Masked epilepsy could exist by itself without any attacks of ordinary epilepsy, though it was by no means less dangerous. On the contrary, patients who, months or years later, also acquired ordinary seizures generally became less violent (41).

Morel and Jules Falret shared many views and at times visited patients together. Falret (42) assigned the mental disorders of epileptics to three categories: There existed passing trouble before, during, or after a convulsive attack, as a mere epiphenomenon of the seizure. Second, there existed disorders ordinarily met in epileptics during the intervals between the attacks, i.e., the epileptic character. The third category comprised the more or less prolonged delirium for which the name "epileptic insanity" ("folie épileptique") was appropriate. Falret correctly differentiated various premonitory preictal symptoms and the more immediate, brief, and stereotyped aura that he recognized as the first symptom of the convulsive attack. He rendered precise descriptions of temporal lobe seizures and postictal states. His main interest, however, was in the third category of mental disorders, epileptic insanity, which he divided into petit mal intellectuel (usually associated with vertigoes) and grand mal intellectuel (usually associated with the convulsive grand mal). "The calm of the movements, the partial lucidity of the ideas, in short, the semblance of reason which are observed in epileptics suffering from petit mal intellectuel contrast in the highest degree with the maniac agitation, the extreme disorder of their actions, and the incessant loquacity of those affected by the grand mal." However, he added, "In reality, only a simple difference of degree exists between these two varieties of epileptic insanity" (42). The delirious types predominantly would follow the attacks rather than precede them; less frequently they appeared in the intervals between the seizures in persons who were recognized as epileptic.

Falret followed Morel's doctrine of larval or masked epilepsy by maintaining that a psychic form could be present when the convulsive form of epilepsy was absent. Violent, automatic, instantaneous, and unmotivated acts committed in a state of postictal delirium, or at times in the course of a petit mal intellectuel, would carry no legal responsibility.

Griesinger's textbook of psychiatry published first in 1845 (43) was known to Falret. In a later publication, Griesinger (44) used the term "psychomotor symptoms" in what he called "epileptoid conditions." These symptoms correspond precisely to those observed in classic psychomotor seizures. It is noteworthy that Griesinger was the first to observe "sexual weakness" in the great majority of his male "epileptoid" patients, as well as "in rare cases longlasting decidedly morbid sexual excitement."

In 1867 Herpin published a book based on his observation of 300 patients from his own private practice (45). The symptoms that preceded the onset of major seizures, the initial symptoms of major attacks, and all the minor attacks appearing in the intervals between complete attacks—in short, the incomplete attacks—were the main objects of Herpin's study. Varied as the initial phenomena and the minor attacks might be, they showed a remarkable constancy in each individual patient. Although this book is famous for the precise delineation of temporal lobe seizures, it also dealt with other forms, including "Jacksonian epilepsy."

Herpin was interested in seizures, and not in the psychiatric aspects of epilepsy. His methods were clinical observation and numerical analysis; his aim was therapy. In 1899 Hughlings Jackson (46) would state: "I wish to show by the quotations from Herpin that statements essentially the same as those I make were made by a great authority long ago." Unlike Jackson, however, Herpin was not interested in any physiologic or pathologic hypotheses.

John Hughlings Jackson (1835–1911). Temkin records the history of Jackson's achievements, from his first publication on epilepsy, "Cases of Epilepsy Associated with Syphilis" (47), in 1861 to his description of the "uncinate group of epileptic fits" in 1898. Some time between 1868 and 1870 it occurred to Jackson that instability of the gray matter of the cerebral convolutions might account for the convulsions. The investigations of Fritsch and Hitzig in *On the Electric Excitability of the Cerebrum* published in 1870 provided early experimental evidence of Jackson's clinical observations and pathologic inferences (48).

The investigators before Jackson began their studies of epilepsy looking at seizures with generalized convulsions and loss of consciousness or at least the minor seizures with dimmed consciousness. Jackson chose the opposite approach, and began his study of epilepsy by investigating unilateral convulsions, the simplest form of epileptic attacks. He disregarded artificial nosologic entities and concentrated on what functional changes in the nervous system might account for the symptoms of the patient. Jackson was led to the following broad definition of epilepsy: "Epilepsy is the name for occasional, sudden, excessive, rapid and local discharges of gray matter" (46, vol 1, p 100). According to this definition there was no single disease called "epilepsy," but many epilepsies, an expression Jackson frequently used. Even "a sneeze is a sort of healthy epilepsy" (43, vol 1, p 121 footnote). Although there were many epilepsies, genuine epilepsy was not essentially different from unilateral epilepsy. In the latter the discharge started in a cerebral area that represented muscular movements and a higher area might become involved. In genuine epilepsy, with sudden loss of consciousness and general convulsions, it was the other way around.

In a somewhat similar way, Jackson explained "temporary mental disorders after epileptic paroxysms" (46, vol 1, pp 119–134), from states of slight confusion to attacks of homicidal mania. Madness in epilepsy, according to Jackson, was postepileptic. All actions performed in such conditions were automatic. Voluntary control was lost and mere automatisms, i.e., unconscious actions, remained. The slighter the paroxysm removing control, the more complex the automatism afterward. In Jackson's opinion, these theories of dissolution of the highest coordinating centers and release of automatic actions paved a way for understanding insanity.

Jackson had an early understanding of the spread of the epileptic activity. As an effect of various pathologic processes, the cells of a discharging lesion suffer from "morbid nutrition" and become diseased. Their morbid condition causes the cells to discharge excessively and too rapidly. These cells become a "mad part," and as the discharge spreads, other "sane cells" are made to "act madly." "The more excessive the discharge, the severer the fit" (46, vol 1, pp 429–433). This principle could explain the varieties of epileptic seizures.

After the cells have discharged, they lose their functions temporarily and form a "negative lesion," resulting in a paralysis of a severity corresponding to that of the preceding discharge. Cells of lower centers, no longer being under control, become overactive.

Hence we have a combination of negative and positive symptoms. A postepileptic paralysis may be associated with increased tendon reflexes. The explanation of postepileptic states formed a pattern for the explanation of insanities in general. In postepileptic states as well as insanities, the actions of the patient, that is, the positive symptoms, are correlated to those layers that have remained intact.

Jackson was fully aware that his distinction of evolutionary levels and layers was schematic and not supported by anatomic data. His concept of "dreamy state," on the other hand, was developed on the basis of careful clinical observations that he was then able to relate to anatomic findings.

In 1888 Jackson confessed that he had formerly underrated the dreamy state (46, vol 1, p 390). Thirteen years earlier he had published a report of an automatism during which the patient mixed an odd concoction in a kitchen pot and had no memory of his actions (46, vol 1, p 126). Jackson had failed to mention that "at the onset of his fits the patient had 'a sort of dreamy state coming on suddenly'." He argued against Falret's concept of masked epilepsy and contended that these automatisms were preceded by epileptic seizures possibly too slight to be noticed. "The highest or controlling centres" having been put out of use, lower nervous centers became overactive (46, vol 1, p 122).

It seems that Jackson accepted the term "dreamy state" from his patients. In 1876 he listed a number of expressions used by patients for the "so-called intellectual aura": " 'Old scenes revert.' 'I fell in some strange place (a boy expressed it—"in a strange country").' 'A dreamy state.' 'A panorama of something familiar and yet strange' " (46, vol 1, p 274). Jackson believed that the dreamy state was not comparable with ordinary warnings, like crude sensations of smell, which resulted from the epileptic discharge of the highest center. Rather, he thought, they were due to overactivity of next lower centers, as yet untouched by the discharge. Careful investigation might reveal various symptoms preceding "these vague 'reminiscences' or 'reveries' " (46, vol 1, pp 274f).

Jackson's distinction between the psychic experience, referred to as "dreamy state," and the crude sensation does not appear well founded. Careful inquiry shows that the "ordinary warnings" of temporal lobe epilepsy, such as epigastric, cephalic, olfactory, or gustatory sensations, tend to be likewise experienced as something very peculiar, a highly specific yet not precisely definable event—something familiar, yet strange. The dreamlike quality of most primictal events (auras) of temporal lobe epilepsy is indeed an important pathognomonic feature.

As necropsy results became available showing involvement of the uncinate gyrus and of a wider area of the temporal lobe, correlated with olfactory sensations or tasting movements with or without mental automatisms, Jackson began to speak of the "uncinate group of epileptic fits" (46, pp 462 and 467).

Idiopathic Genuine Epilepsy. The recognition of Jacksonian epilepsy as a type of seizure associated with gross organic disease of the brain separated it from the majority of cases of epilepsy that did not reveal such disease. The finding of sclerosis in the medial temporal lobe among institutionalized idiopathic epileptics was repeatedly confirmed (49, 50), but was not generally accepted as significant by the time of Gowers (51). Jacksonian epilepsy could be discussed among diseases of the motor cortex of the brain and idiopathic epilepsy among neuroses without known anatomic foundation.

Epilepsy, unaccompanied by visible changes in the brain, whether designated as idiopathic, genuine, or essential, had many causes that had to be considered exciting causes only. Heredity, however, was generally recognized as a predisposing cause. The statistics of the time suggested inheritance in about 30 percent of the cases (51, p 8).

Gowers' *Epilepsy and Other Chronic Convulsive Diseases*, which first appeared in 1881 (51), was based on the study of 1,450 patients who had been under his care, and throughout the book Gowers analyzed this material statistically. He shared many of Jackson's views, but his book was not limited to epilepsy. Epileptic attacks, according to Gowers, were but one class of "the chronic convulsions which are recognized as of 'functional' origin." Hysterical attacks formed the other class. Gowers admitted that it was not always possible, in medical practice, to neatly separate the hysteroid from the epileptic paroxysms.

Epilepsy and Hysteria. Jackson was a strict adherent of the doctrine of psychophysical parallelism. He believed that there was a fundamental difference between physiology and psychology. "There is no physiology of the mind anymore than there is psychology of the nervous system" (46, vol 1, p 367). He categorically made physiology alone the physician's province. Psychologic knowledge was desirable and necessary, but merely in order to recognize symptoms, not in order to understand the patient's behavior. This restriction appeared to pose no problem if one dealt with epilepsy, which was generally believed to be an organic disease, but was not acceptable to neurologists who concerned themselves with hysteria. In the nineteenth century, hysteria was eminently a neurologic problem, and both Charcot and Freud were neurologists.

Charcot accepted many of Briquet's (1796–1881) fundamental concepts. Briquet stated: "To sum up, an attack of hysteria is nothing but the reaction of that part of the brain which receives emotional impressions. The reaction is expressed outwardly by an exaggeration or perversion of those acts through which these impressions are habitually manifested externally" (52, p 398). In hysteria "the convulsions correspond to the expression of the passions, sensations or ordinary acts of life." In epilepsy, on the other hand, "the convulsion is a kind of tetanus without resemblance to the movements which take place under physiological conditions" (52, p 390). While an anatomic substratum for both epilepsy and hysteria was assumed to exist in the CNS, in epilepsy the trend was to look for organic causes that might affect the brain, whereas in hysteria an ever-increasing emphasis was placed upon emotional factors.

Charcot distinguished sharply between epilepsy and hysteria. He admitted the existence of hysteroepilepsy with both types of attacks, but denied the existence of seizures in which the two neuroses were combined (53). Briquet, Charcot, and Richer, among others, all emphasized the contagious nature of hysterical symptoms, and reinterpreted the grand convulsive epidemics of the past as hysterical phenomena.

Crime, Religion, and the Epileptic Character. Falret had pointed out that the epileptic who attempted or committed suicide, homicide, or arson in a state of postictal delirium (grand mal intellectuel) had not the slightest responsibility for "violent acts committed by him in the midst of this completely automatic, though short, delirium" (42, vol 16, p 667). Those afflicted with the lesser degree of epileptic insanity, petit mal intellectuel, characterized by a semblance of reason, "pushed as they say by an invincible force that dominates their will" could still commit all kinds of destructive acts. "They strike mechanically (machinalement), without motivation, without interest, without knowing what they do or, at least, with a very vague consciousness of their actions" (42, vol 18, p 435). In rare exceptions these acts were not free of motives, calculation, and premeditation. "Sometimes, indeed, an attack of petit mal intellectuel suddenly arouses in the heart of an epileptic a feeling of jealousy, of vengeance, or of anger towards a definite person and then pushes him immediately into action, while in his normal state he had succeeded in suppressing this feeling" (42, vol 18, p 436).

Cases illustrative of Falret's notions were then discussed in the literature. Echeverria (54) reported the case of David Montgomery, an industrious, abstemious, religious young cartman, epileptic since childhood, who had killed his wife in her sleep with an ax and had tried to commit suicide afterward. This occurred after a week of repeated seizures had brought about an excited and deluded state. His wife had refused to live with him anymore, and in the course of 4 hrs after the murder, Montgomery made uncontradicted statements about the events: that he had hesitated for 5 min but then had to strike the blow, that he killed her because she had run with other men, and that his temper got the upper hand of him. When he roused from a sleep hours later, he neither knew that he was in jail nor remembered the events.

The very first of Samt's more than 40 cases of epileptic insanity (55) had analogous features, particularly with respect to the memory of an act of violence committed in a state of "psychic equivalent" of epilepsy. Samt, a psychiatrist at the Charité Hospital in Berlin, had adopted the term "psychic equivalents" from Hoffman (56) who had stated in 1862 that insanity may reveal itself by its peculiar symptoms as an equivalent of epileptic convulsions and of the coma. Samt elaborated the theory of psychic equivalents so as to ensure its lasting attention. He praised Falret for having established epileptic insanity as a specific entity, though he did not accept Falret's classification. Instead, Samt divided epileptic insanity into two main forms: postepileptic insanity and psychic equivalents. The latter, which were not bound to any ordinary epileptic manifestations, could be simple, recidivous, or protracted. The diagnosis had to rest solely on symptomatology, development, and course. Stupor with characteristic speech impairment, extreme violence, severe anxious delirium, and multiform defects of memory were the main pathognomonic symptoms. In addition, Samt considered peculiar religious delirious states almost pathognomonic for epilepsy.

Samt's detailed case histories revealed a remarkable concomitance of violence and religious ecstasy. A considerable number of his patients thought they were in heaven; they addressed the physicians and attendants as divine beings and usually ascribed some heavenly status to themselves. He received much information from his patients during the period when their subjective experiences were still fresh in their memory.

Others published similar reports, which show a striking resemblance to medieval and Renaissance tales of epileptics in religious ecstasy. Krafft-Ebing, for example, cites the following case in his textbook of psychiatry (57). A patient was diagnosed as suffering from genuine epileptic attacks followed by a state of mental twilight and confusion. Several times a year, usually before or after an accumulation of seizures, rarely without them, he fell into an irritated and excited state, condemned his godless environment, mistook others for devils, thrashed out, and wished to be crucified for the true faith. At the height of his ecstasy he saw God face to face and declared himself Christ, God's true warrior, prophet, and martyr. Krafft-Ebing added that "consciousness is considerably dimmed during this delirious time, but still amenable to impressions from the external world. Accordingly there is no defect of memory afterwards. The patient remembers his divine visions and does not correct them" (57, vol 2, p 192).

Apart from their twilight states with violent acts and religious ecstasies, the behavior of epileptics between attacks, as well as their emotional and intellectual fate in the course of the disease, came under close scrutiny. As reviewed earlier, Morel had seen irritability as the base of the epileptic character, and suffering produced and magnified it. The epileptic furor could be modified by progressive improvement of the asylums, e.g., separation of epileptics from maniacs, walks in the gardens, and application to work (39). Falret had listed the interictal mental changes together with the transient preictal, ictal, and postictal mental disorders and the more or less prolonged epileptic insanities in his highly modern classification of mental disorders in epilepsy (42).

Maudsley dramatized the mental anguish of epileptics who had to remain institutionalized: "Gentle, amiable, and industrious through their long intervals of lucidity, they hope against hope that each recurring paroxysm will be the last; they eagerly try all remedies, in the hope of curing the disease; they see others leave the asylum restored to health, and confidently anticipate that their turn will also come; but confidence wanes as the attacks recur, the mind is slowly weakened by the storms of fury through which it passes, and they sink finally in the apathy of dementia—a state of mere oblivion, in which they cease to hope or care more" (58, p 228).

Gowers, a neurologist, described the mental state of epileptics in a few terse sentences: "In its slighter form there is merely defective memory, especially for recent acquisitions. In more severe degree there is greater imperfection of intellectual power, weakened capacity for attention, and often defective moral control. Mischievous restlessness and irritability in childhood may develop into vicious and even criminal tendencies in adult life. Every grade of intellectual defect may be met with, down to actual imbecility" (51, p 121).

Samt (55) described habitual peculiarities in the character of some epileptics as follows:

> I have seen such religious martyr faces, epileptics who speak "frank and free from the bottom of their heart," who beat their own chest, "as true as I exist, for emperor and king I have the heart to speak, the dear Lord is with me," epileptics who act like the most pious sufferers, who kneel down and swear as to their angel-like innocence, "yes, I am sometimes a bit mean, but I don't attack, I have a pistol against my head if I do, but I love to live," who, if they are in the wrong, want to be "crucified and condemned," epileptics, who see "dear Jesus" in their dream and recognize a message from "God the father" in a drawing on the wall, and who steal, slug and curse in a most vulgar manner—enough, those poor epileptics, as one might meet them in every institution, who have the prayer book in their pocket, the dear Lord on their lips, yet an excess of viciousness inside.

Samt was one of many writers using words of moral rejection in the description of the epileptic character. Thus, Krafft-Ebing wrote that "bigotry and suffering mien stand in strange contrast to the irritability, quarrelsomeness, brutality and moral defectiveness. . . ." (57, vol 2, p 182).

These descriptions of epileptic behavior came mostly from those caring for epileptics whose functioning in society had become intolerable. The alienists or asylum doctors who observed epileptics at close range in institutions invariably remarked about their unique mental state.

The asylum of the nineteenth century may have been prison to some and a shelter for others. In either case, and regardless of whether a mental disorder was improved or exacerbated, the asylum never caused a mental disorder.

It is reasonable to assume that institutionalized epileptics would not be totally alien from the extramural population. Thus, apart from those who would be found mentally well, one would expect to find a significant population with similar mental traits of lesser degrees of severity than were found intramurally.

In the twentieth century, the documentation of personality and behavior of epileptics was increasingly neglected in favor of the neurologic aspects of epilepsy, as individuals with seizures gradually came under the care of neurologists.

As we end with this review of the *Falling Sickness*, we should pause for a reflection. The changing and recurrent perspectives and paradigms of the disease are somehow less outdated than we may assume, and we can still be truly enlightened by what was observed centuries ago. Naturally, we are pleased to find views that we cherish or that will strike our fancy. Even today, each of us leans toward being an iatrochemist or an animist. But epilepsy challenges our theoretical preferences, confronting us with psychic and biologic aspects, each with a volume that cannot be ignored.

SIGNIFICANT MODERN CONTRIBUTIONS

Hughlings Jackson's Dr. Z: A Case at the Frontier Between Neurology and Psychiatry

> What is notable about Jackson's description of Dr. Z is that although the epileptic experience and the postmortem findings are recorded with meticulous precision there is scant biographical detail and no mention of the circumstances in which Dr. Z came to overdose himself with chloral hydrate. Jackson's account is totally mechanistic and lesion oriented. Despite his avowed interest in the "organ of mind" his separation from the interests of the asylum doctors is total. Thus a case placed at the frontier (and at the division) between neurology and psychiatry symbolises their subsequent parting to their mutual loss [Taylor and Marsh (59)].

The psychiatrists who preceded Hughlings Jackson in describing temporal lobe seizures pioneered the study of the biography of epileptics. However, Morel, Falret, and others who followed in their steps had studied patients in asylums, and the relevance of their findings for the general population of epileptics remained uncertain. Jackson recognized epilepsy as "the name for occasional, sudden, excessive, rapid and local discharges of grey matter" (46, vol 1, p 100), i.e., as a brain disease, and founded a modern epileptology of strictly neurologic focus. Although Jackson studied ictal and postictal mental disorders, he was not interested in understanding the whole epileptic patient.

Jackson's most famous patient, Dr. Z, apparently was never under psychiatric care. Though Dr. Z died of an overdose of chloral hydrate at the age of 42, Jackson never discussed the circumstances of his suicide, which he considered unrelated to epilepsy. David Taylor and Susan Marsh, in an important historic commentary, have revealed the biography of Dr. Z (59). Their contribution is of particular significance, not merely because of the prominence of the individual, but in view of the high incidence of suicide among temporal lobe epileptics. Taylor and Marsh (60) refer to the finding that the incidence of suicide in the series of patients with temporal lobe epilepsy operated on by Murray Falconer at the Guy/Maudsley Neurosurgical Unit is at least 25 times greater than that expected in the general population.

Dr. Z, as chronicled by Taylor and Marsh, was Arthur Thomas Myers, the youngest of three sons of a prominent minister. He lived from 1851 to 1894. Hughlings Jackson's paper of 1888 "On a Particular Variety of Epilepsy" (61) refers to 50 cases and contains an extensive verbatim account written by Dr. Z. This account includes a precise description of Dr. Z's first experience of a temporal lobe seizure at the age of 20, when he was a student at Cambridge. He had his first major seizure 3 years later, with recurrences as long as 18 months apart. Dr. Z's account represents, to this date, the most lucid clinical observation of an individual's temporal lobe seizures and postictal amnesic automatisms.

Hughlings Jackson was his physician for the last 17 years of his life, and Dr. Z took up residence next door to Jackson sometime during the year before his death, in a living arrangement with another physician. Jackson attended the autopsy, which produced the finding of a very small focus of softening in the left uncinate gyrus—a finding congruous with the clinical history, yet perhaps an artefact, as Taylor and Marsh argue persuasively.

Three months before his death, Dr. Z was forced to retire from medical practice. Though the death certificate lists "Asphyxia—Coma—Epilepsy—Bright's Disease of Kidneys, accelerated by a dose of narcotic medicine," suicide must be considered the single plausible cause of death. The obituary, published in the *British Medical Journal* (January 27, 1894), is surprisingly outspoken and renders a sketch of the tragic life of Dr. Z.

As a registrar in the medical wards of St. George's Hospital, Dr. Z had fulfilled the laborious duties of his post

> with singular patience, minuteness, and fidelity, and invented a system of indexing which has since proved of great value. . . . He wrote in the leading journals and contributed various pages of interest, among which may be mentioned the Nervous Sequelae of Smallpox and a Case of Raynaud's Disease. His studies were of late years particularly directed towards abstruse problems connected with nerve diseases, and the subject of hypnotism as a treatment for disease. . . . his bent was largely towards psychological study and the investigation and discussion of the more recondite phenomena of mind. . . . he was much interested in

> some of the problems which the "psychical researchers" aspire to solve. . . . He was a devoted son, and in private life he was of a singularly kind and amiable disposition, given much to acts of hospitality and goodness to others. The slight brusqueness of his address, sometimes remarked by his juniors, was largely due to his infirmity. . . . His history is tinged by a touch of melancholy. . . . Nature had, indeed, worthily designed him as one of those good "all round men" who are the glory of our public school education; but destiny thought fit to inflict upon him that terrible and inscrutable nervous malady which occasionally harassed him in early youth, and of late years advanced with relentless dread, baffling the most devoted medical skill and ultimately involving a fine intellect in ruin and confusion. . . .

The obituary apparently refers to Dr. Z's failed career and suicide, but does not give us a clear picture of the ruin and confusion inflicted upon him by that "terrible and inscrutable nervous malady." We recognize, however, almost all the characteristic traits associated with temporal lobe epilepsy: the minuteness and fidelity of performance; a singularly good-natured and charitable disposition, contrasting with intervening episodes of irritability; and an interest in the supernatural. He was a devoted son and remained unmarried, as one might expect, since temporal lobe epilepsy is so often associated with lack of sexual interest and arousal. For the purpose of inducing sleep, Dr. Z had long been in the habit of taking narcotics, and one may suspect that there was more than "a touch of melancholy" to the history of his later years.

Dr. Z was subject to prolonged postictal automatisms during which he was able to carry out routine activities without recollection. His isolation must have been enhanced by the fact that at least one of his postictal actions was neither routine nor benign. Hughlings Jackson relates, in his 1898 paper (62): "On another occasion there were postepileptic actions by Dr. Z during 'unconsciousness' of a kind which in a man fully himself would be criminal, and must have led to very serious consequences had not, fortunately, his condition been known. What he did was overlooked by those concerned." Was it an act of sexual indecency, as may occur occasionally in the postictal phase (63) and as is perhaps suggested by the Victorian discretion in Jackson's report?

Dr. Z's last paper, "Mind-Cure, Faith-Cure and the Miracles of Lourdes," was coauthored by his brother Frederic and appeared in the year preceding his death (64). Taylor and Marsh describe this 50-page article as rational and not unduly verbose. A personal letter from Dr. Z to his brother Fred, dated 7 years prior to his death, documents the characteristic emotional emphasis and wordiness, as Dr. Z keeps praising his brother's devotion, after disavowing any negative sentiment between them, ever.

> "Dear Fred,
> It is historically and absolutely true that it never entered my head for a moment that you were cool—much less that you were clumsy—or indeed anything but perfectly sympathetic. I have always felt and shall always continue to feel most deeply grateful for your warm brotherly sympathy and affection—it has been over and over again a very great comfort to me—I almost doubt if you can have realised sometimes how great—it may not often express itself in words but there it is—and it cannot be forgotten. Life is unsatisfactory—yes—but you have made me feel it less unsatisfactory.
> Yrs affectionately, A.T.M."

Emil Kraepelin: The Psychiatric Aspects of "Genuine" Epilepsy

In his textbook of psychiatry, Emil Kraepelin deals with the three major categories of insanity recognized by European psychiatry in the first half of our century: dementia praecox and the paraphrenias; epileptic insanity; and manic-depressive insanity. The eighth edition of this influential textbook is the last one edited solely by Kraepelin (65). This summary of his chapter on epilepsy will reflect the specific nature of the psychopathology of epilepsy recognized by Kraepelin, and will permit an appreciation of the remarkable changes brought about by the introduction of the modern anticonvulsants.

Following a flurry of seizures, a psychotic state commonly develops and lasts for days or even a couple of weeks. The postictal psychosis and concomitantly the "epileptic furor" that had been of major concern to psychiatrists became rare as more effective seizure control became possible. The psychopathology associated with epilepsy thus was muted and appeared largely in more subtle forms, which were, however, already recognized by Kraepelin and several of his predecessors.

Kraepelin prescribed bromides, the sole anticonvulsant known during his time, with proper caution to avoid toxic effects. As the long-standing head of a university department treating inpatients and outpatients, he discussed the differences between his population of patients and those observed in institutional settings. The chapter is then based on clinical observations of a unique quality, not distorted by artefacts related to institutionalization or excessive use of any drug, as has sometimes been alleged. The part of the chapter that deals with the physical aspects of epilepsy is not considered here, except for Kraepelin's remarks on the then-well-known neuropathologic marker of genuine epilepsy. Kraepelin referred to the often reported neuropathologic finding of a usually unilateral sclerosis of Ammon's horn in individuals who had suffered from epilepsy. In severe and long-standing cases, Ammon's horn sclerosis was occasionally found bilaterally, and degenerative changes of wider cortical areas could be regularly documented. The significance of Ammon's horn sclerosis was at that time totally unclear, particularly since Ammon's horn was assumed to serve only olfactory functions.

Definition. Kraepelin begins his chapter on epileptic insanity by remarking that epilepsy owes its name to the characteristic, sudden, and repetitive attacks of unconsciousness with convulsions, and then states: "The clinical experience, however, has taught that the initial, extraordinarily impressive pathologic manifestation, the epileptic attack, is an entirely inappropriate characterization of the disease. It has to be emphasized that similar attacks are observed in a great number of diseases which are different from each other, as well as entirely unrelated to the disease process intrinsic to epilepsy." Kraepelin clearly distinguishes the many "symptomatic" forms of epilepsy caused by various coarse cerebral diseases, injuries, tumors, intoxications, and degenerative diseases from "genuine" epilepsy.

Genuine epilepsy involves a disease process. It includes "a large number of symptoms which form an entity by etiology, clinical manifestations, course, and perhaps also by autopsy findings, though its precise delineation is not yet possible to our satisfaction. Even in the absence of convulsions, a case of genuine epilepsy may be recognized by a number of characteristics. Genuine epilepsy is characterized by recurrent endogenous convulsions with loss of consciousness, or by disorders which, from our experience, can be observed frequently in combination or alternation with convulsions." Kraepelin is referring to those paroxysmal manifestations that may precede the convulsion, but may also occur by themselves (as "equivalents"); to episodic ("paroxysmal") mental disorders more or less related to seizures; and to the more chronic interictal personality and behavior changes. "We will see that in a very large number of cases changes peculiar to epilepsy to a certain degree can be demonstrated in the interval between the attacks which may, by themselves, permit the recognition of the disease."

Seizures. Kraepelin describes the characteristic prodromes:

the aura; the major attack; and the postictal phase. He emphasizes the wealth of sensory, psychic, visual, vertiginous, autonomic, and other disorders that may occur, as auras or independently of a major attack as "equivalents."

In discussing the equivalents (a term synonymous with our modern term "complex partial seizures"), Kraepelin states: "All these disorders by themselves may be so equivocal and undefined, that they are not immediately identifiable as symptoms of epilepsy. Only their sudden immediate appearance and fading, their highly stereotyped periodic recurrence and particularly their combination with other signs of epilepsy can reveal their true significance." Along with Gowers, Kraepelin distinguishes the attenuated and shortened attacks as "petit mal" from the "grand mal."

Psychic Epilepsy. Kraepelin designates states with pronounced mental disorders that are somewhat independent of the seizures as "psychic epilepsy." Their relationship to epilepsy is obvious if they are initiated or terminated by a seizure. However, seizures may also occur during the course of this mental disorder, and its differentiation as a pre- or postepileptic disorder is moot. Furthermore, all manifestations of pre- and postepileptic insanity may also occur as independent episodes without connection to seizures, as Samt first clarified. Thus, such forms of psychic epilepsy may represent "equivalents" (analogous to the attenuated attacks) whose relationship to epilepsy can be recognized by clinical characteristics that are identical to those of pre- and postepileptic insanity.

In the middle of the nineteenth century, Jules Falret (42) differentiated between a milder and a severer form of epileptic insanity: *petit mal intellectuel* and *grand mal intellectuel*. Similarly, Kraepelin discusses two main forms of psychic epilepsy: the epileptic dysphorias, or mood changes, and the epileptic twilight states.

Epileptic Dysphorias or Mood Changes

> Periodic dysphorias represent the mildest and most common form of psychic epilepsy. They are brief mood changes, occurring without external trigger factors, with rapid onset and termination, and recurring fairly regularly in an entirely uniform manner. They are not associated with any striking clouding of consciousness. Though they may be observed as preludes to an attack, or occasionally in the aftermath of an attack, they most commonly appear as phenomena independent of the seizures. They may occur with frequency varying from every few days to every few months. A person usually just awakens one day with the dys-

> phoria, but may also have it develop insidiously through the course of a day.

A certain sexual excitement may be experienced initially. The individual suddenly becomes bad tempered, morose, sullen, surly, irritable, and may perceive mistreatment by others. Upon recovery the patient feels remorseful, and some patients may choose to remain in isolation for the duration of their dysphoria.

In other cases the mood changes take on the form of internal unrest and dejection. The epileptics will entertain gloomy thoughts and ideas of having sinned, and may feel that others are being cross with them and are speaking ill of them. Some patients may be seized with intense anxiety, sudden despair, or incomprehensible terror. In such a mood, a marked suicidal intent often develops, and suicide attempts may be carried out. Far more rare than the periodic irritability or dejection is the paroxysmal occurrence of expansive or ecstatic moods with motor excitement and religious preoccupation. A quarrelsome disposition may also become manifest.

As a rule the epileptic dysphoria lasts for 1–2 days, but may dissipate after just a few hours. Consciousness is generally completely clear, though the patients often report feeling somewhat confused and forgetful. Severe headache, perspiration, dilation of pupils, tremor, facial pallor or flushing, tachycardia, nausea, diarrhea, lack of appetite, and insomnia are often present. The episode may be followed by a sense of relief and striking well-being.

During epileptic dysphoria even small amounts of alcohol may lead to complicated states of intoxication, characterized by the combination of marked clouding of consciousness and violent excitement. Alcohol intake may also led to pronounced twilight states. Particularly disastrous is the excessive drinking prompted by epileptic dysphorias, which leads to the characteristic picture of periodic alcoholism (dipsomania).

> It becomes evident, upon more precise inquiry, that the episode [of excessive drinking] regularly begins with a state identical to the epileptic dysphorias, with malaise, sense of oppression, intense sadness, despondency, heightened irritability, giddiness, lack of appetite, insomnia, and at times also an initial sexual arousal. . . . At the same time, the patient becomes possessed with a vehement inner unrest with the consequent impulsive desire to obtain relief by the intake of alcohol. . . .

A further consequence of the epileptic dysphoria is the peculiar restlessness of some patients, with sudden abrupt fugues.

Kraepelin also considers infrequent states with paroxysmal terror and hallucinations, in the absence of significant clouding of consciousness, closely related to the epileptic dysphorias. States of an anxious-irritable mood with hallucinations and pronounced delusions represent a further variation of the dysphoria. These states generally subside after a few days, as abruptly as they began.

> The patient is again affable, goodnatured, harmless, brushes off any references to the 'persecutions,' and laughs about his 'imaginations.' In sporadic cases, however, the auditory hallucinations and delusions may persist for weeks or even months with little fluctuation, so that the state may superficially resemble certain forms of dementia praecox. But such patients, whose consciousness is perfectly clear, are always compelled to doubt their morbid ideas. . . .

Kraepelin then mentions occasional cases in which delusional thinking may not be corrected, and refers here to Buchholz, who had described the combined presence of epilepsy and chronic paranoia. Kraepelin considers such cases to be a form of residual delusions.

Epileptic Twilight States. The second main group of epileptic insanity is associated with a more or less marked clouding of consciousness. These disorders are designated as "twilight states." In twilight states the patients show the disorders of attention, orientation, thought processes, and speech characteristic of confusional states.

> Their mood is highly labile. They are frequently dejected, anxious, despaired, and then again morose, surly, and irritable. In between there may be states of high spirited roguery or ecstatic rapture. . . . Many patients are taciturn, inaccessible, even stuporous, or even cataleptic on occasions; others are intense, threatening, inclined to severe violent acts; again, others are vivacious, anxious or feel a joyful excitement.

Amnesia is frequently present. At times the memory of an episode may be fleeting, fading rapidly upon recovery. Kraepelin compares the recollection of the epileptic twilight states to that of sleep and dreaming, and points out the forensic significance of the findings. He further groups the phenomenon of somnambulism with the epileptic twilight states.

The majority of epileptic twilight states follow the course of a simple, dreamlike confusional state. With the addition of illusions, hallucinations, and incoherent delusions, delirious confusional states frequently develop.

> Ideas with religious content tend to play a large role. The patient believes himself to be in Purgatory, in Heaven, sees God, hears

> the angels sing, wanders upward on the stairway to Heaven, and wants to enter eternity. God speaks to him, he is Saint Peter, has the mission to preach God's word, wants to defend religion; Christ will assist him. Or he believes himself to be God, an angel, Satan; his wife is the Divine Mother, the physician is the Almighty. God does not like him; he is condemned, subject to the temptations of the evil one; he is involved in spiritual battles with sinful thoughts, lives in a sea of torment, or feels so healthy, so free, so fortunate; God has accomplished this; the evil spirit is expelled.

Other grandiose thoughts may occur, and tales of adventurous experiences are common. Characteristically, religious-ecstatic states are intermingled with states of anxiety and violence.

> The mood is variable. The patient experiences much inner pain, is anxious and tense, but soon may be cheerful, elated, or erotically aroused. There is a regular and marked tendency toward grievous deeds of violence. Many patients are quiet, dreamy or morose, sullen, staring straight ahead; others display an aimless unrest, jump around, crawl and roll on the floor, surge forward, speak incessantly in a verbigerant or confused, flighty manner, or preach in babbling monotonous tones; they chant with stereotyped repetition, howl, scream, curse obscenely, behave oddly, theatrically, and rave 'like maniacs.' They suddenly destroy the windows with a nighttable or chair, attempt to rip up the cobblestones, try to stop the streetcar, throw the knife at the spouse or the beer mug in the neighbor's face, plunge at an orderly, choke family members, run after a friend with a pickax, roam around with a drawn knife. . . . One patient thought of setting the house on fire; another lit up his wood cabin; a third spoke of pouring hydrochloric acid in his wife's face, or nailing his child by all four limbs; a female patient wanted to cut open her children's bellies. Sexual assaults may also occur sometimes. As a rule, these acts appear prompted by delusional thoughts. . . . very frequently the violent acts are directed against oneself. . . . In one group of cases the clinical picture is entirely dominated by states of most intense terror with horrifying thoughts. . . . These states are frequently ushered in by specific and regularly-recurring hallucinations; particularly remarkable is the black man and the vision of red objects, blood, flames, figures in a red coat, etc.

The duration of these delirious states is often limited to a few hours, at most to 1 or 2 weeks. The resolution is almost invariably gradual. Some prolonged twilight states, characterized by heavily clouded consciousness and a near-complete absence of activity, are designated as "epileptic stupor." A somewhat rarer form is a delirious state with apparent presence of mind. Its course is slower, and some patients have embarked upon long, aimless journeys during such a state.

The twilight states, like the dysphorias, are often temporally close to major or minor epileptic seizures, usually succeeding them but sometimes preceding them. The patient may have a brief, relatively lucid interval between attack and twilight state. In most instances, however, the disorder evolves without hiatus from post-ictal confusion. Finally, the twilight states may occur as "equivalents" in the absence of any convulsions but associated with other manifestations of epilepsy. In exceptional cases they may occur as the only morbid manifestation, sometimes long before the appearance of attacks, which finally may secure the diagnosis.

During a stay in Java, Kraepelin examined natives who had run amok. He describes "amok" as a twilight state with sudden onset or with onset after a brief period of dysphoria, and likened the condition to an epileptic twilight state. In Kraepelin's opinion, several of the natives examined were undoubtedly epileptic and in others the same diagnosis was suggested.

Aschaffenburg listed twilight states in 36 percent and dysphorias in 64 to 70 percent of his cases. Among institutionalized patients, twilight states were found in 62 percent, somewhat more frequently among female patients. Kraepelin noted twilight states in 16.5, dysphorias in 36.9 and excitatory states (mostly pathologic intoxications) in 13.8 percent of 515 epileptic patients treated in his clinic in Munich.

Epileptic Personality Changes

> In conjunction with the episodic disorders described thus far, the genuine epileptic gradually develops a variably pronounced, but permanent change in his personality, usually within the first five or six years. Indeed, the constant recurrence of endogenous attacks must indicate to us that we have a chronically persistent morbid substrate. Kellner found only 10% of his epileptic patients mentally healthy. . . . On superficial observation, the more permanent epileptic changes are recognizable only in more severe cases. Nevertheless, we can detect a remarkably common type of mental disorder in our patients, which is as diagnostic of epilepsy as the paroxysmally occurring disorders. We will be able to see that, in most cases, the individual traits of this disorder are very mitigated residuals of those upheavels which take place in the paroxysmal psychic disorders. . . . The intellectual performance of our patients may not be disturbed; individual patients may even give the impression of being alert and mentally active. In the preponderant majority of cases, however, there is a remarkable slowing of mental processes which may be determined with a simple stopwatch. . . . In general the patient comprehends questions and impressions correctly but very slowly, and takes a long time to mentally process them and arrive at a response. More complicated impressions give him particular difficul-

> ties. . . . While the details of pictures are easily recognized, the context and the meaning of the whole are difficult for the individual to grasp. Misconceptions and misunderstandings are commonplace. Similarly, single words are often well comprehended, but the sentence is not understood. The patient is unable to follow quick turns of the conversation or to consider several items at the same time. The versatility of his imagination is very limited; new associations are made laboriously and to a modest degree, and external stimuli awaken only a sparse response.
>
> At the same time, orientation, thought associations, and clarity of consciousness almost always remain remarkably intact. . . . Attention is always directed only to the obvious and nearest at hand, while more general references, allusions, witty ambiguities and humorous contrasts elude the patients. The viscosity of mental processes, which is most pronounced in the twilight state, impedes all but the most familiar external stimuli.
>
> The picture of simple epileptic feeblemindedness, which, of course, may be present in widely varying degrees, is best characterized by the term narrow-mindedness. . . . The patient lacks that lucid view of daily events which enables us to separate the important from the trivial, and thus gain general guidelines for our thinking and actions. A consequence is the peculiar *circumstantiality* of the epileptic. The patient begins each narration with particulars which, at first, hardly seem connected to the question, and then accumulates such a mass of totally irrelevant details that his account positively appears not to move from the spot. Each attempt to prompt a more rapid development of the essential, by interpolated questions, usually fails. The patient simply resumes his thread at the point of interruption. Thereby he never loses his continuity, and finally arrives at his goal, albeit via very convoluted paths. . . . The pettiness and meticulousness of his thought processes and the exaggerated neatness in his pursuits are probably related to the preeminence of the particular and the tangible.

Kraepelin refers to authors who observed the greater precision of epileptics, and of feebleminded ones in particular, if compared with healthy individuals.

With more advanced feeblemindedness the memory fails regularly to a considerable degree. The same things are narrated. Pictures and words are poorly recollected, and new impressions are mistaken for familiar ones.

Kraepelin states that simple association experiments carried out by a number of investigators (Sommer, Fuhrmann, Ricklin, Jung, Isserlin, Rittershaus, and others) provide an instructive picture of the thought processes of epileptics.

> Apart from incorrectness of verbal expression, above all, a pronounced slowness and awkwardness of responses, a fixation on one and the same idea and even on the same grammatic form, a trend to respond with sentences, to repeatedly paraphrase the

same thought, and to gesture affirmatively were evident. Associations were frequently meaningless and scant; the verbal expression showed, as was particularly demonstrated by Rittershaus, great clumsiness and pomposity, often even plain paraphrasic compounding of words, and neologisms. Furthermore, in a noticeable manner, there were associations with no recognizable relationship to the stimulus word; such associations seemed to originate from permanent general ranges of ideas which were triggered by the experiment. Their content was connected mostly to the illness or to the personal circumstances of the patient. Jung recorded 31% 'egocentric' associations in a group of his patients. Pure linguistic associations were entirely absent. . . . In Fuhrman's patients, moreover, there appeared a predominant melancholy mood. Ricklin found a marked emotional emphasis of the emerging associations, and Jung concluded, from the pattern of the reaction times, that there was a prolonged aftereffect of the slowly emerging, but intense emotional responses. The number of newly emerging associations from the repetition of an experimental series was remarkably limited; a sign of the uniformity and poverty of ideation. Of course, all the observed mental performances showed marked fluctuations; the disturbances were most pronounced shortly before or after the attacks.

It is natural that with impoverishment of ideation, the importance of the own ego must gradually become enhanced, to an extraordinary degree, in the value system of the patients. Thus, with progressive feeblemindedness, the self esteem of the patients increases, and the content of their orations utlimately becomes limited to the praise of one's self and all that is related to the self. The praise of one's family, the unctuous emphasis on the excellence of the next of kin, is characteristic for such patients. 'The ideal accomplishment of virtue to me is a promenade with my mother alone in the evening', said one patient. . . .

Worries concerning their own physical well-being, bowel movement, sleep, and diet frequently play a large role; minute changes are written down and brought to the physician's attention. At the same time, one often observes a striking optimism concerning their true ailment. . . .

Moreover, religious ideas ('God-nomenclature') are cherished with unusual predilection. In some, peculiar sentiments connected to the attacks may suggest the idea of divine influence; or, the hope for salvation by a supernatural authority may find a particularly fertile soil in these helpless patients. Very often they believe to have a preeminently intimate relationship with heaven, since they had always been so well behaved and had prayed ever so diligently. They often speak of the Divine Father and of the Devil, of the rosary and the Holy Sacraments, have pious faith, do everything because it is ordained by God, submit to his will, ask for bible and catechism, go to church and confession as often as possible, and desire to stay in contact with the clergyman. . . .

The patients often speak of having been wronged. . . . But only in a few cases, as already mentioned, does it develop into paranoid thinking.

The mood of epileptics is sometime oppressed, despondent; sometimes morose, distrustful, irritable; and other times, joyful and contented. With advanced deterioration, the mood often becomes dull and indifferent. Exceptionally common is the development of a permanent intensification of an irritable mood, which reaches its culmination degree during the dysphoria and under the influence of alcohol. The patient becomes sensitive, moody, intransigent about right and wrong, explosive, 'unbearably rude', and may experience fits of intense anger with reckless violence over trifles. He threatens his associates with a knife, destroys objects, and attempts suicide in a fit of rage. One patient shot his dog dead in the street. Others are resentful and vindictive. At the same time, a marked selfishness frequently develops, leading to very vehement resentment of any infringement upon his own rights, yet the sorrow of another concerns him very little. Moreover, the individual may be incredibly stubborn, narrow-minded and obstinate rendering him deaf to all attempts at persuasion. Some patients are malicious, mendacious, spiteful, and represent the most dangerous inmates of asylums and prisons. It must be emphasized, however, that the bad attributes listed here are evident in only a small proportion of the epileptics. Opposite them is a large number of patients who occupy the psychiatrist much less, who are quiet, modest, devoted, amicable and helpful. A certain childlike, trusting friendliness and good nature prevails by a wide margin.

. . . As a rule epileptic patients like to keep themselves occupied, are industrious, thrifty and honest, work with extraordinary slowness but often with pedantic conscientiousness. . . . Many patients display a certain ponderous helpfulness, get involved in everything, attempt to serve as attendants, and to educate their fellow patients. Frequently the patients lead a monotonous, precisely ordered life preoccupied with paltry duties, in utter self-restraint, solitary, sheltered by their families. They are exceedingly well-behaved, though peculiar, narrow-minded and dependent.

Others, however, are unable to achieve lasting employment despite rather well intact abilities; partly because they are repeatedly dismissed because of their attacks, and partly because of their own restlessness. The dysphorias are particularly responsible for incessant job changes. Even apart from that, some patients are inclined to lead a nomadic life. . . . The criminality of some epileptics is seen as due to the calamity brought about by their ailment, their irritability and narrow-minded selfishness, and particularly their frequently being under the influence of alcohol. . . . Epileptics tend to be intolerant of alcohol. They become intoxicated with very small amounts of alcohol, often suffer severe headaches, or even seizures. . . . The drunken state is commonly accompanied by severe excitement with impaired

> consciousness, particularly if the individual was emotionally charged up. In some patients this sensitivity to alcohol exists only during the time of their dysphorias.
>
> Epileptic patients tend to display a certain solemnity, dignified politeness and formality. . . . They are unable to find the correct words, form ponderous, incomplete sentences, are fond of clichés, platitudes, biblical sayings, proverbs. . . . Some patients like to write poetry.

Kraepelin then quotes, as an illustration, a letter from a patient to his priest (the patient later committed murder and suicide in a state of morbid excitement):

> "May the Honorable Reverend allow me to take the liberty to delight the Honorable Reverend with a few lines, as much and how that lies in my power. From the bottom of my heart I am compelled to do so and wish to pronounce in such a way to my most venerated Honorable Reverend my spiritual sentiments and bodily vigour. I have to struggle day and night, now spiritually, now physically, and rejoice at it that it is so, lest much may not be fulfilled what is taught in the Holy Scriptures through our Lord Jesus Christ, therefore I state: who trusts in God has not built his house on sand, for I did perceive it and thus want to share my joy likewise with the Honorable Reverend by stating: I rejoice in Christ, to be able to proclaim with all my heart that all comes from God, about which I have no more doubts by now.
>
> "The selfsame, as I have perceived, is revealed by the Holy Scriptures. Each day I thank God for his mercy everywhere, and rejoice that God has led me to this point, for he has achieved great with me (us) and many mortals, but blessed are those mortals who perceive it. I was enlisted for years in a struggle, saw it and felt it, but was not able to free myself from it, but God be thanked, who gave me (us) the victory through our Lord Jesus Christ. I hope that I will become more vigorous, the restless sleep has improved.
>
> "Thus, I trust confidently in the grace and power of God in Jesus Christ.
>
> "With the most obliging greetings to the Honorable Reverend along with the most highly respected and honored family.
>
> George P."

Kraepelin points out that the described personality and behavior changes of epileptics are present in individual cases to exceedingly variable degrees. Often these may be but faintly expressed, by certain single traits or upon particular occasions. At times these changes may progress to extreme mental infirmity.

Kraepelin renders a lucid elaboration of the writings of his predecessors as he describes genuine epilepsy, a psychiatric disease entity distinct from dementia praecox and manic-depressive disease. He teaches how to recognize temporal lobe seizures, which he terms "equivalents," and focuses on the rich interictal phenomena of the disease. He has no doubt that one should be able to recognize, even in the absence of any seizures, the epileptic nature of the labile and complex mood states termed "dysphorias," which may last merely days or hours. The confusional twilight states are likewise characteristic disorders, but since they usually occur as postictal psychoses, there is less doubt about their diagnosis. Dementia praecox-like psychoses, our "schizophrenia-like psychoses" of epilepsy with consciousness fully intact, were recognized by Kraepelin, but they were a rarity.

We have presented broad, detailed excerpts of Kraepelin's description of the twilight states, even though they are rarely encountered in the era of modern anticonvulsant medication. As indicated, they represent magnified, intense versions of the more permanent and often subtle interictal personality changes. Supernatural rapture, violent outburst, as well as extreme viscosity in these exceptional states correspond to the religious preoccupation, conscientiousness, and irritability, as well as to the slow, circumstantial manner of the more permanent state of mind. Kraepelin was not an asylum doctor, and recognized the large number of epileptics who showed only subtle psychic changes, who were good natured, and who required little psychiatric attention.

Henri Gastaut: Behavior and Personality Changes Associated with Psychomotor Epilepsy—The Temporolimbic Basis of "Genuine" Epilepsy

French psychiatrists of the mid-nineteenth century pioneered the understanding of the psychiatric aspects of epilepsy. One hundred years later, Henri Gastaut, the eminent French epileptologist, defined the cerebral localization and pathophysiology behind the findings of the asylum doctors.

As a result of characteristic electroencephalographic (EEG) findings, the form of epilepsy first studied systematically by Hughlings Jackson (as "dreamy state" or "uncinate group of epileptic fits") was rediscovered in 1938 by Gibbs et. al (66), was named "psychomotor epilepsy," and was gradually defined more clearly in the course of the following decade. Gastaut and his coworkers were the first to experimentally document, from 1951 to 1953, the temporolimbic ("rhinencephalic") origin of psychomotor seizures, and to point out the medial temporal sclerosis as the neuropathologic substrate. Gastaut's group then published a remarkable series of papers on their studies of the behavior of psychomotor epileptics, relating the behavioral findings to their neural basis, on the one hand, and to the extant psychiatric knowledge of epilepsy, on the other. One of the papers in this series (63) detailed the original and startling finding that temporal lobe seizure activity tends to have a profound and chronic suppressing effect on sexual arousal and response.

In spite of the international prominence of Gastaut, his behavioral findings and his efforts to promote a broader perspective of temporal lobe epilepsy were virtually ignored in the English-speaking countries, where few psychiatrists had more than a passing interest in the field of epilepsy.

The Neuropathology of the Epilepsies. In 1954 Gastaut (67) reviewed the state of knowledge concerning the neuropathology of the epilepsies. In the past, the type of epilepsy referred to as "idiopathic," "genuine," "essential," or "chronic" had been opposite of the symptomatic type with seizures clearly related to infectious or toxic disorders, tumors, abscesses, or scars secondary to vascular or traumatic processes. During the preceding century, investigators concentrated on discovering the lesion specific for idiopathic epilepsy among the institutionalized and indeed discovered a "biologic marker": a lesion consisting of a diffuse hemispheric sclerosis predominantly involving the medial temporal lobe and the neighboring limbic structures.

The first systematic neuropathologic study, performed by Bouchet and Cazauvieilh in 1825 (32), had already emphasized the prominence of Ammon's horn sclerosis in the postmortem examinations of institutionalized epileptics. This finding was repeatedly confirmed, and subsequent microscopic studies revealed the loss of neurons and reactive gliosis (responsible for the sclerosis) of Ammon's horn in 30–70 percent of the patients (Table 1). The

TABLE 1. *Frequency of Ammon's horn sclerosis among institutionalized epileptics (microscopic findings)*

Investigators	Frequency (%)
Sommer (1880)	30
Bratz (1899)	50
Alzheimer (1898)	50
Turner (1906)	50
Bratz and Grossman (1923)	40
Spielmeyer (1924–1934)	50
Stauder (1936)	70
Sano and Malamud (1953)	58

presence of a diffuse gliosis of the cerebral cortex without characteristic localization, or of cerebellar lesions was also noted in these patients.

The significance of the neuropathologic findings for the epilepsy had not been realized. They had been looked upon as a puzzle or an oddity at a time when Ammon's horn was erroneously believed to be exclusively an olfactory center, and the presence of lesions to adjoining areas was overlooked. Gastaut paid tribute to Stauder (68), who in 1936, prior to the EEG identification of temporal lobe epilepsy, performed a neuropathologic study of 53 institutionalized epileptics whose clinical history he was familiar with, and concluded that the temporal-hippocampal lesions were indeed characteristic of an *epilepsy with temporal symptomatology.*

Gastaut concluded that the idiopathic epileptics from the asylums in time past had been afflicted with psychomotor or temporal lobe epilepsy. He pointed at recent studies (69–71) that confirmed the very high incidence of temporal lobe epileptics among the institutionalized. The idiopathic epileptics of modern times, as defined by Lennox, Penfield, and Gastaut, are both neurologically and psychiatrically intact; in the absence of any cerebral lesion, they present a genetic-metabolic disorder with a benign course and do not require any hospitalization. These patients had never reached the attention of the asylum doctors. In the third group of epilepsies corresponding to the old symptomatic group, the patients often show chronic neurologic signs (hemiparesis, aphasia, hemianopsia, etc.), but in the absence of limbic involvement are psychiatrically intact.

Interictal Disorders of Activity and of Social Adjustment in Psychomotor Epilepsy. In 1953 Gastaut et al. (72) carried out a comparative psychologic study of 80 epileptics grouped according to rigorous clinical and EEG criteria. Before a patient can be assigned to a pure generalized-functional (or other) subgroup of epilepsy, elaborate evaluations are required, making valid comparison studies very difficult to carry out. We detail here Gastaut's methodology in assigning patients to diagnostic subgroups, because later studies carried out in the United States used much simplified nosologic criteria when selecting patients with generalized seizures as controls for patients with psychomotor epilepsy, and consequently failed to confirm the unique relationship of limbic seizure disorders to behavior, claiming that both groups showed equally high incidences of disturbed behavior (73).

Several EEGs were obtained for each patient, at rest and upon a variety of activation procedures (hyperventilation, intermittent light, sleep, and intravenous Metrazol) until characteristic ictal or interictal discharges were obtained. The neurologist carried out a comprehensive neuropsychiatric evaluation of each case. The psychologic investigation focused on intelligence level, speed of performance, and personality. Neurologist, electroencephalographer, and psychologist were blind to each other's findings. It was only after 2 years of independent studies that the clinical and EEG findings were compared, and only those patients whose findings allowed precisely the same nosologic categorization were then retained for comparison of their psychologic profiles. Individuals unable to maintain a job because of their personality or intellectual limitation were excluded from study. With the employment of such stringent selection criteria, of the average 700 patients with epilepsy examined annually in Gastaut's seizure clinic, only 80 could be retained, of whom only the two groups with psychomotor epilepsy (43 cases) and generalized-functional epilepsy (21 cases) were of sufficient size to permit statistical analyses. The smaller groups with secondarily generalized epilepsy (11 cases) and with partial epilepsy localized to the convexity of the cortex (5 cases) were also included in the study. The patients with generalized-functional epilepsy did not show any of the traits of the "epileptoid constitution." The same was true in the case of the symptomatic epileptics with small surface lesions to the neocortex. Only those patients with seizures secondary to diffuse cerebral lesions involving predominantly diencephalic-rhinencephalic (limbic) areas showed the slowness and impulsivity described by the classic psychiatric authors; most of these patients had psychomotor seizures and EEG abnormalities projected to the temporal lobe region.

In 1955 Gastaut et al. (74) reported further comprehensive studies of psychomotor epileptics. After evaluating 3,000 such patients over a period of 5 years, they carried out a systematic psychologic study of a series of 60 outpatients between the ages of 20 and 50 years, all of average intelligence and educational level. The patients were interviewed and observed during testing and hospital stay, and an inquiry was made with the family whenever possible. They underwent projective testing (Rorschach and Thematic Apperception Test), tests of attention and speed of performance, and intelligence tests including the Wechsler-Bellevue.

The findings led to the distinction of two groups of psychomotor epileptics. Over two-thirds of the patients showed the following syndrome: psychomotor hypoactivity (viscosity); paroxysmal impulsivity manifested by violent outbursts of anger with little provocation; an EEG pattern marked by various degrees of neuronal hypoexcitability. A less prevalent type, present in less than one-fourth of the patients, consisted of a normal activity level, a permanent irritability without violent outbursts, and an EEG pattern more or less marked by neuronal hyperexcitability.

Gastaut points out that patients without psychomotor epilepsy but with generalized seizures secondary to diffuse cerebral changes (e.g., with diffuse diencephalic disorders) present a syndrome identical to that of the first group. The second group shows a relationship to the generalized-functional epileptics, perhaps by reason of an identical inherited predisposition or because of an extension of their lesion to the mesodiencephalic area.

Gastaut emphasizes the paradoxic picture presented by the majority of patients, "who are abnormally calm, or even depressed, [and] whose outbursts of anger occur without valid reason. Indeed, the paradox is even more marked if one considers that during the interval of the unmotivated fits of rage, the psychomotor epileptic often presents a 'hypersocial' character, which makes the presence of the impulsive outbursts even more incomprehensible." He makes light of the hypersocial character by commenting that the loyal attachment of certain epileptics to their families and traditions was merely a manifestation of their basic hypoactivity, adhesiveness, or viscosity.

Gastaut was able to clarify the nature of the violent outbursts among psychomotor epileptics, which he had first considered to be "seizure equivalents." Violent and sometimes dangerous activity may characterize some psychomotor seizures in a few cases, but they are different from the common fits of rage of the interictal phase of psychomotor epileptics. Among several hundred psychomotor seizures reproduced in the laboratory by Metrazol injection, Gastaut observed several violent procursive attacks with amnesia that were identical to the individual's usual attacks. "The patient, totally confused, overturns and breaks everything in his path: this is not a directed aggressivity, but a frenzied agitation in a confusional state." If the path is not obstructed, the agitation gradually diminishes and the confusion clears after some automatic activities. If the patient is restrained, marked violent behavior may result in serious injury to others.

On the other hand, interictal outbursts of rage typically directed at someone with little provocation and with consciousness and memory intact could not be reproduced with Metrazol injection, despite 100 trials. Finally, in rare instances, EEG recordings were obtained during spontaneous outbursts of rage, and these distinguished themselves by their absence of epileptiform discharges.

Gastaut further documented the incidence of behavioral changes characteristic of psychomotor epileptics among nonepileptic individuals who presented a paroxysmal temporal lobe focus in their EEG examination. One of his illustrative cases follows.

> *Case 9.* A non-epileptic 60-year-old woman, of particularly amiable disposition, two or three times yearly when mildly reprimanded by her husband, explodes in a state of rage with extreme violence, lasting one to two hours. For two or three days prior to the outburst she is particularly taciturn, and a depressive period of about one week follows the episode. The EEG shows a sharp wave focus in the right temporal region.

The behavioral changes characteristic of psychomotor epileptics (viscosity and irritability), however, tend to become manifest only after a minimum of 2 years following the clinical onset of seizures.

The direct relationship of the behavioral changes to the irritative temporolimbic lesions explains two phenomena. So often the patient's behavior gradually deteriorates in the interval between the attacks, reaching a peak just prior to an attack, and diminishes after the attack, thus corresponding to the cycle of focal excitability of the limbic structures. If, on the other hand, the seizures are suppressed, the behavior may be aggravated, since the cyclic palliative effect of the neural exhaustion afforded by the ictus has been eliminated.

Gastaut concludes that there is no contradiction between his findings and those of the psychiatric observers of idiopathic or genuine epilepsy, because they were made on the same patients: those with psychomotor epilepsy. However, he noted that a minority of psychomotor epileptics do not present the characteristic behavioral picture.

Changes of Sexual Behavior in Psychomotor Epilepsy. The fact that Griesinger (44) in 1868 made a brief notation of the "sexual weakness" of epileptics can hardly detract from the originality of Gastaut and Collomb's comprehensive study (63) of the sexual behavior of patients with epilepsy. While references to abnormal sexual acts among epileptics can be found in older psychiatric texts, Gastaut and Collomb established a proper perspective on such occasional occurrences. Their striking finding was that of a chronic global hyposexuality among a majority of patients with psychomotor epilepsy.

This finding has by now been amply confirmed and is discussed further in Chapters 6 and 9 of this volume. Patients with psychomotor seizures secondary to diffuse limbic lesions may also present, in rare cases, paroxysmal sexual manifestations of three types: priapism associated with loss of consciousness and amnesia, occurring in psychomotor attacks with predominant autonomic (hypothalamic) effects; episodes of sexual arousal, with awareness and memory maintained, in reaction to seizures with abnormal genital sensations; and less rare episodes of sexual excitement, sometimes resulting in sexual indecencies, accompanied by loss of awareness and amnesia, occurring in the course of, or following, certain psychomotor attacks.

The findings concerning sexual changes in other types of epilepsy made by Gastaut and Collomb can be summarized as follows: (a) Patients with generalized-functional epilepsies never show any sexual changes related to their seizure disorder. The same can be said of those with partial epilepsies related to lesions in the convexity of the hemispheres, except for very rare cases with an irritative lesion involving the paracentral lobule (with its cortical representation of the genitals); such a lesion may lead to paroxysmal sexual sensations. (b) Generalized seizure disorders secondary to a mesodiencephalic lesion may rarely be associated with sexual manifestations, either in paroxysmal form with priapism (seizure discharges in the autonomic zones of the floor of the third ventricle) or in chronic form with modification of sexual activity and with endocrine disorders (according to the presence of a seizure disorder in the respective autonomic zones).

The authors further point out that anticonvulsants are not responsible for the hyposexuality. Rather, by eliminating seizure activity, the drugs may restore sexual arousal and response. The hyposexuality becomes established 2 years after onset of clinical seizures. On the other hand, it may be present even though clinical seizures occur rarely, and can be observed in individuals with a temporal lobe seizure focus who never had any overt clinical seizures.

Case 28. A 21-year-old male suffered a severe head injury with loss of consciousness for three days. Over the following months he developed the complaints typical of a posttraumatic syndrome. An EEG showed right temporal theta waves associated with a flurry of sporadic sharp waves of modest amplitude. Two years later, the patient returned complaining of a loss of sexual arousal which developed gradually over the past few months and had become nearly complete. This impotence concerned him much more than his headaches and dizzy spells, because it had led to a misunderstanding on his wife's part, who believed he was cheating on her. The wife confirmed these statements, and related her husband's recent personality changes as further evidence of her misfortune: "He can't stand me anymore; all I say goes on his nerves; he then has dreadful fits of rage . . . and finally, he doesn't want to have sex with me anymore." The patient never had any symptoms suggestive of seizures. The EEG now showed bilateral independent foci of spikes and slow waves.

The Temporal Lobe Syndromes after Bilateral Ablation and in Temporal Lobe Epilepsy. Gastaut compared his behavioral findings with those of the well-known ablation experiments in animals (75). The cited interictal behavior disorders of temporal lobe epileptics represent exact opposites of the hypervigilance with short attention span (hypermetamorphosis), placidity, and hypersexuality observed as characteristic traits of the Klüver-Bucy syndrome after bilateral temporal ablations (Table 2). Gastaut suggests that this is not a surprising finding if one considers that interictally, owing to the effect of the irritative lesions, the temporal lobe epileptic must present a state of excitation and not a state of depression of the temporolimbic system. The ictal and interictal discharges in psychomotor epileptics affect the temporolimbic system with its diffuse connections to hypothalamus and mesencephalon, and result in specific profound behavioral changes. These findings are more fully discussed in Chapter 9 of this volume.

We finally must mention Gastaut's study of Vincent Van Gogh's illness (76). In his late life, Van Gogh suffered from temporal lobe epilepsy with psychotic episodes. He had been correctly diagnosed as epileptic by the French psychiatrists who cared for him and who were very familiar with what Morel and Falret taught about the psychiatric aspects of epilepsy.

Vincent Van Gogh was the son of a preacher and had once embarked on a career as a missionary to the poor before devoting his life to painting. He had become agnostic, and was astounded by the intrusion of religious experiences in his mind during his illness. He showed the full range of extraordinary personality and behavioral traits associated with temporal lobe epilepsy, notably, an enormously enhanced and labile emotionality, with outbursts of anger, on the one hand, and cosmic-religious raptures, on the other. He committed suicide at a time when both the seizures and the psychotic state had remitted.

Carbamazepine: Psychotropic Effects of an Anticonvulsant—A Drug in Search of a Disorder

Psychiatrists have increasingly observed that the tricyclic anticonvulsant drug carbamazepine may bring about marked, even

TABLE 2. *Comparison of human behavioral findings with those from ablation experiments in animals*

Modifications of *animal* behavior after bilateral rhinencephalic ablations (principally basal) (KLÜVER and BUCY, 1937–1939; PRIBRAM and BAGSHAW, 1953; SCHREINER and KLING, 1953).	Disorders of *human* behavior in the interval between psychomotor attacks, from questioning, observation, and psychometric studies of 100 patients. (H. GASTAUT, J. ROGER and N. LESÈVRE, 1952–1954).
A. Modification of general activity *It is augmented;* the animal does not stop moving around in its cage; it is interested in and touches everything, since everything retains its attention in a transitory manner ("hypervigilance" of attention).	A. Modification of general activity *It is diminished;* the patient is slow in his movements, gestures, changes of facial expression, speech, ideation, deliberation, and association or recall of ideas. Psychometric tests express this slowness, which is accompanied by precision if the intelligence is normal.
B. Modification of social behavior *It is improved;* the animal becomes placid, displays a grooming reaction; it loses its fighting behavior and exhibits defensive or aggressive reactions, only with difficulty.	B. Modification of social behavior *It becomes worse;* the patient becomes impulsive, aggressive, and inclined to violent, angry reactions, sometimes dangerous. Sometimes perverted character traits are associated with irritability and hypocrisy, making the patient intolerable in the social and even the family milieu.
C. Modification of sexual behavior *It is augmented;* the animal tries incessantly to have sexual relations with any other animal, regardless of its age, sex, or species.	C. Modification of sexual behavior *It is diminished:* many patients become progressively impotent or indifferent, or both.
D. Modification of eating behavior It is not modified quantitatively, but rather qualitatively; the animal puts everything in its mouth to feel or taste it; it ingests unusual foods.	D. Modification of eating behavior It is neither modified quantitatively nor qualitatively.

From Gastaut (75).

dramatic, and lasting improvements in certain otherwise intractable patients. These are often said to be patients with atypical affective, schizoaffective, or schizophrenia-like syndromes with or without signs of epilepsy. Some have been lumped in the category of borderline states. No specific psychiatric syndrome has been identified, however, which would reliably respond to the anticonvulsant.

In Chapter 8 Jonathan Himmelhoch defines a syndrome of major mood disorders related to epileptic changes. His is an important discovery. The syndrome of excessive and labile emotionality, with alternating enhanced anger and remorse, sudden, brief depressive moods, sometimes fleeting beatitudes, and religious preoccupation, is indeed found in patients with temporal lobe epilepsy. Obsession with trivial details is common in these patients, and transient paranoid ideation may occur, whereas sexual arousal is usually muted, but in rare cases excessive. The wide range of mental changes characteristic of temporal lobe epilepsy is present here and tends to be confusing to the clinician who is not familiar with the syndrome. Kraepelin's description of the epileptic dysphorias or mood changes, which is included in this chapter, conforms precisely to what we can observe here, and Kraepelin never related these peculiar dysphorias to manic-depressive illness. These patients respond to carbamazepine and, to a lesser degree, phenytoin because their primary disorder is epileptiform. The mood changes are secondary, just as the thought disorders are secondary to epilepsy in the related schizophrenia-like psychosis of epilepsy.

Psychiatric interest in carbamazepine has been stimulated by the observation that it appears to have therapeutic effects in affective illness. Following earlier Japanese reports, Post and Ballenger (77, 78) with their group at the National Institute of Mental Health have shown that carbamazepine may have significant antimanic and some antidepressant properties. The reports by Post's group do not include clinical case studies, and leave unanswered the question of whether their patients suffered from classic mania—or perhaps rather from atypical "rapid-cycling" affective syndromes that had not responded to standard antimanic treatment, in which case they may belong to the group described by Himmelhoch. Nevertheless, the studies carried out by Post's group have been most interesting in many respects.

The psychotropic effects of carbamazepine have been documented in several groups of patients (77). Dalby (79) finds that in 40 reports about 50 percent of 2,500 epileptics improved psychiatrically. The behavioral changes characteristic of temporal lobe seizure disorders, in particular, have been shown to improve: slowness of thought, viscosity, lability of mood, irritability, and fits of rage, as well as states of anger and depression (79–95). A few reports comment on dramatic and lasting improvements afforded by carbamazepine in affective and schizophrenia-like syndromes associated with epilepsy (83, 85, 86, 96, 97). Furthermore, nonepileptic patients with nonspecific EEG abnormalities who suffer from often marked psychiatric disorders have been shown to respond favorably to this drug (92, 93, 98–110). In this group improvements in violent behavior, irritability, emotional lability, depression, agitation, and apathy have been reported.

To epileptologists experienced in treating difficult cases of temporal lobe epilepsy, carbamazepine's psychotropic properties are often not as clearly evident. Unlike phenobarbital and primidone, carbamazepine admittedly does not tend to impair cognition and behavior. In our experience there can be definite beneficial psychotropic effects when carbamazepine is prescribed for patients with epilepsy. But the more striking psychopharmacologic effects occur in patients whose temporal lobe epilepsy disorder is very subtle, as Himmelhoch has postulated.

Within a couple of years, a patient who has temporal lobe epilepsy or a seizure disorder with limbic involvement tends to develop some characteristic personality and behavioral changes, though these may remain very subtle. If these changes are bothersome, and carbamazepine was not prescribed as the drug of first choice, it should now be used as the drug with the best psychotropic effect. Phenytoin (Dilantin) may also have psychotropic effects, but to a lesser degree. The barbiturates (phenobarbital, primidone) generally should be avoided. Only one anticonvulsant should be used, if at all possible. Monotherapy has many advantages; e.g., carbamazepine prescribed alone at 600–800 mg daily tends to result in a good blood level, whereas with the concomitant administration of phenytoin, considerably higher doses may still leave the patient below the optimal therapeutic level. While a complete control of seizures may also result in much improved behavior, this is not always the case, and patients need to be treated individually. Some patients whose subclinical seizure activity persists may be emotionally more stable if they have an occasional seizure. Ernst Rodin deals with the medical treatment of patients with epilepsy in Chapter 4.

Of clinical significance for the psychiatrist is the fact that temporal lobe epilepsy frequently remains undiagnosed (see Chapter 2). If a patient presents with characteristic emotional and behavioral changes, a careful inquiry into the presence of seizures needs to be undertaken, and treatment should be carried out accordingly. This is illustrated by the following case.

Case 1
Subtle Temporal Lobe Seizures with Marked Personality Changes and Emotional Lability

A 42-year-old homemaker sought help for marked mood swings, feeling tense "like a spring," and increased irritability with frequent loss of temper. She admitted to drinking too much and felt much remorse for what she was putting her family through. She also complained of pains in her neck and knees and experienced feelings of numbness. A depressive episode of 2-week duration had first occurred 3 years ago. She cried easily, "over nothing," e.g., when listening to a hymn in church or when seeing small children walk by. It was an effort for her to get moving in the morning, and for the past 2 years it took her twice as long to get things done. Recently, she often reached a point where she didn't care if she lived.

She related that 2 years ago she had awakened "with the worst sore throat" and felt weak and clammy; as she went for some aspirin, she fainted and fell down the steps, splitting her scalp. She remained unconscious for 20 min and was unable to speak for 30 min after the episode. The family physician sutured her laceration and asked no questions, perhaps assuming that she had been drinking. This, however, was not the case. One year later there was a similar, but milder, episode of sudden nausea and feeling faint.

An EEG indicated the presence of an irritative and potentially epileptiform disturbance in the left anterior and midtemporal areas. With the prescription of 200 mg carbamazepine three times daily, her mood swings, irritability, and use of alcohol ceased. She had no further episodes, and her grateful family was pleased that her "bad personality" had changed so much for the better.

The EEG can be very helpful, but the physician has to be guided by the clinical findings. If a routine EEG with sleep is unremarkable in a patient suspected to have temporal lobe disorders, at least one repeat EEG after a night of sleep deprivation and/or with special leads (nasopharyngeal or sphenoidal) should be requested. EEG findings may be minimal, and at times may remain absent. Specific psychiatric findings are decisive in determining the use of carbamazepine. The following cases illustrate how patients' characteristic psychopathology may respond exceedingly well to carbamazepine in the absence of seizures, and even with minimal, inconclusive EEG findings.

Case 2
Temporal Lobe Spiking, Questionable Minor Seizures, and Atypical Psychotic State with Enhanced and Labile Emotionality

A 46-year-old homemaker had to be admitted to a psychiatric hospital for 9 months because of marked mood swings from excited euphoric states with religious coloration to sometimes nearly stuporous depressive states. She also experienced a heightened intensity of her emotions with marked verbosity, fluctuating paranoid delusions, obsessions with trivial details, a childlike dependence on others, and somatic complaints. Her condition had gradually worsened over a period of a few years. Because of the unusual clinical picture and the occurrence of sudden brief interruptions of consciousness and visual distortions, a neurologic investigation was undertaken. Her EEG revealed left temporal spiking.

After trials of phenytoin, phenobarbital, and primidone, carbamazepine was prescribed, resulting in a calming of her emotionality and clearing of her thinking. She continued to be preoccupied with minute details, so imipramine was prescribed on a trial basis, resulting in further improvement. Following her hospitalization, she was successfully maintained for 5 years on Tegretol 200 mg three times daily and Tofranil 50 mg twice daily. Because of the absence of a convincing history of seizures, her medications were finally tapered off. She then gradually relapsed into a state reminiscent of that which had required her hospitalization. Prompt remission was obtained upon resumption of her medication.

This case documents the usefulness of combining a modest dose of an antidepressant with carbamazepine, as Himmelhoch also points out (see Chapter 8).

Case 3
Mild Paroxysmal EEG Findings with Severe "Borderline State" Marked by Heightened and Labile Emotionality

An 18-year-old girl had been experiencing rapid mood changes over the preceding 4 years. She began to overeat and had gained about 70 lbs over the last 2 years. She was overly sensitive, and would alternate between intense anger and a very good-natured attitude, appearing to her parents as being "like two persons." Treatment with three different therapists had no impact. She had begun to feel suicidal and would bang her head against the floor in times of despair. Her parents felt unable to cope with her any longer and sought a consultation, with an urgent request for hospitalization.

It was learned that just prior to the onset of her illness she had, on two occasions, suffered what appeared to be a convulsion, upon undergoing, respectively, bronchoscopy and venipuncture. An EEG was negative at that time. The episodes were felt to be perhaps of a vasovagal nature, and no medication was prescribed. A current EEG showed minimal evidence of potentially paroxysmal tendencies (a single slow sharp wave complex projected from deep or midline sources to the frontal regions) and was judged inconclusive.

In view of the characteristic clinical syndrome, she was not hospitalized, but was promptly started on carbamazepine 200 mg three times daily. Within a few days, she felt at ease, even-tempered, and in control of herself. Two months later her blood level dropped clearly below therapeutic range and the dosage was increased to 1,000 mg. She maintained her improvement without any psychotherapeutic support, was able to lose her excess weight, and entered college away from home. Her mother had sometimes fantasized a "magic wand" to solve her daughter's problems and felt that carbamazepine made her fantasy a reality.

Following excessive use of depressant substances, the well-known withdrawal seizures may occur. In certain patients the withdrawal phase, or the intermittent prolonged use or abuse of the substances, may be marked by characteristic psychiatric syndromes related to the emergence of seizure activity. Ballenger and Post (111) and Himmelhoch (112) have described these events, which must be considered of considerable clinical significance yet are still generally ignored.

Case 4
EEG with Mild Bitemporal Dysrhythmia, "Panic Attacks" Following a Bout of Excessive Drinking

A 40-year-old insurance agent, accustomed to imbibing one to five martinis daily, celebrated a certain occasion by going on a 3-day drinking spree. After <2 h of sleep following the last drink, he suddenly awoke with a funny feeling and an intense, panicky restlessness. He was overcome with bizarre thoughts, fear of losing control, a clammy sensation, dryness of the throat, and chest pain. The episode lasted almost 48 h. One week later he *had a recurrence of this attack after having four or five drinks the evening before. He forced himself to take a scheduled plane trip, but once on the plane he was in panic, afraid of doing something horrible, and, in fact, had a strong impulse to jump out of the plane. He never drank again, but still had a third recurrence 1 week later. Terrified, he checked himself into a hospital for the third time.*

An EEG showed mild bitemporal dysrhythmia. He had rapid mood swings and lacked any sexual arousal during the 6 weeks since onset. It was learned that 6 years prior to this illness, he had suffered two episodes of loss of consciousness, the first following an injection of cortisone and adrenaline and the second during the course of an attack of urticaria after eating shellfish. For 1 year before, he had begun to be irritable and abusive after alcohol intake, and had been overeating, gaining about 15 lbs.

Dilantin 300 mg daily and Xanax 0.5 mg four times daily were prescribed, but he still had brief episodes of anxiety and felt tired. He remained fearful of a recurrence of his severe attacks and had to be persuaded to carry out another scheduled plane trip. Both drugs were phased out, and 10 weeks after the onset of his attacks carbamazepine was started. Before the drug reached a satisfactory level, he had another episode of panic lasting 30 min while sitting in a barber's chair, fearing a loss of control—that he might grab the barber or suddenly run. Thereafter his condition stabilized and he began to feel like his former self.

The emotional lability, intense impulsivity, and loss of any sexual arousal are characteristic traits.

Subclinical seizure activity may be ongoing for prolonged periods following removal of the offending substance. Carbamazepine, as the drug of first choice for psychiatric disturbances related to a subictal disorder, may sometimes have to be continued for an extended period.

Carbamazepine is generally well tolerated. Serious hematologic complications of carbamazepine, in the form of rare pancytopenia, persistent leukopenia, and isolated thrombocytopenia, are uncommon (see Chapter 4). There is a major discrepancy between the manufacturer's recommendations for expensive laboratory monitoring and the routine practice of most clinicians. Hart and Easton (113) have made the following sensible recommendations: (a) Reports of serious hematological complications of carbamazepine must be submitted to the manufacturer to establish the incidence and benefit of laboratory monitoring as well as other characteristics of these complications. (b) Blood and platelet counts should be performed before the initiation of carbamazepine therapy. Patients with abnormalities on these tests and those taking other myelotoxic drugs should be considered at special risk. Carbamazepine therapy in these groups should be monitored closely or avoided. (c) Complete blood counts should be made every 2 weeks for the first 2 months. If no abnormalities appear, counts should be obtained quarterly or with the appearance of symptoms or signs of bone marrow suppression. Patients should be instructed to contact their physician immediately if petechiae, pallor, undue weakness, fever, or infection occurs. (d) If leukopenia develops, it should be monitored at 2-week intervals, seeking the expected return to baseline. The drug dose should be reduced if possible, and the presence of infection or severe leukopenia ($<3,000$ white blood cells/mm^3 or $<1,500$ neutrophils/mm^3) calls for immediate cessation of carbamazepine use.

Before lithium was discovered as the first specific antimanic drug, the diagnosis of schizophrenia had been indiscriminately made in many cases in the United States. The presence of the new drug forced the diagnostic process to be honed, and many cases that superficially looked like schizophrenia were then recognized as manic cases.

With carbamazepine we apparently have a drug effective not only for generalized seizures and for temporal lobe (complex partial) seizures, in particular, but for the range of characteristic psychiatric disorders that occur on the basis of temporolimbic seizure involvement and that this volume attempts to define and interpret. We are addressing an admittedly complex yet distinct and actual problem.

Psychiatrists may be hesitant to trust their clinical senses and are understandably concerned that even expert use of EEG findings will often not provide an answer to their questions. There is hope that the modern spectroscopic methods may soon permit laboratory measures of even those seizure disorders that are inaccessible by current EEG methods.

Leopold Szondi: The Paroxysmal Factor—An Integration of Genetic and Psychodynamic Findings

The tradition of European psychiatry dating back to the nineteenth century had provided the natural frame of reference for Kraepelin's description of a psychopathology of genuine epilepsy distinct from the two other major forms of mental illness, dementia praecox and manic-depressive illness. From the same familiar background, Gastaut made his brilliant synthesis of psychiatric data with the modern neurologic findings of temporal lobe epilepsy.

We may be convinced that the descriptions of specific personality and behavior traits, labile mood states, and even psychoses found in association with epilepsy are correct. We may be further impressed by the persistent finding among "genuine" epileptics, i.e., temporal lobe epileptics, of the coexistence of two trends—to pent up and explosively release anger, on the one hand, and to be remorseful, conscientious, and often hyperreligious, on the other—a finding suggesting the dynamic interaction of two opposite tendencies. Many of these patients show subtle psychic changes and may present as slight caricatures of, or identical to, a personality type that can be found among healthy individuals.

Can all of this be reduced to the accident of an epileptogenic lesion in the temporolimbic system, or could a genetic factor play a significant etiologic role? Lennox (114) found that the prevalence of seizures for the near relatives of probands with epilepsy symptomatic of a focal lesion was 3.6 times higher than for the near relatives of nonepileptics. Although a number of studies did not find a genetic predisposition in symptomatic epilepsy, when further studies were done using EEG data, the prevalence of convulsions and/or epileptiform cerebral dysrhythmias among parents and siblings of hemiplegics with convulsions was observed to be significantly higher than for the parents and siblings of hemiplegics without convulsions, suggesting strongly a familial predisposition, probably owing to genetic factors (115). Among the near relatives of surgically treated patients with partial epilepsy, the majority of whom underwent surgical treatment for temporal lobe epilepsy, there was a prevalence of epileptiform EEGs nearly three times greater than that found in the control group (116). The common febrile convulsions are usually transmitted as a dominant trait, and are thus more genetically determined than other seizure disorders (117). They may leave anoxic scars leading to manifest temporal lobe seizures in later life. In this manner, inheritance may play an indirect role in focal seizures.

Metrakos and Metrakos (118) believe that the epilepsies have more in common than division at the clinical seizure level would imply, and speak of a common genetically controlled predisposing factor in divergent forms of epilepsy. Andermann (119) postulates a multifactorial inheritance of the epilepsies, whereby one or more major genes or polygenes interact with maturational and endocrine factors (resulting in age and sex differences) as well as with various exogenous factors and produce the variety of clinical and EEG findings encountered. She assumes three thresholds in increasing order of liability: one for epileptiform EEG abnormalities; one for a history of one or more seizures; and one for chronic epilepsy. Accordingly, separate heritabilities could be calculated for each seizure type.

In a recent review, Reynolds (120) cites the sole finding of Slater and coworkers (121) who documented the absence of a genetic background for schizophrenia in the schizophrenia-like psychosis of epilepsy and states that there is an extraordinary lack of information about genetic factors in relation to personality and psychiatric disorders in epilepsy. This is not entirely correct.

Szondi (122) refers to the extensive European literature on the inheritance of mental disorders, which was accumulated prior to World War II and subsequently forgotten in the wake of the tragic abuses of psychiatric genetics by facist ideology. Though genetics is still far removed from precisely determining the mode of inheritance of the major mental disorders, three major spheres of independently inheritable psychiatric disorders have been recognized: the schizophreniform; the manic-depressive (circular); and the epileptiform (paroxysmal) hereditary sphere. To these he added the sphere of sexual disorders.

Through extensive pedigree studies, Szondi has shown that migraine, stuttering, and a series of minor disorders are genetically closely related to epilepsy. He postulates that there is no sharp dividing line between the illness and the norm; they are merely different points on the same continuum. Thus, the manifestation of the gene groups that determine schizophreniform reactions has a very wide range of variation of which the socially adjusted extreme is the schizothymic constitution and the psychopathologic extreme is schizophrenia. Between these two one finds a great many neurotic phenomena.

Szondi considers the major mental illnesses to be disorders of specific drive needs that are based on specific, qualitatively different drive genes. The variety of phenomena within a specific drive need is based on quantitative differences in the multiple alleles of a specific gene. Drives are composed of opposite pairs of needs, and needs of opposite pairs of tendencies. The dynamic tension characteristic of drives is based on this polarity of specific needs and tendencies. Szondi constructs a drive system composed of opposing pairs of drives that, on the one hand, occur in each individual and, on the other, show an exact correspondence to the psychopathologic hereditary spheres. In accordance with the four major psychiatric disorders, there are four drives: the sexual drive; the paroxysmal drive; the ego drive; and the contact drive. Thus, manic-depressives suffer from a disorder of their contact needs, and schizophrenics from a disorder of their ego needs. Since each of the four hereditary spheres has two clinically and genetically separable forms of manifestation (Table 3), Szondi arrives at a total of eight specific drive needs (Table 4).

Here we will limit our focus to the paroxysmal drive. How does this drive function in the normal and in the ill individual, and what does Szondi's concept contribute to our understanding of epilepsy?

TABLE 3. *Hereditary spheres and the eight basic inheritable psychiatric disorders*

I. Sexual disorders	1. Homosexuality (*h*) 2. Sadism (*s*)	
II. Paroxysmal disorders	3. Epilepsy (*e*) 4. Hysteria (*hy*)	
III. Schizoform disorders	5. Katatonic (*k*) 6. Paranoid (*p*)	Schizophrenia
IV. Circular disorders	7. Depression (*d*) 8. Mania (*m*)	

From Szondi (122).

TABLE 4. *The eight basic drive factors*

1. *h*-drive factor:	Need for affection, love, femininity
2. *s*-drive factor:	Need for activity, aggression, sadism, masculinity
3. *e*-drive factor:	Need to pent up crude emotions: anger, hate, rage, jealousy, envy, vengefulness
4. *hy*-drive factor:	Need for attention and recognition
5. *k*-drive factor:	Need to constrict the ego, ego-systole (the critical, material, or possessive ego)
6. *p*-drive factor:	Need to expand the ego, ego-diastole (the spiritual ego)
7. *d*-drive factor:	Need to search for and acquire objects
8. *m*-drive factor:	Need to cling to acquired objects (attachment)

From Szondi (122).

In his later writings (123,124), Szondi terms the paroxysmal-epileptiform drive factor (*e*) "the ethical factor." It determines the penting up of the crude affects of anger, hate, vengefulness, envy, and jealousy to the point of sudden and explosive discharge. On the other hand, the same factor, with its opposite tendency, determines the awakening of conscience, tolerance, justice, altruism, and piousness. Szondi refers to the penting up of crude affects to the point of murderous intent as the "Kain complex." Moses, who had killed an Egyptian, fled, had religious visions, then heard the voice of God and became his prophet, bringing to his people the commandments. In Moses both poles of the ethical factor are clearly evident (125).

The epileptiform or ethical factor thus determines the forces of "good" and "evil," the paroxysmal nature of humans, which can be observed in three phases: the penting up of crude affects; the explosive discharge or attack; and the phase of making up—the ethical-religious phase. This process of general significance tends to be most dramatically expressed in certain epileptic disorders. Thus follows the paradoxic finding of the "two-faced epileptic" or the "Jekyll-and-Hyde" nature of many patients. Although many patients appear stabilized in the hyperethical phase, the paroxysmal force of the process tends to be episodically destabilizing and frequently results in marked emotional lability.

A very positive personality type could be described at the normal extreme of the spectrum: individuals who are conscientious, law abiding, and devout. The very just, however, may tend to be angered by injustice and intolerant of the unfaithful. A caricature of this personality type can be found among some temporal lobe epileptics. The sexual needs tend to be of limited significance in the entire group.

The ethical attitude reflects the human inner conscience, and can be differentiated from the moral attitude determined by how one is viewed by others and society. The latter is a central issue of the hysteric patient. Contrary to popular belief, the explosive discharge in epilepsy is not primarily destructive. Destructive-sadistic acts are basically related to the extremes of the drive factor determining activity-aggressivity (*s*-factor).

Szondi's concepts attempt to organize our understanding of very complex findings. A genetic predisposition plays a major role in the cerebral events. Every individual has the potential to react with a seizure, and the emotionality of certain epileptics merely represents extraordinary variants of the norm. Human ethical and religious attitudes are obviously of central importance and may be better understood in the light of new concepts.

At the biologic level, the study of pedigrees can be carried out, e.g., to determine if atypical or subictal psychoses bear a kinship to disorders from the epilepsy spectrum (seizures, migraine, stuttering, epileptiform personality) or to the spectrum of disorders related to manic-depressive disease. At the psychodynamic level, very individualized studies are called for.

The original thesis that epilepsy was a hereditary disease seated in the brain and capable of affecting the mind was stated by the Hippocratic physicians. The scientific inquiry proceeds meticulously by studying but fragments at a time, and the specialist tends to lose sight of the whole picture. A disorder as complex as epilepsy requires not only differentiation but also major steps toward a synthesis, as have beeen undertaken by Szondi. His concepts give a new meaning to the old term the *Sacred Disease*, though we are aware that there are many variations to the disorder called epilepsy.

REFERENCES

1. Temkin O: *The Falling Sickness.* Baltimore, The Johns Hopkins Press, 1971
2. Hippocrates: *Oeuvres complètes d'Hippocrate.* 10 vols. Edited by Littré E. Paris, 1839–61
3. Plato: *Plato, VII, Timaeus, etc.*, English transl. by Bury RG. Loeb Classical Library, 1929
4. Caelius Aurelianus: *On Acute Diseases and on Chronic Diseases.* Edited and transl. by Drabkin IE. Chicago, The University of Chicago Press, 1950
5. Pliny: *Naturalis historia.* Rec. by Janus L. Leipzig, vol 1, 1870; vols 2–6, 1856–65
6. Euripides: *Euripides, Vols 2 and 3.* English transl. by Way AS. Loeb Classical Library, 1929–30
7. Aretaeus: *The Extant Works of Aretaeus, the Cappadocian.* Edited and transl. by Adams F. London, The Sydenham Society, 1856
8. Galen: *Opera Omnia.* Edited by Kuhn CG. Leipzig, 1821
9. Aristotle: *The Works of Aristotle. Vol 9, Ethica Nicomachea.* Edited and transl. by Ross WD. Oxford University Press, 1925
10. Philodemus: *De ira liber.* Edited by Wilke C. Leipzig, Tuebner, 1914
11. Plutarch: *Plutarch's Moralia.* English transl. by Babbitt FC. Loeb Classical Library, 1927
12. St. Hildegard: *Causae et curae.* Edited by Kaiser P. Leipzig, Teubner, 1903
13. Abulqasim: *De chirurgia, Vol 1.* Edited by Channing J. Oxford, 1778
14. Taxil J: *Traicté de l'épilepsie, maladie vulgairement appellée au pays de Provence, la gouttete aux petits enfans.* Tournon, 1602
15. Guainerius A: *Practica Antonii Guainerii papiensis doctoris preclarissimi, Impressum opus mandato et expensis heredum quondam domini Octaviani Scoti civis Modoetiensis et Sociorum.* 1516
16. Steeghius G: *Ars medica.* Frankfurt, 1606
17. Benivenius A: *De abditis nonnullis ac mirandis morborum et sanationum causis.* Florence, 1507
18. Sylvius FD: *Opera medica.* Geneva, 1693
19. Willis T: *Dr. Willis' Practice of Physick, Being the Whole Works of That . . . Physician.* London, 1684
20. Wepfer JJ: *Cicutae aquaticae historia et noxae.* Basel, 1679
21. Stahl GE: *Theoria medica vera.* 3 vols. Edited by Choulant L. Leipzig, 1831–33

22. Hunter R, Macalpine I: *Three Hundred Years of Psychiatry 1535–1860.* London, Oxford University Press, 1963

23. De Haen A: *Pars quinta rationis medendi in nosocomio practico.* Vienna, 1760

24. Tissot SA: *Traité de l'épilepsie, faisant le tome troisième du traité des nerfs et de leurs maladies.* Paris, 1770

25. Tissot SA: *L'onanisme, dissertation sur les maladies produites par la masturbation, nouvelle edition.* Lausanne, 1782

26. Maisonneuve JGF: *Recherches et observations sur l'épilepsie, présentées à l'école de médecine de Paris.* Paris, 1804

27. Calmeil L-F: *De l'épilepsie, étudiée sous le rapport de son siège et de son influence sur la production de l'aliénation mentale.* Thése de Paris, 1824.

28. Esquirol E: *Des maladies mentales.* 2 vols. Paris, 1838

29. Mead R: *De imperio solis ac lunae in corpora humana, et morbis inde oriundis.* London, 1746

30. Prichard JC: *A Treatise on Diseases of the Nervous System, Part the first.* London, 1822

31. Meyer L. Ueber Mania transitoria. *Virchows Arch* 8:192–210, 1855

32. Bouchet and Cazauvieilh: De l'épilepsie considérée dans ses rapports avec l'aliénation mentale. Recherches sur la nature et le siège de ces deux maladies. *Arch Gen Med* 9:510–542, 1825; 10:5–50, 1826

33. Herpin T: *Du prognostic et du traitement curatif de l'épilepsie.* Paris, 1852

34. Reynolds JR: *Epilepsy: Its Symptoms, Treatment, and Relation to Other Chronic Convulsive Diseases.* London, 1861.

35. Bravais LF; *Recherches sur les symptômes et le traitement de l'épilepsie hémiplégique.* Paris, 1827

36. Bright R: Cases illustrative of the effects produced when the arteries and brain are diseased. *Guys Hosp Rep* 1:9–40, 1836

37. Bright R: *Reports of Medical Cases, Vol 2, Part 2.* London, 1831

38. Lasègue C: Morel—sa vie médicale et ses oeuvres. *Arch Gen Med* 1:589–600, 1873

39. Morel BA: *Etude cliniques. Traité théorique et pratique des maladies mentales considérées dans leur nature, leur traitement, et dans leur rapport avec la médecine légale des aliénés.* 2 vols. Nancy, Paris, 1852–53

40. Morel BA: *Traité des maladies mentales.* Paris, 1860

41. Morel BA: D'une forme de délire, suite d'une surexcitation nerveuse se rattachant à une variété non encore décrite d'épilepsie (Épilepsie larvée). *Gazette Hebdomadaire Med Chir* 7:773–775, 819–821, 836–841, 1860

42. Falret J: De l'état mental des épileptiques. *Arch Gen Med* 16:661–679, 1860; 17:461–491, 1861; 18:423–443, 1861

43. Griesinger W: *Die Pathologie und Therapie der psychischen Krankheiten.* Stuttgart, 1845

44. Griesinger W: Ueber einige epileptoide Zustände. *Arch Psychiatr Nervenk 1:320–333, 1868–69*

45. Herpin T: *Des accès imcomplets d'épilepsie.* Paris, 1867

46. Jackson JH: *Selected Writings of John Hughlings Jackson.* 2 vols. Edited by Taylor J. London, Hodder and Stoughton, 1931–32

47. Jackson JH: Cases of epilepsy associated with syphilis. *Med Times Gazette* 1:648–652, 2:59–60, 1861

48. Fritsch G, Hitzig E: *Ueber die elektrische Erregbarkeit des Grosshirns.* Berlin, n.d. (reprinted from Reichert's und du Bois-Reymond's Archiv, Heft 3, 1870)

49. Meynert T: *Der Bau der Gross-Hirnrinde und seine örtlichen Verschiedenheiten, nebst einem pathologisch—anatomischen Corollarium.* Neuwied-Leipzig, Heuser (Separat-Abdruck aus der Vierteljahrsschrift für Psychiatrie etc.), 1872

50. Sommer W: Erkrankung des Ammonshirns als aetiologisches Moment der Epilepsie. *Arch Psychiatr Nervenkr* 10:631–675, 1880

51. Gowers WR: *Epilepsy and Other Chronic Convulsive Diseases.* London, 1881

52. Briquet P: *Traité clinique et thérapeutique· de l'hystérie.* Paris, 1859

53. Charcot J: *Leçons sur les maladies du système nerveux (oeuvres complètes, I).* Rec. and published by Bourneville TI. Paris, 1886

54. Echeverria MG: Criminal responsibility of epileptics, as illustrated by the case of David Montgomery. *Am J Insanity* 29:341–425, 1872–73

55. Samt P: Epileptische Irreseinsformen. *Arch Psychiatr Nervenkr* 5:393–444, 1875; 6:110–216, 1876

56. Hoffman F: Ueber die Einteilung der Geisteskrankheiten in Siegburg. *Allgemeine Z Psychiatr Psychischgerichliche Med* 19:367–391, 1862

57. Krafft-Ebing RV: *Lehrbuch der Psychiatrie auf klinischer Grundlage.* 2 vols. Stuttgart, 1883

58. Maudsley H: *Responsibility in Mental Disease.* New York, 1874

59. Taylor DC, Marsh SM: Hughlings Jackson's Dr. Z: the paradigm of temporal lobe epilepsy revealed. *J Neurol Neurosurg Psychiatry* 43:758–767, 1980

60. Taylor DC, Marsh SM: Neuropathology and social pathology: the effects of small lesions in the temporal lobe, in *Proceedings on*

Tegretol in Epilepsy. Newark, NJ, Geigy Pharmaceuticals, 1977, p 21

61. Jackson JH: On a particular variety of epilepsy ("Intellectual Aura"), one case with symptoms of organic brain disease. *Brain* 11:179–207, 1880

62. Jackson JH, Colman WS: Case of epilepsy with tasting movements and 'dreamy state'—very small patch of softening in the left uncinate gyrus. *Brain* 21:580–590, 1898

63. Gastaut H, Collomb H: Étude du comportement sexuel chez les épileptiques psychomoteurs. *Ann Med Psychol (Paris)* 112:657–696, 1954

64. Myers AT, Myers FWH: Mind-cure, faith-cure and the miracles of Lourdes. *Proc Soc Psychol Res Lond* 9:160–209, 1893

65. Kraepelin E: *Psychiatrie, Vol 3.* 8th edition. Leipzig, Johann Ambrosius Barth, 1923

66. Gibbs FA, Gibbs EL, Lennox WG: Epilepsy; a paroxysmal cerebral dysrhythmia. *Brain* 60:377–388, 1937

67. Gastaut H: État actuel des connaissances sur l'anatomie pathologique des épilepsies. *Act Neurol Psychiatr Belq* 56:5–20, 1956

68. Stauder KH: Epilepsie und Schläfenlappen. *Arch Psychiatr Nervenkr* 104:181–212, 1936

69. Liddel DW: Observations on epileptic automatism in a mental hospital population. *J Ment Sci* 99:732–748, 1953

70. Roger A, Dongier M: Corrélations électrocliniques chez 50 épileptiques internés. *Rev Neurol* 83:593–596, 1950

71. Sano K, Malamud N: Clinical significance of sclerosis of the cornu ammonis. *Arch Neurol Psychiatry* 70:40–53, 1953

72. Gastaut H, Roger J, Lesèvre N: Différenciation psychologique des épileptiques en fonction des formes électrocliniques de leur maladie. *Rev Psychol Appl* 3:237–249, 1953

73. Blumer D: Temporal lobe epilepsy and its psychiatric significance, in *Psychiatric Aspects of Neurologic Disease.* Edited by Benson DF, Blumer D. New York, Grune & Stratton, 1975 pp 171–198

74. Gastaut H, Morin G, Lesèvre N: Étude du comportement des épileptiques psychomoteurs dans l'intervalle de leurs crises. *Ann Med Psychol (Paris)* 113:1–27, 1955

75. Gastaut H: Interpretation of the symptoms of psychomotor epilepsy in relation to physiological data on rhinencephalic function. *Epilepsia* 3:84–88, 1954

76. Gastaut H: La maladie de Vincent Van Gogh envisagée à la lumière des conceptions nouvelles sur l'épilepsie psychomotrice. *Ann Med Psychol (Paris)* 114:196–238, 1956

77. Ballenger JC, Post RM: Therapeutic effects of carbamazepine in

affective illness: a preliminary report. *Commun Psychopharmacol* 2:159–175, 1978

78. Post RM, Uhde TW, Ballenger JC, et al: Carbamazepine, temporal lobe epilepsy, and manic-depressive illness. *Adv Biol Psychiatry* 8:117–156, 1982

79. Dalby MA: Behavioral effects of carbamazepine, in *Neurology, Vol 11*. Edited by Penry JK, Daly DD. New York, Raven Press, 1975, pp 331–343

80. Kristof M, Kolinova M: Antiparoxysmal and psychotropic effect of carbamazepine in the pharmacotherapy of epilepsy. *Act Nerv Super (Praha)* 15:176–177, 1973

81. Dodrill CB, Troupin AS: Psychotropic effects of carbamazepine in epilepsy: a double-blind comparison with phenytoin. *Neurology (Minneap)* 27:1023–1028, 1977

82. Marjerrison G, Jedlicki SM, Keogh RP, et al: Carbamazepine: behavioral, anticonvulsant and EEG effects in chronically-hospitalized epileptics. *Dis Nerv Syst* 29:133–136, 1968

83. Lehmann HE, Ban TA: Studies with new drugs in the treatment of convulsive disorders. *Int J Clin Pharmacol* 1:230–234, 1968

84. Bonduelle M: My study of Tegretol in the treatment of epilepsy, in *Tegretol in Epilepsy*. Edited by Wink CAS. Manchester, C Nicholls, 1972, pp 80–88

85. Dalby MA: Antiepileptic and psychotropic effect of carbamazapine (Tegretol) in the treatment of psychomotor epilepsy. *Epilepsia* 12:325–334, 1971

86. Mamoli A: La carbamazepina nel trattamento prolungato dell'epilessia nelle sue manifestazioni sia comiziali che psicopatologiche. *Riv Neurol* 42:1–19, 1972

87. Simpson GM, Kunz E, Watts TPS: Behavioral and anti-epileptic effects of an amino-stilbene derivative, in *Scientific Proceedings of the Fourth Congress Collegium Internationale Neuro-Psychopharmacologicum, Birmingham, 1964*. Amsterdam, Elsevier, 1964, pp 442–448

88. Smyth VOG: The use of Tegretol in temporal lobe epilepsy, in *Tegretol in Epilepsy*. Edited by Wink CAS. Manchester, C Nicholls, 1972, pp 48–53

89. Visentin B, Mattiuzzi D, Galvagni V: Osservazione cliniche sull'attività anticomitiale e psichotropa della carbamazepina. *Riv Neurol* 41:18–33, 1971

90. Steinbrecher W: Die Therapie zerebraler Anfallsformen mit Tegretol. *Med Welt* 25:1381–1385, 1966

91. Rett A: The so-called psychotropic effect of Tegretol in the treatment of convulsions of cerebral origin in children, in *Epileptic Seizures—Behavior—Pain*. Edited by Birkmayer W. Stuttgart, Huber, 1975, pp 194–204

92. Kuhn R: The psychotropic effect of carbamazepine in nonepileptic adults, with particular reference to the drug's possible mechanism of action, in *Epileptic Seizures—Behavior—Pain.* Edited by Birkmayer W. Stuttgart, Huber, 1975, pp 268–271

93. Groh C: The psychotropic effect of Tegretol in non-epileptic children, with particular reference to the drug's indications, in *Epileptic Seizures—Behavior—Pain.* Edited by Birkmayer W. Stuttgart, Huber, 1975, pp 259–263

94. Knauel H, Grüter W: Über psychotrope Wirkungen des Tegretal. *Zbl Gesamte Neurol Psychiatr* 188:18, 1967

95. Spreafico G: Anticonvulsant and psychotropic effects of Tegretol in a group of irregularly behaved mentally deficient epileptic children. *Minerva Pediatr* 19:465–467, 1967

96. Garcia-Pardo Gonzalez M: Contribution to the treatment of the psychiatric symptoms of epileptic origin. The value of Tegretol. *Acta Luso Esp Neurol Psiquiatr* 3:246–260, 1964

97. Hellekson C, Buckland R, Price T: Organic personality disturbance: a case of apparent atypical cyclic affective disorder. *Am J Psychiatry* 136:833–835, 1979

98. Monroe RR: *Episodic Behavioral Disorders.* Cambridge, Harvard University Press, 1970

99. Treffert DA: The psychiatric patient with an EEG temporal lobe focus. *Am J Psychiatry* 120:765–771, 1964

100. Williams D: Neural factors related to habitual aggression. Consideration of differences between those habitual aggressives and others who have committed crimes of violence. *Brain* 92:503–520, 1969

101. Hill D, Fenton GW: The temporal lobe: EEG and disorders of behaviour. *Br J Psychiatry* 4:49–54, 1969

102. Monroe RR: Anticonvulsants in the treatment of aggression. *J Nerv Ment Dis* 160:119–126, 1975

103. Maletzky BM: The episodic dyscontrol syndrome. *Dis Nerv Syst* 34:178–185, 1973

104. van Krevellen DA, Maresca A, Schreurs-Dijkstra M: Evaluation of Tegretol in the treatment of behaviour disorders in children. *Acta Paedopsychiatr (Basel)* 37:222–234, 1970

105. Castaño GR: Uso de carbamazepina en niños con trastornos de la conducta. *Prensa Med Mex* 37:215–220, 1972

106. Remschmidt H: The psychotropic effect carbamazepine in non-epileptic patients, with particular reference to problems posed by clinical studies in children with behavioural disorders, in *Epileptic Seizures—Behavior—Pain.* Edited by Birkmayer W. Stuttgart, Huber, 1975, pp 253–258

107. Farago F, Nikolic V: Electroclinical analysis of behaviour disorders with special consideration of the effect of Tegretol, in *Excerpta*

Medica International Congress Series, No 94: Proceedings of the Eighth International Congress of Neurology, Vienna, 1965. Amsterdam, Elsevier, 1965, pp E162–E163

108. Donner M, Frisk M: Carbamazepine treatment of epileptic and psychic symptoms in children and adolescents. *Ann Paediatr Fenn* 11:91–97, 1965

109. Tunks ER, Dermer SW: Carbamazepine in the dyscontrol syndrome associated with limbic system dysfunction. *J Nerv Ment Dis* 164:56–63, 1977

110. Puente RM: The use of carbamazepine in the treatment of behavioural disorders in children, in *Epileptic Seizures—Behavior—Pain.* Edited by Birkmayer W. Stuttgart, Huber, 1975, pp 243–247

111. Ballenger JC, Post RM: Kindling as a model for alcohol withdrawal syndromes. *Br J Psychiatry* 133:1–14, 1978

112. Himmelhoch JM: Mixed states, manic-depressive illness, and the nature of mood. *Psychiatr Clin North Am* 2:449–459, 1979

113. Hart RG, Easton JD: Carbamazepine and hematological monitoring. *Ann Neurol* 11:309–312, 1982

114. Lennox WWG: The heredity of epilepsy as told by relatives and twins. *JAMA* 146:529–536, 1951

115. Rimoin DL, Metrakos JD: The genetics of convulsive disorders in the families of hemiplegics. Proceedings of the Second International Congress on Human Genetics, 1964, pp 1655–1658

116. Andermann E, Metrakos JD: *EEG Studies of Relatives of Probands with Focal Epilepsy Who Have Been Treated Surgically.* New York, American Epilepsy Society, 1968

117. Lennox-Buchthal MA: Febrile convulsions, in *Handbook of Clinical Neurology, Vol 15: The Epilepsies.* Edited by Vinken PJ, Bruyn GW. New York, American Elsevier, 1974

118. Metrakos K, Metrakos JD: Genetics of epilepsy, in *Handbook of Clinical Neurology, Vol 15: The Epilepsies.* Edited by Vinken PJ, Bruyn GW. New York, American Elsevier, 1974

119. Andermann E: Multifactorial inheritance in the epilepsies, in *Advances in Epileptology, the XIth Epilepsy International Symposium.* Edited by Canger R, Angeleri F, Penry JK. New York, Raven Press, 1980

120. Reynolds EH: Biological factors in psychological disorders associated with epilepsy, in *Epilepsy and Psychiatry.* Edited by Reynolds EH, Trimble MR. Edinburgh, Churchill Livingstone, 1981

121. Slater E, Beard AW, Glithero E: The schizophrenia-like psychoses of epilepsy. *Br J Psychiatry* 109:95–150, 1963

122. Szondi L: *Schicksalsanalyse.* 3rd edition. Basel, Schwabe & Co., 1965

123. Szondi L: *Schicksalsanalytische Therapie.* Bern, Huber, 1963

124. Szondi L: *Lehrbuch der Experimentellen Trebdiagnostik.* 3rd edition. Bern, Huber, 1972

125. Szondi L: *Moses. Antwort auf Kain.* Bern, Huber, 1973

2

Epidemiologic Overview of Epilepsy: Morbidity, Mortality, and Clinical Implications

Janusz J. Zielinski, M.D., D.Sci.

Epidemiology is a branch of medicine concerned with the frequency and distribution of disorders, diseases, disabilities, and deaths in human populations. It is also concerned with identifying biologic, chemical, physical, and social factors related to the occurrence, course, and outcome of disease.

As a result of the epidemiologic approach, it is sometimes possible to learn how to prevent a disease even when its actual cause remains unknown. In London in the 1840s, John Snow (1) showed how cholera spreads and how to prevent the disease nearly 30 years before the discovery of the causative factor, *Vibrio cholerae*. More recently, a strong association between tobacco smoking and lung cancer has been found. The epidemiologic approach can be especially valuable with disorders of uncertain, multiple, or multidimensional etiologic factors (e.g., schizophrenia and epilepsy, along with many other psychiatric and neurologic disorders).

Epidemiology not only tells us the frequency and distribution of disorders in a given population, but also helps to identify specific segments of the population that have a high risk of being affected by a disorder. Finally but significantly, during field surveys, undiagnosed and untreated cases of a disease can be identified that otherwise would not have come to clinical attention.

EPIDEMIOLOGIC METHODS

Of the three basic epidemiologic methods, the oldest and most widely used is descriptive epidemiology, which usually deals with the reported frequency of various health phenomena in different populations at various times. Routine medical statistics, hospital records, sick leaves, and death certificates are often used. This methodologic approach is the easiest and least expensive, but the results are often not sufficiently accurate or reliable. For instance, if the frequency of hospital admissions with a diagnosis of psychiatric disorder appears very low in some area, several possibilities may be considered. The low hospitalization rate may reflect an above-average socioeconomic status in the population, a lack of psychiatric service, or a limited number of hospital beds in the area. Although routine medical statistics are biased to some extent, they are readily available and may be useful for purposes of health policy and organization.

Analytic epidemiology verifies hypotheses generated by descriptive studies by means of specially designed research programs. These are more expensive but provide more reliable results that can often be applied directly in clinical medicine. Retrospective studies are aimed at finding possible causative factors in samples of inhabitants who are already ill (e.g., history of exposure to head trauma or meningitis in patients with epilepsy). Prospective studies, which are the most valuable but usually expensive, are based on the long-term follow-up of samples of the population, some of which are or have been exposed to a probable causative factor (e.g., tobacco smoking, head trauma, etc.) and others that have not. Finally, the incidence of a disease is compared between exposed and nonexposed (control) individuals.

Experimental epidemiology is concerned with finding the extent to which the results of a prospective study are influenced by the introduction of an intervening factor. Two good examples would be the effect of vaccination upon the incidence of a contagious disease, and the effect of speed limits or obligatory use of seat belts upon the incidence of posttraumatic epilepsy caused by auto accidents.

FINDING AND DEFINING "EPILEPSY CASES"

In any epidemiologic study of disease, the definition of what constitutes a case of the disease is crucial to the quality of the study's results. Epilepsy is a purely clinical diagnosis based on the presence of recurrent seizures.

Unfortunately, the physician rarely witnesses a seizure and usually must rely on a description of them from a witness whose ability to observe is limited. If the patient suffers from partial seizures, establishing a correct diagnosis may depend upon the experience of the physician in interviewing about the manifestation.

Defining a case of psychosis, schizophrenia, etc. may also be difficult even when there are no differences in diagnostic criteria among various psychiatric schools. Serious difficulties may be met in attempts to define a "psychiatric case." Perhaps the most useful definition would be "everyone who was seen by a psychiatrist." But what about those who should have seen a psychiatrist but failed to do so? Gruenberg said, "Everyone knows that the longer time you will spend with a psychiatrist, the more likely he is to find something wrong with you" (E. Gruenberg, personal communication, 1974). Thus, structured psychiatric examinations, psychometric methods, or questionnaires are employed in order to provide comparative diagnoses or levels of intensity of symptoms such as anxiety or depression.

It is the dream of the epidemiologist that every person contracting a disease would immediately consult a doctor who would not only make a correct diagnosis but properly complete a statistical form. Unfortunately, the opposite frequently happens. This author has met many patients with a seizure disorder who did not consider their symptoms morbid or dismissed them as unimportant (2).

A girl with previously undiagnosed absence seizures commented, "These blackouts are so brief, they have occurred as long as I can remember—They do not bother me—I think everyone may experience something like that."

Another woman with quite typical but brief and nongeneralized complex partial seizures stated, "These are clearly neurotic symptoms; I do not think I need any treatment for them."

Among epileptic patients at 17 general practices in London, only one-fifth suspected that they had epilepsy before they decided to consult a doctor (3). The same may be true of children; 20–25 percent of those suffering from various types of seizures never sought medical advice (4). Among 98 Warsaw inhabitants whose epilepsy was discovered during the survey, 26 percent of a 0.4 percent random sample of the population had not been previously diagnosed (2, 5).

If diagnosing epilepsy is so difficult and uncertain in outpatients, why not base epidemiologic estimates on hospitalized patients or those seen in highly specialized centers? Surely their diagnoses would be more accurate and reliable—as reliable as it would be to estimate the average height in a population by measuring, for example, customers of a department store for tall people! However, data originating in hospitals or special centers may be very useful for estimations of the proportion of people with poorly controlled seizures, associated neurologic or psychiatric problems, low socioeconomic status, etc.

Those in whom epileptic seizures have ceased for a longer time (i.e., $\geqslant$5 years) constitute another problem. Should they be classified "epileptic" per the axiom "Once epileptic—always epileptic?" (6). In more representative samples of persons with epilepsy, the proportion of such cases may reach $\geqslant$30 percent (5, 7).

As previously mentioned, the oldest and most popular method of case finding is based upon the review of medical records. The diagnosis of epilepsy then depends exclusively upon diagnostic criteria used by the doctors who have seen the patients. Accuracy of diagnosis can be substantially improved if a sample of patients can be reexamined. This method was used in Iceland and in Warsaw (5, 8).

More reliable data can be obtained through compiling a special register containing information on all cases of epilepsy currently diagnosed in a given population (i.e., a city, county, or country). Epidemiologic studies of epilepsy and febrile convulsions in Rochester are based on the medical files of the Mayo Clinic and affiliated medical units (7, 9). A special register of epilepsy cases has also been established in Aarhus, Denmark (10).

Another approach is a specially designed study of a chosen population. This type of study provides the most accurate basis for estimating the actual frequency of epilepsy. Such studies were carried out in Guam, Carlisle, Warsaw, and Bogota (15, 11–13). In Carlisle and Warsaw, a parallel survey of medical files was performed.

INCIDENCE OF EPILEPSY

Incidence rates reflect "new cases" of epilepsy per the formula:

$$\text{Incidence} = \frac{\text{New cases occurring during a year}}{\text{Size of population in the middle of a year}} \times 100{,}000.$$

A study based upon analyses of records of medical facilities can be termed "first attendance rate." It is known that several years may elapse between the occurrence of a first seizure and attendance at a medical facility (7, 9).

Table 1 lists selected epidemiologic studies of epilepsy done in various countries. In general, epilepsy was defined as "more than

TABLE 1. *Incidence rates for epilepsy (of selected studies)*

Country	Authors	Case ascertainment method	Population studied	Annual incidence per 100,000
Denmark	Juul-Jensen and Ipsen (10)	Medical records, epilepsy register	Aarhus, Denmark	30
Great Britain	Brewis et al. (12)	Medical records, central register of patients	Carlisle, England	30
Guam	Stanhope et al. (11)	Records of neurologic clinic	Guam	23
	Stanhope et al. (11)	Field survey	Guam, same area	46
Iceland	Gudmundsson (8)	Medical records, reexamination	Iceland	26
Japan	Sato (14)	Medical records	Niigata	17
Norway	Krohn (15)	Medical records	Northern Norway	11
Poland	Grudzinska (16)	Records of epilepsy clinic	Industrialized urban area, Zabrze	22
	Zielinski (5)	Records of neurologic and psychiatric facilities	Warsaw	20
United States	Hauser and Kurland (7)	Records of Mayo Clinic	Rochester, MN	
			1955–1964	54
			1965–1967	46
			1935–1967	49

one afebrile seizure." The value of field survey as a case-finding method was demonstrated in the Guam study where the incidence rate was double the findings in some studies based only on medical records (11).

In the United States, a combined annual incidence rate for recurrent and single seizures was reported as high as 120 per 100,000 (7), and still the incidence of single and afebrile seizures seems underestimated. Using the above data, the Commission for the Control of Epilepsy and Its Consequences accepted an average weighted incidence of epilepsy for the U.S. population of 46.2 per 100,000. Thus, in 1970, 95,700 new cases of epilepsy were expected to appear in the United States (17).

Most authors agree that the incidence of epilepsy is higher among males than females in virtually all age groups. As far as age is concerned, incidence rates are highest within the first decade of life (and the highest in the first few years of life), become lower in the second decade, and remain at a low level until the end of the fifth or sixth decade. Beginning at age 60, a considerable increase in the incidence rate has been found, especially in the Rochester, Minnesota, and Warsaw studies. An increased rate in the older age groups does not necessarily reflect a higher incidence of brain tumor or cerebrovascular disease, since in 70 percent of new cases of epilepsy occurring in people over 60 years of age, no definite causative factors could be found (7).

PREVALENCE OF EPILEPSY

Prevalence constitutes another morbidity index. It describes the frequency of all current cases of epilepsy in a given population, and is frequently estimated for a given day (point prevalence), usually per 1,000 population, according to the formula:

$$\text{Prevalence} = \frac{\text{Number of people with epilepsy}}{\text{Size of population at that time}} \times 1{,}000.$$

Occasionally, prevalence rates are calculated more extensively, for the average expected life span (total prevalence). The values obtained are then close to the so-called "cumulative incidence rates," which show that cases of epilepsy, like those of other chronic disorders (including many psychiatric conditions), tend to accumulate in the population. We can say that prevalence (P) is a function of incidence (i) and time (t) according to the formula: $P = i \times t$.

Thus, although incidence rates for epilepsy are low, its prevalence rates are high, owing to the usually long survival of the victims.

Some of the many prevalence studies from around the world are presented in Table 2. Prevalence rates range from 1.5 per 1,000 in Japan to 19.5 per 1,000 in Colombia. In younger age groups prevalence rates are usually higher than those for all ages. Over the third and fourth decades of life, they remain relatively stable and tend to fall afterward. Only in Rochester and Warsaw were the prevalence rates in older age groups definitely higher, whereas in Aarhus they were higher only in the sixth decade of life. This seems to be due to more effective case-finding methods with the consecutive accumulation of cases in Rochester and Warsaw.

As with incidence, the prevalence of epilepsy among males is usually higher than among females. There are various speculations regarding the reasons, including more frequent substance abuse and risk of head trauma among males. A higher prevalence of chronic alcoholism among males, including those with epilepsy, is well known.

As for head trauma, in a random sample of the Warsaw popu-

TABLE 2. *Prevalence rates for epilepsy*

Country, area studied	Authors	Rate per 1,000	Comments
Chile			
Melipilla	Chiofale et al. (18)	27.6 (range 27.1–31.9)	Children aged 9 years; method and definition similar to those of Washington County study of Rose et al. (24; see below)
Colombia			
Bogota	Gomez et al. (13)	19.5	No Fs or Ss cases
Denmark			
Aarhus	Juul-Jensen and Ipsen (10)	6.9	Including 1.1 for "observation of epilepsy"
Great Britain			
England and Wales			
Carlisle	Brewis et al. (12)	5.5 (known) 6.0 (household survey)	"Lifetime"; no Fs, Ss, or symptomatic epilepsy
Isle of Wight	Rutter et al. (19)	7.2	Including 5.4 for "uncomplicated" epilepsy; children aged 4–15 years
	Pless and Graham (20)	8.9	Including 6.4 for "uncomplicated" epilepsy and 4.9 for having seizures in last year; children aged 10–12 years
Iceland	Gudmundsson (8)	3.4 (active) 5.2 (lifetime)	No Fs or Ss cases

TABLE 2. *Continued*

Country, area studied	Authors	Rate per 1,000	Comments
Japan			
Niigata	Sato (14)	1.5	Symptomatic seizures excluded
Mariana Islands			
Guam	Mathai et al. (21)	2.3 (active) 4.4 (total)	No Fs or Ss cases
	Stanhope et al. (11)	5.3 (field survey) 3.1 (known cases)[a]	No Fs or Ss cases—"active" cases only; high proportion of symptomatic epilepsy
Norway			
Northern	De Graaf (22)	3.5	Subartic, large area; difficult traveling
Poland			
Zabrze	Grudzinska (16)	3.4	No Fs or Ss cases; highly industrialized area
Warsaw	Zielinski (5)	4.3 (known cases)[a]	No Fs or Ss cases
		7.8 (active)	Field survey
		9.2 (lifetime)	Field survey
Sampled Poland Areas	Zielinski (23)	2.8	One-year attendance; diagnosed epilepsy; various facilities
United States			
Rochester, MN	Hauser and Kurland (7)	5.3 for 1950 6.2 for 1960 5.7 for 1965	Recurrent, afebrile seizures; "active" cases of epilepsy
Washington County, MD	Rose et al. (24)	18.6 (range 14.1–20.1)	Third grade schoolchildren, aged 8–9 years; cases of Fs and Ss with EEG changes or positive family history of epilepsy included; response rate 91 percent

TABLE 2. *Continued*

Country, area studied	Authors	Rate per 1,000	Comments
Multnomah County, OR	Meighan et al. (25)	9.7 (range 7.8–12.8)	Third grade schoolchildren, aged 8–9 years; cases of Fs with EEG changes or positive family history of epilepsy included; response rate 76 percent
New Haven, CT	Shamansky and Glaser (26)	9.5—M, white 9.1—F, white 19.6—M, nonwhite 15.0—F, nonwhite	Cumulative incidence; children up to 15 years old, by sex (M, F) and race (white, nonwhite; rates for nonwhite females estimated by J.J.Z.)

Fs, febrile seizure; Ss, single seizure; EEG, electroencephalographic.
[a]Diagnosed epilepsy cases identified during review of the medical files.

lation, 2.2 percent of children and 4.0 percent of adults reported at least one previous hospital admission because of acute head injury. A history of more severe head trauma prior to onset of seizures was noted nearly twice as often in males as in females (30 vs 16 percent). The overall prevalence rate of posttraumatic epilepsy was found to be 1.0–1.5 per 1,000 population (15).

LIFETIME (TOTAL) PREVALENCE AND CUMULATIVE INCIDENCE OF EPILEPSY

Incidence and prevalence rates show that epilepsy is at least twice as frequent among younger people as among adults. These differences could be explained only if a great proportion of children with epilepsy died before reaching adulthood. Although mortality rates among people with epilepsy are higher than expected for the general population, they do not seem high enough to explain the decline in the presence of epilepsy in the middle age groups. The only other possibility is that in a considerable proportion of children, the seizures cease for an indefinite length of time. According to Kurtzke (27), "Epileptic seizures like old soldiers fade away with age."

The overall prognosis in epilepsy, when based on longitudinal studies of more representative, unselected samples of patients, again looks optimistic. Twenty years after diagnosis 70 percent of Rochester patients were seizurefree for at least 5 years, including 20 percent who continued to take anticonvulsants and 50 percent not taking antiepileptic drugs. The prognosis was best in cases of generalized epilepsy of unknown etiology (80–85 percent were seizurefree 20 years after diagnosis). The outcome was less favorable in patients with complex partial seizures and in adult-onset cases and poorest for those neurologically handicapped from birth (28).

On follow-up of Warsaw patients, 37 percent had been seizurefree for >5 years and >60 percent for at least 2 years. Information was obtained in most cases from multiple sources (the patient, family member, doctor, etc.). It is noteworthy, however, that patients who are seizurefree for a longer time are frequently unwilling to provide any information during the follow-up interview. Many consider themselves "completely cured" and do not wish to be reminded about their past disorder (29). This explains why the more benign forms of epilepsy are underrepresented in the medical case series. In 1968 Rodin (30) concluded, "The majority of patients who attend clinics regularly do so because their seizures are not satisfactorily controlled." Similarly, Turner's opinion (31) that "there is a direct association between the frequency of seizures and the mental state, for the more frequent the attacks, the greater degree of mental impairment and vice versa" remains valid.

In a number of studies, not only remission but also relapse rates have been calculated. In Rochester the percentage of those who relapsed after achieving the "remission state" (i.e., 5-year seizurefree status) was estimated at 15 percent by 10 years after remission and 24 percent by 20 years (28). The 5-year follow-up in Warsaw revealed relapse after at least 2 years of seizure freedom in 5.4 percent of "known" (i.e., listed in files of various medical facilities) epileptic patients (group K) and in 2.9 percent of those found in the population sample (group F). At the same time, however, the percentage of individuals in these two groups who were seizurefree for at least 5 years increased from 12 to 18 percent and from 15 to 37 percent, respectively. Moreover, in groups K and F, only 5 and 8 percent, respectively, resumed treatment during the follow-up, while 22 and 7 percent, respectively, discontinued anticonvulsants at the same time (29). Thus, in both studies the tendency toward improving and achieving a remission state prevailed over the frequency of relapses.

A better estimate of risk of contracting epilepsy during a lifetime is the accumulated incidence. This is calculated by the summation of the incidence in various age groups. For example, if the annual incidence rate per 100,000 for the 0–4 age group is 80 and it is 50 for the 5–9 age group, then the total number of patients at the end of the first decade of life will be $(5 \times 80) + (5 \times 50) = 650$ per 100,000 = 6.5 per 1,000 = 0.65 percent. Several authors (10, 26) used this method to calculate the accumulated incidence. Hauser and Kurland (7), assuming that the average life expectancy for a Rochester inhabitant is 70 years, estimated that 6 percent of the general population may have had at least a single afebrile epileptic seizure, and that almost 4 percent may have had recurrent seizures (epilepsy) at some period in their lives. This estimate has been considered as the "lifetime" or "total" prevalence rate of epilepsy.

UNDIAGNOSED EPILEPSY CASES

As with many other chronic disorders, it is difficult, if not virtually impossible, to discover all the cases of epilepsy in a surveyed population. This is due to the varying clinical appearance of seizures, long-term remissions, inaccurate or insufficient case-finding methods, social attitudes toward epilepsy (the tendency to conceal socially "stigmatizing" disorders), and so on.

To illustrate part of the difficulty that may occur during a field survey in a population, let us use this author's study of the epidemiology of epilepsy in Warsaw (5). Records of various medical and social facilities were reviewed, and a random sample of these patients was examined. At the same time a random sample of 0.4 percent (4,500 inhabitants) of the general population of Warsaw was interviewed by a specially trained team of interviewers. In addition, household members constituted a cluster sample of 10,600 for a total of 15,000 subjects. Six questions about various manifestations of epileptic seizures, mixed with another six questions dealing with other sudden events, such as attacks of heart palpitation or shortness of breath, were included in the questionnaire. There were also direct inquiries about epilepsy and current or past use of anticonvulsants. If the information obtained suggested that the interviewed person has or had seizures, he or she was interviewed again by the neurologist from the team. If the suspicion still existed, a detailed medical history was taken, and the person was thoroughly examined. Finally, two groups of persons with epilepsy were compared: those known to medical and social services (group K) and those found during the field survey (group F). The prevalence rates per 1,000 population estimated according to the distribution of basic clinical variables in these two groups are shown in Table 3.

In the sample of the general population, some of those who refused to be interviewed were identified from lists of epileptic patients known to medical facilities, indicating that epilepsy may have been the direct reason for declining the interview. If these refusals are included, the "total" prevalence rate of epilepsy reaches 10.4 per 1,000 or 1 percent. It is also interesting that 37 percent of individuals with epilepsy in group F had never been treated in spite of easily obtainable and free medical care (2, 5). This estimate is very close to Gudmundsson's 35 percent in Iceland (8).

Finally, among the 98 Warsaw inhabitants with epilepsy found in the primary and cluster samples, 25 percent had never been diagnosed as having epilepsy. The majority of them had experienced brief partial seizures, mostly of temporal lobe origin, which they considered unworthy of treatment even if they had had sporadic major motor seizures in the past. Thus, cases of mild, nongeneralized temporal lobe seizures may be far more prevalent than expected (2). They can also be easily missed during a questionnaire survey of the general population sample. Of the people with epilepsy living in a given area at a given time, only 30–40 percent may consult a physician. Some 25 percent were treated sometime in the past; of the > 35 percent who were never treated, 25 percent were never even diagnosed as having epilepsy.

Based on the results of epidemiologic studies on epilepsy done

TABLE 3. *Prevalence rates per 1,000 population in the Warsaw study*

	Prevalence per 1,000 population	
Clinical variables	**Group K**	**Group F**
In remission for 5 years	0.5	1.4
On anticonvulsants when examined	3.3	3.2
On anticonvulsants now or anytime in the past	3.9	5.2
"Active" epilepsy (seizures during last 5 years)	4.2	7.8
Total prevalence rate	4.3	9.2

Group K, patients with epilepsy known to medical and social services, group F, patients with epilepsy found during the field survey. From Zielinski (5).

in the United States and other countries, including the estimate of undiagnosed cases of the disorder, the Commission for the Control of Epilepsy and Its Consequences estimated the number of persons with epilepsy in the United States in 1975 at 2,135,000 (17). And, 34 percent (725,900) would not have been identified!

HOSPITAL ADMISSIONS AND LONG-TERM INSTITUTIONALIZED PATIENTS WITH EPILEPSY

As previously mentioned, routine medical records are seldom sufficient or adequate sources for epidemiologic estimates of epilepsy and many other chronic diseases as well. It is known, for instance, that admission rates for psychiatric disorders may significantly depend upon the number of beds available or the distance between the patient's residence and the hospital facility. Analyses of hospital admission rates give a very crude estimate of the number of patients actually admitted, unless the analysis is limited to first admissions.

It is known that the severer the course of the epilepsy or psychiatric disorder, the higher the chance of admission and readmission (especially multiple) to a hospital or outpatient clinic. Thus, finding that patients with epilepsy constitute some 3–10 percent of all mental hospital admissions provides little epidemiologic information (32).

Short-stay hospital admissions with a diagnosis of epilepsy in 1974 were calculated in the United States at 59 per 100,000 population, including 30 for "first listed epilepsy" (i.e., single diagnosis or the first one among multiple diagnoses). "Other or unspecified epilepsy" was diagnosed in almost half of the admissions, "major epilepsy" in another 35 percent, and "status epilepticus" in 4 percent. The category of "convulsions" (770.3—*International Classification of Diseases, 8th Revision*) or psychiatric disturbances in epilepsy was not considered (33).

Among the Warsaw residents with epilepsy found during the field survey (group F), 31 percent had a history of at least one neurologic admission and 1 percent a psychiatric one, whereas in group K, 41 percent had a history of admission to a neurology department and 11 percent to a psychiatric one (5). These findings may give a rough estimate of the varying frequency of hospitalization of epileptic individuals.

Inpatients with epilepsy in mental hospitals and chronic care institutions in Poland were estimated to be 3 percent of all patients with epilepsy known to the medical services. In all those cases, severe mental, intellectual, or neurologic handicaps were directly responsible for the institutionalization (34, 35). This concurs with estimates for Great Britain (36) and the Federal Republic of Germany (37). Higher figures were found in Norway: 10 percent of all patients with diagnosed epilepsy (38). The Commission for the Control of Epilepsy and Its Consequences gives the following estimated rates (per 1,000 general population) for the United States (17): total prevalence of epilepsy, 10.00; "unidentified" cases, 3.40; cases in nursing homes, 0.09; cases in institutions for mentally retarded, 0.17; cases in state mental hospitals, 0.09; cases in other facilities, 0.01; needing residential care but not yet admitted, 0.32. Thus, some 78,000 people with a seizure disorder (5.5 percent of known cases) remain in various long-term care facilities in the United States and another 68,000 (4.8 percent) need such care.

SEIZURE TYPE

The distribution of seizure types is usually analyzed in more or less select groups of patients with epilepsy found in various clinics, departments, or electroencephalography (EEG) laboratories. Unfortunately, only very few epidemiologic surveys yield comparable data (Table 4).

The proportion of individuals with primary generalized seizures was similar in the Rochester (7), Warsaw (5), and Gastaut et al. (40) case series (34–38 percent). Individuals with temporal lobe seizures constituted the highest percentage of Warsaw's group F

TABLE 4. *Relative frequency of generalized and partial seizures in case series of epileptic patients and individuals with epilepsy found during selected epidemiologic studies*

	Epidemiologic surveys				Case series	
Type of seizure	Rochester, 1960[a]	Warsaw[b]		Bogota[c]	10,840 epileptic patients in EEG department[d]	4,590 private patients with epilepsy[e]
		Known cases	Field survey			
Generalized	34	48	35	73	67	38
Partial	66	52	65	27	33	62
Complex partial	(27)	(34)	(43)	—	(25)	(40)

Values are percentages. EEG, electroencephalography.
[a]Hauser and Kurland (7).
[b]Zielinski (5).
[c]Gomez et al. (13).
[d]Gibbs and Gibbs (39).
[e]Gastaut et al. (40).

and of Gastaut's patients, and the lowest in the Rochester and in the Gibbs and Gibbs sample (39). Thus, the proportion of those with temporal lobe seizures may reach at least 40 percent of the total population of people with epilepsy.

The frequency of complex partial seizures without secondary generalization in the general Warsaw population was 12 percent in group F versus 4 percent in group K, whereas the percentage of cases with secondary generalized complex partial seizures was similar in both K and F groups (30 percent each). This shows that temporal lobe seizures, if not secondarily generalized to grand mal seizures, may be very difficult to discover. Moreover, although several cases of "inactive" epilepsy were found among those with a history of major motor seizures, virtually all identified patients with nongeneralized complex partial seizures had them at the time of the questionnaire interview. The alternative explanation may be either that temporal lobe seizures are the most permanent or that only people currently suffering from those seizures reveal their presence during a questionnaire interview.

INCIDENCE OF PSYCHIATRIC MANIFESTATIONS IN EPILEPSY

If defining epilepsy for epidemiologic purposes was found rather difficult, then attempts to define "psychiatric manifestations" would seem far more complicated. The vast majority of epileptic seizures may be defined as psychiatric manifestations, including various levels of impairment of consciousness and a variety of psychopathological symptoms: illusions, hallucinatory experiences, ictal dysmnestic or oneroidal phenomena, etc.

Because epilepsy is considered a relatively frequent disorder, there must also be a higher chance of it coinciding with other frequent disorders. There are many papers on the frequency of various psychiatric disorders in case series of epileptic patients selected from various neurologic, psychiatric, and other facilities. This topic was recently reviewed by Blumer (41), Betts (42), and Parnas and Korsgaard (43). Unfortunately, in most of the epidemiologic studies of epilepsy, psychiatric manifestations have not been considered. Both Gudmundsson in Iceland (8) and this author in Warsaw (5) did not employ structured psychiatric examinations. The difficulties in obtaining consistent results of psychiatric evaluations of the patients are best illustrated in the Iceland study. Among the patients examined by Gudmundsson, 55 percent showed some mental abnormalities, but only 30 percent showed abnormalities among those examined by other physicians.

All in all in Gudmundsson's national sample of people with epilepsy, of 916 patients who had not been psychotic, 50 percent revealed a "normal" personality, 24 percent were "ixoids," 8 percent were "ixothymics" (equivalent to "viscous" and "epileptic" personality traits), and 18 percent were neurotics. Males appeared more frequently ixoids or ixothymics, whereas more females were neurotic. The discrepancies between Gudmundsson's diagnoses and those of the other examining physicians were most significant in the categories of "normal personality" (46 vs 70 percent) and "neurotic personality" (19 vs 5 percent). A total of 71 people (7 percent) were diagnosed as psychotic. Among them, more were females. Among patients with psychosis, ixoid or ixothymic personality was diagnosed in almost 70 percent. Less than 5 percent of all the patients had a history of admission to a mental hospital. This is half as much as in the Warsaw sample of known epileptic patients (group K), but almost five times more than in the Warsaw population sample (group F).

In the Warsaw study (5) the sample of known epileptic patients (group K) was examined by psychiatrists other than this author who personally examined all those in group F. Only 2 percent of patients in group F were diagnosed psychotic compared with 3 percent in group K. No mental abnormalities were discovered in 32 percent of the patients in group K and in 42 percent in group F. Mental dullness or retardation was diagnosed in 17 and 19 percent, mental deterioration symptoms in 30 and 14 percent, and behavioral problems in 22 and 25 percent, respectively. It should be stressed, however, that the severity of mental abnormalities varied significantly and that generally there were difficulties in classifying the patients, especially in the field survey, some of whom were seen only once.

Mental deterioration (dementia) in most cases was felt to be due to head trauma, meningoencephalitis, and often aging or cerebral arteriosclerosis. Features of the so-called "epileptic characteropathy" or "epileptic dementia" were found in 11 percent of the cases in group K and 6 percent in group F. It is worth mentioning that the percentage of such cases in Alstrom's study (44) was estimated at 7 percent, but in another psychiatric-epidemiologic study in the same country, it was at 30 percent (45).

Difficulties in defining the term "epileptic character" or "epileptic personality" have been discussed by many authors and are extensively reviewed by Blumer and Benson (46) and Betts (42). Some of the symptoms originally thought to be typical for epileptic personality are currently being attributed to dysfunction of the temporal lobes. It is highly probable that the chronic use of some anticonvulsants also contributes to the development of subacute or chronic encephalopathy including mental and behavioral abnormalities (47–49).

Among individuals classified under "behavioral problems" in groups K and F of Warsaw, hysterical traits or emotional immaturity was diagnosed in 6 and 14 percent, respectively (5). In 14 percent of males from group K and 20 percent from group F, the tendency toward alcohol abuse was discovered. A similar observation was previously published by Oleanders and Steinwall (50). One should bear in mind, however, that in an unstructured psychiatric evaluation of people known to have epilepsy, examiners may be more likely to attribute their findings to the disorder first of all.

The frequency of intellectual impairment has been analyzed in select case series of epileptic patients. Again, there are only a few epidemiologic studies that consider the distribution of this feature.

Because in the Warsaw study (5) the scales used for measuring the intelligence quotient in epileptic patients had not been validated for the general population, control groups were examined for comparison. Controls were matched according to age, sex, and educational level (in children, education of parents) from the interviewed sample of Warsaw inhabitants without epilepsy. From the data presented in Table 5, it may be concluded that in both

TABLE 5. *Intelligence levels of epileptic patients found in epidemiologic studies in Iceland[a] and Warsaw[b]*

		Warsaw[b]				
		Children		Adults		
Intellectual level	**Iceland[a]**	**Known sample**	**Controls**	**Known sample**	**Field sample**	**Controls**
Average or higher	71.2	83.7	94.5	74.3	76.0	95.7
Dull normal (inferior)	14.8	3.6	5.5	21.2	20.0	3.9
Retarded (deficient)	6.9	12.7	—	4.6	4.0	0.4
Demented	7.1	X	X	X	X	X
No. examined	987	55	55	237	75	236

Values are percentages.
[a]Gudmundsson (8).
[b]Zielinski (5).

adult epileptic samples in Warsaw, the category "dull normal" (or "borderline normal") was the most prevalent (20 percent), whereas mental retardation was more frequently diagnosed in children with epilepsy (13 percent). "Dementia" had not been considered in Warsaw, but in both of the above-discussed studies, the subjects with epilepsy had a greater prevalence of mental subnormality than the general population.

Rutter et al. (19) examined a general population sample of 2,193 children of the Isle of Wight. Using a "clinical-diagnostic approach," 6.8 percent of all children were found to have a "psychiatric disorder." Children with chronic disorders that were not of neurologic origin had nearly twice this percentage of psychiatric disorders. However, 34 percent of the children with epilepsy showed psychiatric disorders, and in those in whom seizures were associated with permanent neurologic disorders, as many as 58 percent had psychiatric disorders. Among 63 children with "uncomplicated epilepsy," a neurotic disorder was diagnosed in 8 (12.7 percent) compared with only 1.9 percent in the general population of children. Antisocial or conduct disorder was diagnosed in 9.5 and 1.9 percent and "mixed disorder" in 4.8 and 1.2 percent, respectively. A hyperkinetic syndrome was found in 1.6 percent of children with epilepsy. In their later study (51) the authors found a significantly higher percentage of children and adolescents with psychiatric disorders in the general population of children aged 10–14 years (11 to 13 percent).

EPIDEMIOLOGY OF PSYCHIATRIC DISORDERS: A CHANCE OF INCIDENTAL COEXISTENCE WITH SEIZURE DISORDER

A number of studies have shown quite a wide range of prevalence rates. Data in Table 6 show that the prevalence rates for all psychoses expectedly vary depending upon the diagnostic method employed. Similarly, as in epilepsy, the cohort analysis gave one of the highest estimates for lifetime prevalence (44 per 1,000 population in Bornholm), whereas most of the point prevalence estimates varied between 3.9 and 6.7 per 1,000. Most of the studies done in the United States provide results in that range. Prevalence rates for schizophrenia were the highest in Bornholm and northern Sweden (9 and 9.6 per 1,000, respectively), whereas in the United States they varied between 1.0 and 2.9 per 1,000. Babigian (56) gives an estimation between 2.3 and 4.7 per 1,000.

Depression is not only one of the most frequent psychiatric conditions, but it also seems to be one of the most difficult to

TABLE 6. *Results of selected psychiatric-epidemiologic studies*

Country, area	Authors	Studied population (× 10³)	Prevalence per 1,000: Schizophrenia	Prevalence per 1,000: Psychosis	Total psychiatric disorders
United States					
Baltimore	Lemkau et al. (52)	55	2.9	6.7	60.5
Tennessee, rural area	Roth and Luton (53)	25	1.7	6.3	69.4
Hutterites, rural	Eaton and Weil (54)	—	1.0	6.2	23.2
New Haven, urban area	Hollingshead and Redlich (55)	237	—	6.1	—
Monroe County, NY	Babigian (56)	716	4.7	—	—
Denmark					
Bornholm	Fremming (57)	5 (cohort)	9.0	44.0	—
Sweden					
North, rural	Book (58)	9	9.6	—	—
West, rural	Sjögren (59)	9	4.6	11.0	19.1
Poland					
Urban and rural	Henisz (60)	3 (sample)	—	7.2	140.1
England					
18 general practices	Shepherd et al. (61)	15	—	5.9	102.1

define. In the 1930s the prevalence of depression in the United States population was estimated at 0.8–0.9 per 1,000 (52, 62). On the other hand, Roth and Luton (53) found the rates 0.7 per 1,000 for psychotic depression alone and 1.4 per 1,000 for depressive neurotic reaction alone. Leighton et al. (63) estimated the prevalence of depression in Canada at 3.0 per 1,000. A longitudinal survey of a U.S. urban community (64) showed that "major depression" was diagnosed in 3.7 percent, "minor depression" in 2.0 percent, and "depressive personality" in an additional 4.5 percent. A review of studies on psychiatric morbidity in general medical practices showed that the proportion of patients at risk for acquiring various psychiatric conditions (neuroses, anxiety states, other psychiatric disorders) varied between 4 and 13 percent in a 1-year period of the survey (61). Psychiatric morbidity, estimated by means of patient consulting rates, was found as high as 102 per 1,000, including 5.9 per 1,000 for psychoses, 2.3 for mental subnormality, 1.4 for dementia, 88.5 for neuroses, and 5.5 for personality disorders. Organic illness with psychiatric overlay accounted for an additional 15 per 1,000 (61). In a random sample of the population in an area in Poland, the presence of psychiatric disorders amounted to 140 per 1,000 or 14 percent (60).

The mailed questionnaire inquiry is another approach. The results are less reliable because only some of the questionnaires are returned. The question as to whether one can find more or fewer people with psychiatric problems among nonrespondents often remains unanswered. Nevertheless, a recently published study of D'Arcy (65) in Canada showed that about 15 percent of those responding to Goldberg's General Health Questionnaire suffered from nonpsychotic psychiatric symptoms.

Finally, a high frequency of psychiatric disorders, including more or less overt depression, was found among adolescents. An epidemiologic study on the Isle of Wight (66) showed that in the age group of 10–14 years, the rate of adolescents with a diagnosed psychiatric disorder varied between 11 and 13 percent, whereas 7–9 percent reported suicidal ideation and up to 23 percent self-depreciation. Sadness was observed in 13–15 percent of those examined. It may be worth remembering that the prevalence rates of epilepsy are also high for that age.

Although some psychiatric conditions, such as mental retardation and other organic brain syndromes, are more likely to be associated with epileptic seizures (which often result from the same brain injury that led to mental deterioration), the actual frequency of psychoses and depression among individuals suffering from epileptic seizures remains an open question.

Slater and Beard (67) have acknowledged that if the risk of developing schizophrenia is calculated at 0.008 (considering the prevalence rate of this condition at 8 per 1,000 population at risk) and the rate for epilepsy at 0.005, then the two disorders could be expected to occur together purely by chance at 0.00004, i.e, in 4 cases per 100,000 population. The authors calculated that in their catchment area (Greater London), some 148 cases were expected. They collected and examined 69 inhabitants with chronic psychotic states associated with temporal lobe epilepsy. The clinical picture of those psychoses only resembled schizophrenia. Parnas and Korsgaard (43) found that the coexistence of epilepsy and schizophrenia may be by chance and that Slater's method of estimation is inaccurate. It is worth remembering that among individuals with epilepsy, the "average risk" of acquiring a coexisting psychiatric disorder may be similar to that in the general population.

Other than biologic factors can also be involved. Whitman et al. (68), analyzing prevalence rates of epilepsy in families with various levels of income, have pointed out that the lower the income, the higher the frequency of seizure disorder (5.7 in families with income lower than $5,000, and only 2.1 when incomes reached $10,000 or more). Poor socioeconomic conditions thus may be associated not only with a higher frequency of psychiatric disorders (55, 69), but also with higher prevalence rates of epilepsy.

MORTALITY RATES FOR EPILEPSY

Our knowledge about mortality and the causes of death in epileptic patients has been based mostly upon the analysis of routine mortality statistics and studies of selected case series of known patients, i.e., those whose epilepsy was diagnosed sometime before their death. "Death of a person with epilepsy" must be considered separately from "death due to epilepsy." When death results from a disease in which epileptic seizures are only one of several symptoms (brain tumor, hematoma, encephalitis, etc.), the diagnosis of epilepsy frequently does not appear on the death certificate.

Although only a fraction of those with a seizure disorder may be identified during analysis of death certificates, routine mortality statistics are the easiest and most readily available source of data that may be used for various comparisons. In most European countries in the 1970s, the average annual mortality rates for epilepsy varied between 1 and 2 per 100,000. Generally, rates were highest in Chile, Mexico, Portugal, and Colombia (3–4 per 100,000) and lowest in the United States, Japan, Denmark, and Iceland (< 1 per 100,000). These differences can be due in part to local variations in the routine completion of death certificates (70).

In most countries death rates are higher for males than for females. They are usually high in the first year of life, and then stay low until the fifth and sixth decades, when they begin to rise again (70).

A detailed analysis of death due to epilepsy in the United States (27) shows that it is significantly higher for nonwhites than for whites. This pertains particularly to males (the total mortality rate for males is three times higher in nonwhites and over five times higher in the 25- to 50-year age groups). This may be due to a higher frequency of epilepsy-related fatalities in nonwhites, to a greater chance of nonwhite victims having a diagnosis of epilepsy on the death certificate, or to both.

Death rates are significantly higher for those who are single than for those who are married. This was thought to reflect a more regulated life for married persons (systematic treatment, abstinence from street drugs and alcohol, lower risk of head traumas, etc.). On the other hand, persons with more severe epilepsy, especially if associated with psychiatric disorder, clearly have a lesser probability of getting married. Thus, epilepsy determines the prognosis for marriage rather than marriage determining the prognosis for epilepsy.

Death certificates are not a sufficiently reliable source for evaluating mortality and causes of death in epilepsy (5, 9, 71) because of underreporting and inappropriate coding of the cause of death. In Rochester only 10 percent of death certificates of known epileptics showed the diagnosis of epilepsy (9).

In the Warsaw study only 29 percent of the death certificates of 218 deceased epileptic patients known at one of the reviewed facilities contained the diagnosis of epilepsy (5). This diagnosis was found more often if the patient had died in a psychiatric hospital (75 percent) or in a neurology department (40 percent), but less often if death occurred in other departments or at home (20 and 18 percent, respectively). Of deaths that were determined, in the course of the study, to be due to epilepsy, only 74 percent of the certificates showed this diagnosis as the cause of death. If death was due to an accident that clearly resulted from a seizure, epilepsy was cited in only 43 percent, as the physician completing the certificate may not have been informed about the victim's epilepsy. Interestingly, epilepsy was frequently reported on the death certificates of persons who died from pneumonia. Thus, if one attempts to analyze the causes of the deaths of epileptics based on death certificates, deaths in a mental hospital, from pneumonia, or from epilepsy predominate (71).

There are only a few population-based studies of mortality rates and causes of death for epileptic individuals. Henricksen et al. (72) have followed up a series of epileptic patients, most of whom were examined in a neurology department. Epilepsy due to brain tumor or cerebrovascular accident was excluded. Death rates were 2.9 times higher for epileptic patients than for the controls (insurance policy holders). Thus, the mortality rate was 2.9 (3.7 for males and 2.2 for females). After excluding cases with frequent seizures, the rate fell to 2.0.

In the Warsaw survey there were 218 deaths in the known epileptic population, excluding brain tumor and cerebrovascular accident cases. The mortality rate based on the total death number was 1.8, but for those who died by the age of 50, it was as high as 3.5. It may then be concluded that younger epileptic patients carry a greater risk of death (71).

Survivorship ratios, mortality rates, and causes of death were analyzed in the case series of Rochester residents with epilepsy (7, 9). The total mortality rate was found to be 2.3. Cases of idiopathic generalized grand mal seizures had a high mortality rate (3.5), especially during the first 5 years after diagnosis. Patients with temporal lobe epilepsy (including those with secondary grand mal seizures) showed a relatively low mortality rate (1.5) through 30 years. A high rate (4.1) was found in cases of myoclonic seizures. One of the most striking results of the study was a persistently high mortality rate (2.0) among patients remaining seizurefree for at least 5 years. Five years after diagnosis, the survival rate was 95 percent, at 10 years 90 percent, and at 15 years 89 percent. Thus, death is most likely during the first decade following the diagnosis of epilepsy. Unfortunately, no data are provided as to how many patients actually died from epilepsy (9). It is only mentioned that in five cases, diagnosis of epilepsy appeared on the death certificate as an underlying cause of death. How many of the 12 fatalities due to accidents (6.5 percent of total deaths) were related to epileptic seizures is also unknown. Another 32 deaths (17.3 percent) were due to stroke and 4.9 percent to influenza or pneumonia. Suicide was noted in only 1.6 percent.

Causes of death were studied in epileptic patients in the Warsaw survey and in epileptic patients of a psychiatric hospital in Poland (5, 73). Every effort was made to obtain all possible information about the circumstances and type of death, including review of hospital and other medical records, postmortem studies, police records, and interviews with family members and with family physicians when necessary. Of a total of 218 deaths noted in the Warsaw study, 14 percent were due to epilepsy, 16 percent to heart diseases, 15 percent to brain tumors, and 7 percent to suicides. The miscellaneous causes included cancer (9 percent), stroke (12 percent), and deaths more or less associated with acute alcohol intoxication (3 percent, mostly in patients with severe behavior problems and organic brain syndrome). Extremely high percentages of death due to status epilepticus (18 percent) and pneumonia (25 percent) in a psychiatric hospital are fully consistent with the findings of other authors who studied epileptic series in psychiatric facilities (71).

In the world literature there are four series of deaths in epileptics collected by means of comparable methodologic approaches (71–73). A comparison of the distribution of causes of death is presented in Table 7, which shows that the frequencies of various causes of death were very similar in these studies. It also suggests that milder cases of epilepsy were underrepresented. The findings of Lennox (6) were based on somewhat differently collected material, but with the exception of sudden death and accidents not due to seizures they also look similar.

As previously mentioned, suicides in the Rochester series were noted in only 1.6 percent of deaths (9). In the Warsaw, West German, and Lennox series and in the Denmark series, the percentages of death by suicide were 10 and 26 percent, respectively. An extensive review of suicide and epilepsy was recently published by Matthew and Barabas (75). The authors estimate the average frequency of death by suicide in epileptic patients at 5 percent,

TABLE 7. *Causes of death of epileptic patients in four selected samples*

Cause of death	United States[a]	Denmark[b,c]	West Germany[d]	Poland[c,e]
Status epilepticus	9	—	10	6
Sudden death	18	—	6	13
Accident due to seizure	9	—	8	5
Epilepsy total	36	26	24	24
Suicide	10	22	10	12
Accident not due to seizure	18	11	3	7
Heart diseases	} 36 (Heart diseases, Carcinoma, Miscellaneous combined)	11	9	8
Carcinoma		6	10	12
Miscellaneous		17	18	27

Values are percentages.
[a]Lennox (6).
[b]Henriksen et al. (72).
[c]Brain tumor and cardiovascular accident cases excluded.
[d]Haltrich, cited in Janz (74).
[e]Zielinski (5, 71).

i.e., over three times as frequent as in the U.S. general population (1.4 percent). Overall, the observed deaths by suicide in epileptic patients are at least three to five times higher than expected.

CONCLUSIONS

The results of epidemiologic studies of epilepsy may serve not only for the estimation of the number of people suffering from various types of epileptic seizures, but also to determine clinical and social implications, including the frequency of various psychiatric disorders. By means of epidemiologic methods, the actual dimension of these problems can be estimated. Up to 4 percent of the general population may suffer from recurrent epileptic seizures for a period in their lives; roughly one-fourth of them may never be diagnosed despite easily accessible, efficient, and even free medical help. An epidemiologic approach broadens our knowledge of the general medical prognosis in epilepsy in terms of seizure control, mental and social functioning, and survival. At the same time, we can identify the size of those groups of patients who, because of a poor prognostic outlook, need special attention and care. These patients are most easily found among those attending highly specialized centers and among inpatients of mental hospitals and various other institutions. Findings made in these case series, however, cannot be generalized to those seen only by their family practitioners or even those who remain untreated.

Because of the relatively high prevalence rates of both psychiatric disorders and epilepsy, the possibility of their coexistence is also high. The proportion of people with epilepsy suffering from psychiatric disorders, as well as the proportion of people with psychiatric problems who also have seizures, have not been precisely defined yet. Therefore, the psychiatric findings in selected case series of patients with epilepsy may not be safely generalized unless compared with control groups or samples of the population from which the patients originate. For instance, the finding that déjà vu, a symptom considered typical for complex partial seizures, may occur as frequently among patients with epilepsy as among nonepileptic psychiatric cases and even in "normal" people (76) illustrates the usefulness and role of an epidemiologic approach in evaluating the accuracy of clinical definitions and diagnostic criteria.

Similarly, the relationship between variables, such as effectiveness versus side effects of anticonvulsants in patients with rare seizures, and the occurrence and pathogenetic correlates of psychotic or behavioral manifestations in epilepsy, can be evaluated best by epidemiologic methods. Also, by these means we are capable of finding adequate control groups, including untreated or undiagnosed people with epilepsy. From the results of epidemiologic studies, it is also known that even when biologic correlates look almost indisputable (i.e., between temporal lobe lesions and behavioral disorders), economic and psychosocial factors still may play an important role in triggering or decreasing the possibility of the appearance of psychiatric symptoms. Moreover, socioeconomic factors may influence both the frequency and the course of epilepsy.

Finally, the analysis of mortality data shows the high risk of death in epileptic patients from the disorder itself and from suicide. The latter may be considered an indirect indication of the prevalence of severe depression, especially in younger people with epilepsy. Many of these fatalities may be prevented if we do not limit our attention merely to seizures.

Epidemiologic data may occasionally seem boring or tedious. They must be very specific and may not always be easily conclusive. The clinician, however, may frequently find much useful information for clinical research and practice in that data that is unobtainable by any other avenue of investigation.

REFERENCES

1. Schoenberg BS, Mann RG, Kurland LT: Snow on the water of London. *Mayo Clin Proc* 49:680–684, 1974
2. Zielinski JJ: People with epilepsy who do not attend doctors, in *Epileptology. Proceedings of the Seventh International Symposium on Epilepsy.* Edited by Janz D. Stuttgart, Georg Thieme, 1976, pp 18–23
3. Hopkins A, Scambler G: How doctors deal with epilepsy. *Lancet* 1:183–186, 1977
4. Miller FJ, Court SD, Walton WS, et al: *Growing Up in Newcastle Upon Tyne. A Continuing Study of Health and Illness in Young Children with Their Families.* London, Oxford University Press, 1960
5. Zielinski JJ: *Epidemiology and Medical-Social Problems of Epilepsy in Warsaw.* Washington, DC, US Department of Health, Education, and Welfare, 1974
6. Lennox WG: *Epilepsy and Related Disorders.* London, Churchill Livingstone, 1960
7. Hauser WA, Kurland LT: The epidemiology of epilepsy in Rochester, Minnesota, 1935 through 1967. *Epilepsia* 16:1–66, 1975
8. Gudmundsson G: Epilepsy in Iceland: a clinical and epidemiological investigation. *Acta Neurol Scand* 25(suppl 43):1–124, 1966
9. Hauser WA, Annegers JF, Elveback LR: Mortality in patients with epilepsy. *Epilepsia* 21:399–412, 1980
10. Juul-Jensen P, Ipsen J: Prevalence and incidence of epilepsy in Greater Aarhus, in *Epileptology. Proceedings of the Seventh International Symposium on Epilepsy.* Edited by Janz D. Stuttgart, Georg Thieme Verlag, 1976, p 10
11. Stanhope JM, Brody JA, Brink E: Convulsions among the Chamorro people of Guam, Mariana Islands. I. Seizure disorders. *Am J Epidemiol* 95:292–298, 1972
12. Brewis M, Poskanzer D, Rolland C, et al: Neurological disease in an English city. *Acta Neurol Scand* 42 (suppl 24):9–89, 1966
13. Gomez JG, Arciniegas E, Torres J: Prevalence of epilepsy in Bogota, Colombia. *Neurology (Minneap)* 28:90–94, 1978
14. Sato S: An epidemiologic and clinicostatistical study of epilepsy in Niigata City [Japanese]. *Clin Neurol* 4:461–471, 1964
15. Krohn W: A study of epilepsy in Northern Norway, its frequency and character. *Acta Psychiatr Scand* 150 (suppl 36):215–225, 1961
16. Grudzinska B: Epidemiology of epilepsy in population of a large industrial city. Incidence and prevalence [Polish]. *Neurol Neurochir Pol* 8:175–180, 1974
17. Commission for the Control of Epilepsy and Its Consequences: *Plan*

for Nationwide Action on Epilepsy, Vol 1. Washington, DC, DHEW, Pub Hlth Serv, NIH, DHEW Pub No (NIH) 78-276, 1978

18. Chiofale N, Kirschbaum A, Fuantes A, et al: Prevalence of epilepsy in children in Melipilla, Chile. *Epilepsia* 20:262–266, 1979
19. Rutter M, Graham P, Yule W: *A Neuropsychiatric Study in Childhood. Clin Develop Med 35/36, 1970*. London, Spastics International Medical Publications in association with William Heinemann Medical Books, 1970
20. Pless B, Graham P.: Epidemiology of physical disorder, in *Education, Health and Behaviour*. Edited by Rutter M, Tizard J, Whitmore K. London, Longman, 1970, p 285
21. Mathai KV, Dunn DP, Kurland LT, et al: Convulsive disorders in the Mariana Islands. *Epilepsia* 9:77–85, 1968
22. De Graaf AS: Epidemiological aspects of epilepsy in Northern Norway. *Epilepsia* 15:291–299, 1974
23. Zielinski JJ: Epidemiology of epilepsy in Poland on the basis of visits to physicians [Polish]. *Przegl Epidemiol* 29:123–132, 1975
24. Rose SW, Penry JK, Markush RE, et al: Prevalence of epilepsy in children. *Epilepsia* 14:133–152, 1973
25. Meighan SS, Queener L, Weitman M: Prevalence of epilepsy in children of Multnomah County, Oregon. *Epilepsia* 17:245–256, 1976
26. Shamansky SL, Glaser GH: Socio-economic characteristics of childhood seizure disorders in New Haven area: an epidemiological study. *Epilepsia* 20:457–474, 1979
27. Kurtzke JF: Mortality and morbidity data on epilepsy, in *NINDS Monograph No 14: The Epidemiology of Epilepsy: A Workshop*. Edited by Milton A, Hauser WA. Washington, DC, US Department of Health, Education, and Welfare,, 1972, p 21
28. Annegers JF, Hauser WA, Elveback LR: Remission of seizures and relapse in patients with epilepsy. *Epilepsia* 20:729–737, 1979
29. Zielinski JJ, Kuran W, Witkowska-Olearska K: The course of epilepsy and drug taking in randomly selected groups of patients in the light of 5 year follow-up [Polish]. *Pol Tyg Lek* 33:1927, 1978
30. Rodin EA: *The Prognosis of Patients with Epilepsy*. Springfield, Charles C Thomas, 1968
31. Turner WA: *Epilepsy. A Study of the Idiopathic Disease*. London, Macmillan, 1907
32. Slater E, Roth M: *Clinical Psychiatry*. 3rd edition. London, Baillière, Tindall and Cassell, 1969
33. Jerath BK, Kimbell BA: Hospitalization rates for epilepsy in the United States, 1973–1976. *Epilepsia* 22:55–64, 1981
34. Zielinski JJ: Social prognosis in epilepsy. *Epilepsia* 13:133–140, 1972

35. Zielinski JJ, Okolowicz-Zielinska I, Kuligowski ZW: Long-term epileptic patients of psychiatric hospitals and nursing care institutions [Polish]. *Neurol Neurochir Pol* 7:515–521, 1973

36. Pond DA, Burden GS: Review of the social and medical services for the epileptic patient in England and Wales. *Epilepsia* 4:77–89, 1963

37. Janz D: Social prognosis in epilepsy especially in regard to social status and the necessity for institutionalization. *Epilepsia* 13:141–147, 1972

38. Henriksen GF: Psychiatric aspects of epilepsy [Norwegian]. *Tidsskr Nor Laegeforen* 89:972–974, 1969

39. Gibbs, FA, Gibbs EL: *Atlas of Electroencephalography*. Cambridge, Addison-Wesley, 1964

40. Gastaut H, Gastaut JL, Gonçalves E, et al: Relative frequency of different types of epilepsy: a study employing the classification of the International League Against Epilepsy. *Epilepsia* 16:457–461, 1975

41. Blumer D: Temporal lobe epilepsy and its psychiatric significance, in *Psychiatric Aspects of Neurologic Disease*. Edited by Benson DF, Blumer D. New York, Grune & Stratton, 1975, pp 171–198

42. Betts TA: Psychiatry and epilepsy, in *A Textbook of Epilepsy*. London, Churchill Livingstone, 1982, pp 227–270

43. Parnas J, Korsgaard S: Epilepsy and psychosis. *Acta Psychiatr Scand* 66:89–99, 1982

44. Alstrom CH: A study of epilepsy in its clinical, social and genetic aspects. *Acta Psychiatr Scand* [Suppl] 63:1–284, 1950

45. Essen-Moller E: Individual traits and morbidity in a Swedish rural population. *Acta Psychiatr Scand*, [Suppl] 100:1–160, 1956

46. Blumer D, Benson DF: Personality changes with frontal and temporal lobe lesions, in *Psychiatric Aspects of Neurologic Disease*. Edited by Benson DF, Blumer D. New York, Grune & Stratton, 1975, pp 151–170

47. Reynolds EH: Chronic antiepileptic toxicity: a review. *Epilepsia* 16:319–352, 1975

48. Reynolds EH: Biological factors in psychological disorders associated with epilepsy, in *Epilepsy and Psychiatry*. Edited by Reynolds EH, Trimble MR. London, Churchill Livingstone, 1981, pp 264–290

49. Fenton GW: Personality and behavioural disorders in adults with epilepsy, in *Epilepsy and Psychiatry*. Edited by Reynolds EH, Trimble MR. London, Churchill Livingstone, 1981, pp 77–91

50. Oleanders S, Steinwall O: Preliminary evaluation of early prognostication in epilepsy. *Acta Neurol Scand* 41 (suppl 13):509–516, 1965

51. Rutter M, Graham P, Yule W: *A Neuropsychiatric Study in Childhood*. London, Spastics International Medical Publications in association with William Heinemann Medical Books, 1972

52. Lemkau P, Tietze C, Cooper M: Mental hygiene problems in an urban district. *MH* 25:624, 1941

53. Roth WF, Luton FH: Mental health program in Tennessee. *Am J Psychiatry* 99:662, 1943

54. Eaton JW, Weil RJ: *Culture and Mental Disorders.* Glencoe, The Free Press, 1955

55. Hollingshead AB, Redlich FC: *Social Class and Mental Illness.* New York, John Wiley & Sons, 1958

56. Babigian HM: Schizophrenia: epidemiology, in *Comprehensive Textbook of Psychiatry.* Edited by Freedman AM, Kaplan HI, Sadock BJ. Baltimore, Williams & Wilkins, 1975, pp 860–866

57. Fremming KH: *Expectations of Mental Infirmity in a Sample of the Danish Population.* London, Cassell Ltd, 1951

58. Book JA: A genetic and neuropsychiatric investigation of a North Swedish population with special regard to schizophrenia and mental deficiency. *Acta Genet (Basel)* 4:345–414, 1953

59. Sjogren T: Genetic statistical and psychiatric investigation of a West Swedish population. *Acta Psychiatr Neurol,* supplement 52, 1948

60. Henisz J: *Zesz Bad Reg Uprzem, No 4: Psychiatric and Social Study of Plock Community* [Polish]. Warsaw, P.A.N., 1963, pp 137–168

61. Shepherd M, Cooper B, Brown AC, et al: *Psychiatric Illness in General Practice.* 3rd edition. Oxford, Oxford University Press, 1981

62. Cohen BM, Fairbank RE: Statistical contributions from the mental hygiene study of the Eastern Health District in Baltimore. II. Psychosis in the Eastern Health District. *Am J Psychiatry* 94:1377–1395, 1938

63. Leighton DC, Harding JS, Macklin DB, et al: Psychiatric findings of the Stirling County Study. *Am J Psychiatry* 119:1021–1026, 1963

64. Weissman MM, Myers JK, Harding PS: Psychiatric disorders in a U.S. urban community: 1975–1976. *Am J Psychiatry* 15:459–462, 1978

65. D'Arcy C: Prevalence and correlates of nonpsychotic psychiatric symptoms in the general population. *Can J Psychiatry* 4:316–324, 1982

66. Rutter M, Tizard J, Yule W, et al: Research report: Isle of Wight studies, 1964–1974. *Psychol Med* 6:313–332, 1976

67. Slater E, Beard AW: The schizophrenia-like psychoses of epilepsy. *Br J Psychiatry* 109:95–150, 1963

68. Whitman S, Coleman T, Berg B, et al: Epidemiological insight into the socioeconomic correlates of epilepsy, in *A Multidisciplinary Handbook of Epilepsy.* Edited by Hermann BP. Springfield, Charles C Thomas, 1980, pp 243–271

69. Langner TS, Michael ST: *The Midtown Manhattan Study, Vol. 2: Life-Stress and Mental Health.* London, Free Press, 1963

70. Zielinski JJ: Epidemiology, in *A Textbook of Epilepsy*. Edited by Laidlaw J, Richens A. London, Churchill Livingstone, 1982, pp 16–33
71. Zielinski JJ: Epilepsy and mortality rates and causes of death. *Epilepsia* 15:191–201, 1974
72. Henriksen PB, Juul-Jensen P, Lund M: *Social Studies in Epilepsy, No 5: The Mortality of Epileptics. Epilepsy and Insurance.* London, International Bureau for Epilepsy, 1967
73. Kahl-Kunstetter J, Zielinski JJ: Causes of deaths of epileptic patients-inmates of a mental hospital [Polish]. *Neurol Neurochir Pol* 22:847–853, 1972
74. Janz D: *Die Epilepsien*. Stuttgart, Georg Thieme Verlag, 1969
75. Matthew WS, Barabas G: Suicide and epilepsy: a review of literature. *Psychosomatics* 22:515–524, 1981
76. Neppe VM: Is déjà vu a symptom of temporal lobe epilepsy? *S Afr Med J* 60:907–908, 1981

3

Neurologic Aspects of the Epilepsies

Ernst Niedermeyer, M.D.

Epileptic seizure disorders used to be a psychiatric domain. Neurologists and internists may have been unwilling to deal with these disorders because of the mysterious and uncanny nature of epileptic manifestations. During the second half of the nineteenth century, Hughlings Jackson developed a strictly neurologic approach to the epileptic seizure disorders (1–3), but his work did not break the psychiatric hegemony until the middle of the twentieth century. This was particularly true in the German-speaking countries. Psychiatry textbooks of this epoch (4–6) have large sections on epilepsy, whereas neurology textbooks treat the epilepsies in the vicinity of hysteria and the neuroses (7, 8). In 1948 a textbook of neurology and psychiatry (9) discussed epilepsy in the psychiatric section.

In those earlier days, the diagnosis of epilepsy had to be supported by the observation of a spontaneous seizure. While around-the-clock observation was available in a psychiatric ward, chances were that a physician would scarcely arrive in time to witness a seizure, so that an attendant (quite often inept for this task) had to make a descriptive report. In most of these cases, the differential diagnosis was limited to the question of grand mal epilepsy versus hysteria.

The advent of electroencephalography (EEG; 10) and the discovery of typical EEG correlates of the major epileptic seizure types (11, 12) represent major milestones in the neurologic approach to the epilepsies. Since the beginning of the second half of this century, this development has given the epilepsies a firm place in the field of neurology. The assessment of the epilepsies, however, must never degenerate into a tug-of-war between neurology and psychiatry. The fascinating psychiatric aspects of a large number of epileptic patients have to be evaluated in an amicable collaboration of the two specialties.

Such waves of fluctuating psychiatric and neurologic emphasis never existed with regard to childhood epilepsies; they were and remain a pediatric domain, except that pediatric subspecialties in neurology and epileptology have developed. Epileptic seizure disorders are most prevalent in childhood, and an epileptologist for adult cases ought to be thoroughly familiar with childhood epilepsies because of their repercussions on seizure disorders of adulthood.

"THE EPILEPTIC NEURON": NEUROPHYSIOLOGIC-NEUROBIOCHEMICAL CONSIDERATIONS

Electrophysiologic events are epiphenomena of neurobiochemical changes. The latter appear to be of primary significance, but their documentation is technically very difficult. On the other hand, electrophysiologic phenomena are relatively easily documented with amplifying electronic equipment.

Modern research has focused on single neuron behavior recorded with intracellular microelectrodes. The existence of "epileptic neurons" has been stressed (13, 14). Autonomous and sustained abnormal firing as well as increased electrical excitability have been considered major features of an epileptic neuron (15). Instability of the membrane, producing paroxysmal depolarization shifts, has been ascribed to the epileptic neurons (16).

What causes the "epileptic behavior" (i.e., the massive firing) of such neurons? Ionic changes play a major role. A strong influx of calcium ions is now considered a crucial factor (17–19). With calcium influx, potassium moves out, and the augmentation of extracellular potassium will depolarize the cell. With further potassium outflow, the neurons can no longer be repolarized, denoting the breakdown of membrane stability control.

An epileptogenic focus contains both strongly and weakly epileptic cells (group 1 and group 2 epileptic neurons). The strongly epileptic cells generate the epileptic activity, while the weaker cells gradually follow the lead and produce synchronous epileptic firing (20), similar to human political behavior in which hard-core revolutionaries may lead a mass of followers.

The abnormal synchronization of paroxysmally firing neurons is presumably carried out by synaptic mechanisms. At this stage the decline of antagonistic and seizure-preventing inhibitory mechanisms becomes evident. A dramatic scenario of events (21) shows itself in microspikes in the scalp EEG (in contrast to the axosomatic microspikes in single neurons). These have been attributed to facilitation and disfacilitation processes of upper cortical laminae (22, 23).

Normally, inhibitory mechanisms are found in almost every CNS level (24), particularly in the cerebellar cortex. However, in the turmoil of epileptic events, inhibitory mechanisms temporarily break down. A seizure is terminated when these inhibitory impulses restore themselves, not simply as a result of metabolic exhaustion as one might suppose.

TYPES OF EPILEPTIC SEIZURES

The types of epileptic seizures must be well understood for pragmatic as well as theoretical reasons. It must be kept in mind that certain seizure types require special anticonvulsive therapy. Thorough familiarity with the types of epileptic seizures naturally is very helpful in the differential diagnosis between epileptic and nonepileptic seizures. Further information is found in Chapter 5 of this book and in the work of Gastaut and Broughton (25).

Almost two centuries have elapsed since Esquirol differentiated the "grand mal" from minor attacks called "petit mal." Astute clinical observation and eventually the use of the EEG made possible the distinction of a number of seizure types.

Classification of seizures has been an area of considerable con troversy. A rather conservative classification is presented in Table 1. A modern international classification (Table 2) has been the result of painstaking work of a special commission headed by Dreifuss (27), partly superseding an earlier similar classification promoted by Gastaut (28). These modern classifications have not yet been universally accepted. In the following, older customary terms will be used together with the modern terms (usually indicated in parentheses).

Grand Mal (Tonic-Clonic Seizures)

The grand mal is presumably the most common seizure type. It can occur at any age except during the first six months of life.

TABLE 1. *Types of epileptic seizures*

Grand mal
- With focal initiation (aura)
- Without focal initiation (primary generalized)

Petit mal absence

Psychomotor seizures
- Automatism
- Experience (psychosensory)

Focal motor and other focal seizures

Myoclonic seizures

Special type associated with infantile spasms
- Jackknifing

Special types associated with Lennox-Gastaut syndrome
- Atonic drop attacks
- Tonic seizures
- Clonic seizures

From Niedermeyer (26), reprinted with permission.

TABLE 2. *Proposal for revised seizure classification (Commission on Classification and Terminology, 1981)*

I. Partial (focal, local) seizures

A. Simple partial seizures (consciousness not impaired)

1. With motor signs
   (a) Focal motor without march
   (b) Focal motor with march (Jacksonian)
   (c) Versive
   (d) Postural
   (e) Phonatory (vocalization or arrest of speech)

2. With somatosensory or special sensory symptoms (simple hallucinations; e.g., tingling, light flashes, buzzing)
   (a) Somatosensory
   (b) Visual
   (c) Auditory
   (d) Olfactory
   (e) Gustatory
   (f) Vertiginous

3. With autonomic symptoms or signs (including epigastric sensation, pallor, sweating, flushing, piloerection, and pupillary dilatation)

TABLE 2. *(Continued)*

4. With psychic symptoms (disturbance of higher cerebral function). These symptoms rarely occur without impairment of consciousness and are much more commonly experienced as complex partial seizures
   (a) Dysphasic
   (b) Dysmnesic (e.g., déjà-vu)
   (c) Cognitive (e.g., dreamy states, distortions of time sense)
   (d) Affective (e.g., fear, anger)
   (e) Illusions (e.g., macropsia)
   (f) Structured hallucinations (e.g., music, scenes)

B. Complex partial seizures
(with impairment of consciousness; may sometimes begin with simple symptomatology)

1. Simple partial onset, followed by impairment of consciousness
   (a) With simple partial features (A.1–A.4) followed by impaired consciousness
   (b) With automatisms
2. With impairment of consciousness at onset
   (a) With impairment of consciousness only
   (b) With automatisms

C. Partial seizures evolving to secondarily generalized seizures (generalized tonic-clonic, tonic, or clonic)

1. Simple partial seizures evolving to generalized seizures
2. Complex partial seizures evolving to generalized seizures
3. Simple partial seizures evolving to complex partial seizures evolving to generalized seizures

II. Generalized seizures (convulsive or nonconvulsive)

A. Absence seizures

1. Typical absences
   (a) Impairment of consciousness only
   (b) With mild clonic components
   (c) With atonic components
   (d) With tonic components
   (e) With automatisms
   (f) With autonomic components
   (b–f may be used alone or in combination)
2. Atypical absences
   (a) May have changes in tone that are more pronounced than in A.1
   (b) Onset and/or cessation that is not abrupt

TABLE 2. *(Continued)*

B. Myoclonic seizures
Myoclonic jerks (single or multiple)

C. Clonic seizures

D. Tonic seizures

E. Tonic-clonic seizures

F. Atonic seizures
(Astatic)

(combinations of the above may occur, e.g., B and F, B and D)

III. Unclassified epileptic seizures

IV. Addendum

With respect to occurrence of seizures (cyclic, fortuitous) or precipitation by triggering events.

From Niedermeyer (26), reprinted with permission.

Its sequence of a tonic and a clonic phase is well known. The duration of the seizure ranges from 40 to 90 s. Massive generalized spiking in the EEG characterizes the tonic stage, and bursts of spikes are separated by slow waves in the clonic stage. Abrupt cessation of the clonic motion and temporary EEG flatness mark the termination of the attack. Profound coma is present during the entire attack and usually subsides within minutes after the seizure (along with restoration of the "baseline" EEG).

Tongue biting is fairly common (in the early clonic phase). Loss of urinary sphincter control occurs less frequently. Life-threatening complications such as asphyxia (food particles, etc.) are extremely rare.

The major convulsion may be generalized from the start (primary grand mal) or may occur with focal initiation (secondary grand mal). A focal (partial) seizure may quickly or gradually evolve into a grand mal. If the preceding focal seizure is experienced subjectively (sensory, visual, olfactory, auditory, emotional phenomena), the term "aura" is often used. One must keep in mind that an aura is nothing but a focal attack that may evolve into a grand mal if there is sufficient spread of the epileptic activity.

Petit Mal Absences

The petit mal attack consists of a brief absence of 5- to 30-s duration with a highly characteristic and practically diagnostic 3–3.5/s spike-wave pattern. There is very little motor accompaniment. Petit mal absences are generalized events from the EEG viewpoint, notwithstanding the fact that their clinical manifestations are mild.

Petit mal absences usually occur in childhood between the ages of 4 and 12 years; they seldom persist through adolescence into adulthood. The prevalence of petit mal absences is relatively low (5–10 percent of childhood epilepsies and almost negligible in adulthood).

Psychomotor (Complex Partial) Seizures

Psychomotor seizures consist mainly of automatisms with stereotyped movements such as chewing, swallowing, lip smacking, etc. These are associated with loss of consciousness while postural functions are almost always preserved (the patient usually does not fall). In the postictal phase, more complex "automatic" behavior may occur, such as fumbling with clothes. Typically there is no recollection for the observable (automatic) seizure events. These seizures last from 30 s to 5 min. The duration may be longer if there is a protracted postictal phase.

Psychomotor seizures frequently consist of, or begin with, experienced (remembered) ictal phenomena. Common are peculiar epigastric sensations or a "déjà vu" experience. The déjà vu consists of heightened familiarity of a certain situation. The present is experienced as though it has been going on for eons. Thus, the seizure interferes with the past-present relationship. These ictal experiences are frequently tinged with emotions, fear being the most common (29–32).

The aura or experienced form of psychomotor seizures also encompasses hallucinations and misperceptions in all senses. Visual misperceptions are complex rather than elementary. Particularly well known are olfactory sensations (usually a very bad odor); in such cases a neoplastic etiology should be ruled out with particular care.

Experienced psychomotor seizures (also called "psychosensory") are usually of shorter duration than attacks with observable events (psychomotor automatisms), and some of these sensations are even flashlike. Patients with automatisms usually have a more severe and therapeutically less responsive form of seizure disorder than those with experienced attacks alone.

Almost all psychomotor (complex partial) seizures originate in the temporal lobe; a few arise from adjacent frontal structures. Limbic structures, especially the amygdala, play a leading role, as has been impressively demonstrated (33, 34).

Ictal psychic phenomena and the frequent association of psychiatric disorder (35) have heightened speculation about the relationship between the temporal lobe and uncontrolled behavior such as violence. This idea has been thoroughly investigated by Rodin (36, 37). In fact, most cases of rage attacks show no EEG evidence of temporal lobe epilepsy (38).

The EEG of temporal lobe epilepsy with psychomotor seizures is characterized by anterior temporal sharp waves or spikes in the interictal interval (39), which are more likely to occur in sleep. The discharge may be unilateral or bilateral. Often, the discharge is not readily demonstrable, and it may take several repeat tracings to produce EEG evidence. The ictal EEG shows a highly variable discharge type (40).

Psychomotor seizures occur in childhood and adolescence, but mostly in adulthood. The earliest manifestations in childhood may consist of sudden fear and are not easily diagnosed.

The prevalence of psychomotor seizures is high and may exceed that of grand mal (especially in institutions for chronic epileptics). The response to anticonvulsants is often poor, and the prognosis is guarded for this reason.

Focal Motor and Other Focal Seizures (Elementary Partial Seizures)

The character of focal motor and other focal seizures depends on the cortical zone of origin. The most common attacks arise in the motor cortex and consist of contralateral twitching in limited body regions: fingers, hand, arm, leg, etc. The gradual spread of these clonic manifestations is known as the "Jacksonian march." The patient remains conscious during the clonic motions, but the attack may eventually progress into a full-blown grand mal convulsion.

Massive and extensive focal motor seizure activity may be followed by a transient hemiparetic deficit known as "Todd's paralysis." This phenomenon is more common in childhood.

Focal motor attacks may occur at any age and are less common than grand mal and psychomotor seizures. Because of their local cortical origin, the etiology should be carefully assessed. Parasagittal meningiomas and arteriovenous malformations are notable among the various etiologies.

Much less common are sensory seizures arising from the postcentral gyrus and consisting of paresthesias (seldom pain) in the involved contralateral extremities. Turning (adversion) of the head to the side contralateral to the focus is a rather frequent seizure manifestation that arises chiefly from the frontal lobes (with loss of consciousness from anterior foci; without loss of consciousness from foci located closer to the motor strip).

Focal seizures may originate from other cortical projection areas. Elementary visual hallucinations (sparks, a ball of fire, etc.) are experienced in occipital lobe epilepsy, which also may produce nystagmoid eye movements. Auditory, gustatory, and vertiginous sensations are much less common. Olfactory attacks are more frequent and fall into the category of psychomotor seizures (temporal lobe epilepsy).

Myoclonic Seizures

Myoclonus may be epileptic or nonepileptic in character. It denotes a brief jerk of essential bilateral character; such jerks may be quite massive. Myoclonic seizures are more common in children, but may occur at any age.

Other Types of Seizures

Further seizure types will be discussed under Age-Determined Epileptic Conditions (especially infantile spasms and Lennox-Gastaut syndrome).

Unclassifiable Seizures

There are many complex seizure manifestations that defy taxonomic categorization.

ETIOLOGIES OF EPILEPTIC SEIZURE DISORDERS

It is impossible to list all the conditions that can give rise to epileptic seizure disorders. The majority of the causes can be dated back to the prenatal, perinatal, and early postnatal periods. Various types of brain damage sustained early in life will prove to be epileptogenic even though the first seizure may occur after considerable delay (years or decades). Cerebral palsy in its various forms may be associated with seizures in 30–70 percent of cases (41). There are also progressive degenerative brain diseases of infancy and childhood with epileptogenic character; Tay-Sachs disease and cerebromacular degenerations (Batten's disease, etc.) belong in this category. Many others could be added, especially the hereditary progressive myoclonus epilepsy (Lafora-Unverricht) with progressive myoclonus, grand mal, ataxia, and dementia. Table 3 shows the most common etiologies of epileptic seizures, listed according to their age at onset.

Certain forms of seizure etiologies have special characteristics. *Alcohol withdrawal seizures* are found in chronic alcoholics and consist of grand mal attacks following heavy drinking. Hypomagnesemia and blood alkalosis are found in this stage (42). In a second stage, delirium tremens may develop (usually 72–96 h after cessation of drinking).

Posttraumatic epilepsy must be broken down into a variety of forms. A grand mal may occur a few seconds after an acute head

TABLE 3. *The most common causes of epileptic seizures according to age at onset (listed in presumed order of importance)*[a]

First Week

Perinatal asphyxia
Perinatal trauma (often with intracranial bleeding)
Very early CNS infection
Cerebral malformation
Hypocalcemia
Hypoglycemia
Other early metabolic changes

Second Week

Early CNS infection
Extracranial infection (with electrolyte derangement)
Hypocalcemia (alimentary)
Kernicterus
Cerebral malformation

3rd week to 3 months

CNS infection
Subdural collection following CNS infection
Cerebral malformation

4 months to 2 years

Febrile convulsions (triggered by trivial febrile diseases)
CNS infection
Residual epilepsy due to early CNS damage (cerebral palsy)
Cerebrovascular problems: arterial occlusion, venous thrombosis
Inborn errors of metabolism
Neurocutaneous disorders

Note: In predisposed children, seizure disorder may appear as infantile spasms or Lennox-Gastaut syndrome.

TABLE 3. *(Continued)*

3–10 years
Benign Rolandic epilepsy (dysfunction-predisposition)
Primary generalized epilepsy (dysfunction-predisposition)
Residual epilepsy due to early CNS damage (cerebral palsy)
Trauma
Inborn errors of metabolism
CNS infection
CNS poisoning (lead, etc.)
Neurocutaneous disorders
Note: In predisposed children, seizure disorder may appear as Lennox-Gastaut syndrome.
11–20 years
Primary generalized epilepsy (dysfunction-predisposition)
Trauma
Residual epilepsy due to early CNS damage (cerebral palsy)
CNS infection
Arteriovenous malformation
21–40 years
Trauma
Brain tumor
Chronic alcoholism
Residual epilepsy due to early CNS damage (cerebral palsy)
Arteriovenous malformation
41–60 years
Brain tumor
Chronic alcoholism (in certain areas, leading cause)
Trauma
Cerebrovascular disease (also vasculitis)
60 years and older
Cerebral arteriosclerosis
Brain tumor, primary
Brain tumor, metastatic

[a]Cause frequently remains unknown. In tropical and subtropical countries, CNS parasites may be the leading cause. From Niedermeyer (26), reprinted with permission.

injury (immediate posttraumatic seizures) often without further neurologic or epileptologic consequences. In a severe cerebral contusion or in an epidural, acute subdural, or intracerebral hematoma, seizures (grand mal, focal) may develop on the second day after the trauma, usually at the height of cerebral edema. Late posttraumatic epilepsies with an onset of seizures between 3 months and 2 years after the injury are most typical. This form is caused mostly by cerebral laceration (open brain wounds) with brain-dura scar formation. Naturally, these conditions occur mainly in wartime. Chronic subdural hematoma as a late sequela of a (frequently trivial) trauma in older individuals is often associated with focal seizures or grand mal.

In severe *CNS infections*, epileptic seizures may occur during the acute stage but may also develop as a sequela of the disease. This is true for most forms of encephalitis and meningoencephalitis, regardless of viral, bacterial, or rickettsial etiology. Herpes simplex encephalitis is a typical example of a viral disease that is frequently associated with or followed by seizures.

Brain tumors are an important cause of seizures, especially in adulthood. Epileptic seizures occur in 50 percent of the tumors affecting the cerebral hemispheres and in about one-third of all intracranial tumors (43). The highest epileptogenicity is found in oligodendrogliomas (90 percent), followed by astrocytomas (69 percent), metastatic tumors (41 percent), meningioma (37 percent), and glioblastoma multiforme (34 percent). Slowly growing tumors in the vicinity of the rolandic cortex are particularly epileptogenic. The epileptogenicity of intracranial tumors decreases with the increasing distance of the tumor from the cerebral cortex (basal ganglia, thalamic tumors) and is virtually nonexistent in cases of tumors located between the third ventricle and the cerebellum.

The role of brain tumors as a cause of epileptic seizures varies according to the composition of an epileptic population and ranges from 0.74 to 15 percent. In childhood, brain tumors are uncommon causes of a seizure disorder, but with seizure onset in adulthood, the possibility of a brain tumor should be ruled out with greatest care using structural tests, especially the computed tomographic (CT) scan.

Brain abscesses are highly epileptogenic. This is also true for chronic subdural hematoma, chronic granulomatous lesions (tuberculoma, syphilitic gumma—now extremely rare), and, especially in tropical countries, intracranial parasites (with cysticercosis being a leading cause of epileptic seizures in some South American regions).

Cerebrovascular disorder may give rise to a variety of pathological changes. Seizures are associated with strokes (cerebrovascular accidents) in 12.5–20 percent of cases. These attacks are mostly of focal motor (elementary partial) character. "Premonitory" seizures may precede a stroke by weeks or months (44). In about 4 percent of cases of chronic arteriosclerosis with strong cerebral involvement, epileptic seizures may occur; this is a common etiology of seizures beginning in old age. Epileptic seizures may occur during subarachnoid bleeding from intracranial aneurysms and in the wake of aneurysm surgery. Arteriovenous malformations are also a well-known cause of seizures (mostly focal motor or grand mal). Seizures may also occur in cortical venous thrombosis, hypertension (especially in the malignant type), systemic lupus erythematosus, and sickle cell anemia with neurologic complications.

Metabolic encephalopathies may prove to be acutely or chronically epileptogenic. Hypoglycemia has a particularly pronounced epileptogenic effect, producing massive myoclonus and grand mal. These manifestations are common in hyperinsulinism (functional, or neoplastic with islet cell tumor), insulin-induced coma in diabetic patients, and naturally also during Sakel's insulin treatment of schizophrenics with induced hypoglycemia. Hyperglycemia is much less epileptogenic, except for nonketotic hyperglycemic states, which tend to give rise to prolonged focal motor seizures. Hypocalcemia is highly epileptogenic; grand mal usually develops at calcium serum levels of 5.0–6.0 mg/100 ml. Seizures are much less common in hypercalcemic states. Convulsions may emerge in hyponatremic states, especially in severe forms of adrenocortical insufficiency (Addison's disease). The central form of intermittent porphyria is sometimes associated with seizures.

Renal failure gives rise to renal encephalopathy. About one-third of patients with acute renal failure develop seizures (45), usually caused by water-electrolyte imbalance (46). Myoclonus is very common in acute and chronic uremic states. The disequilibrium syndrome in dialyzed patients enhances the epileptic manifestations. Renal disturbance also occupies a pivotal position in eclampsia gravidarum, which is usually associated with hypertension and grand mal attacks occurring intrapartum. Much less epileptogenicity is found in hepatic encephalopathy.

Toxic encephalopathies of acute or chronic character may cause epileptic seizures. Heavy metals such as lead or manganese must be mentioned in this context, but only a limited number of causes can be cited in this overview.

For the psychiatrist the long-term use of phenothiazines is a particularly important etiology of seizures. Chlorpromazine is presumably more epileptogenic than other phenothiazines. The seizure-inducing effect is unrelated to the syndrome of tardive dyskinesia.

Tricyclic antidepressants such as imipramine (Tofranil) and amitriptyline (Elavil) may give rise to grand mal, even in subtoxic dosages, but presumably in predisposed individuals only.

Electroconvulsive treatment (electroshock) given in excessive amounts may be the cause of spontaneous grand mal attacks.

The role of *genetic factors* must be neither under- nor overrated. The relationship between genetic factors and epilepsy is complex. First, disease genes must be correctly recognized, i.e., the presence of a strictly genetic disease producing seizures. This pertains to Tay-Sachs disease, essential myoclonus epilepsy, and a host of other diseases.

The role of "threshold genes" that determine the degree of predisposition to epileptic seizures is very interesting. Unfortunately, very little is known about the nature of these genes, which undoubtedly exist. Let us suppose that two healthy individuals of the same age sustain the same type of craniocerebral trauma but only one of them develops posttraumatic epilepsy. This would be an example of individual predisposition.

Every human being (and also every member of the animal kingdom) is capable of exhibiting epileptic reactions to epileptogenic stimulation or irritation. This is axiomatic for the use of electroconvulsive treatment that (like Metrazol) generates a grand mal response in every individual, but with differences of threshold (i.e., parameters of electrical stimulation).

AGE-DETERMINED EPILEPTIC CONDITIONS

The relationship of epileptic seizure disorders to specific age groups is not yet widely appreciated, but its significance is enormous for several reasons. Certain epileptic conditions, usually characterized by certain types of seizures but often of polyetiologic origin, emerge in infancy and childhood. Most importantly, some of these conditions are basically benign, whereas others are severe and recalcitrant in character. Thus, the prognosis depends heavily on the type of epileptic condition. These seizure disorders usually evolve during the first two decades of life, but their repercussions may extend into adulthood. The first years of life are of crucial importance for adult health, in the view of psychodynamically oriented psychiatrists and also epileptologists.

Age-determined epileptic conditions are usually characterized by: certain types of seizures; particular paroxysmal EEG patterns; and a typical course and prognosis. The etiologies, however, are many. Figure 1 shows the relationship between the seizure types and certain age-determined epileptic conditions. A longitudinal view of the course is shown in Figure 2.

Neonatal Convulsions

Neonatal convulsions comprise benign and severe forms. Severe (malignant) forms are associated with brain damage and foreshadow mental retardation, cerebral impairment, and continuing seizure problems. The most common causes of the severe forms are severe asphyxia at birth, congenital CNS malformations, and massive early CNS infections. Lombroso (47) has detailed these conditions more thoroughly.

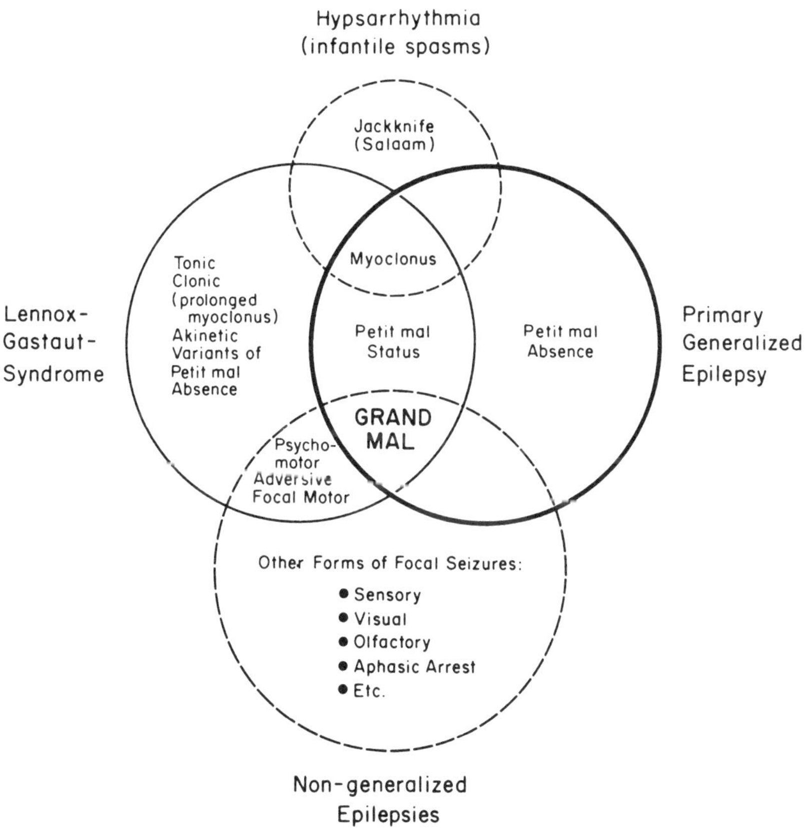

FIGURE 1. Types of seizures, age-determined epileptic conditions, and all forms of focal (partial) epilepsies. (From Niedermeyer [26], reprinted with permission.)

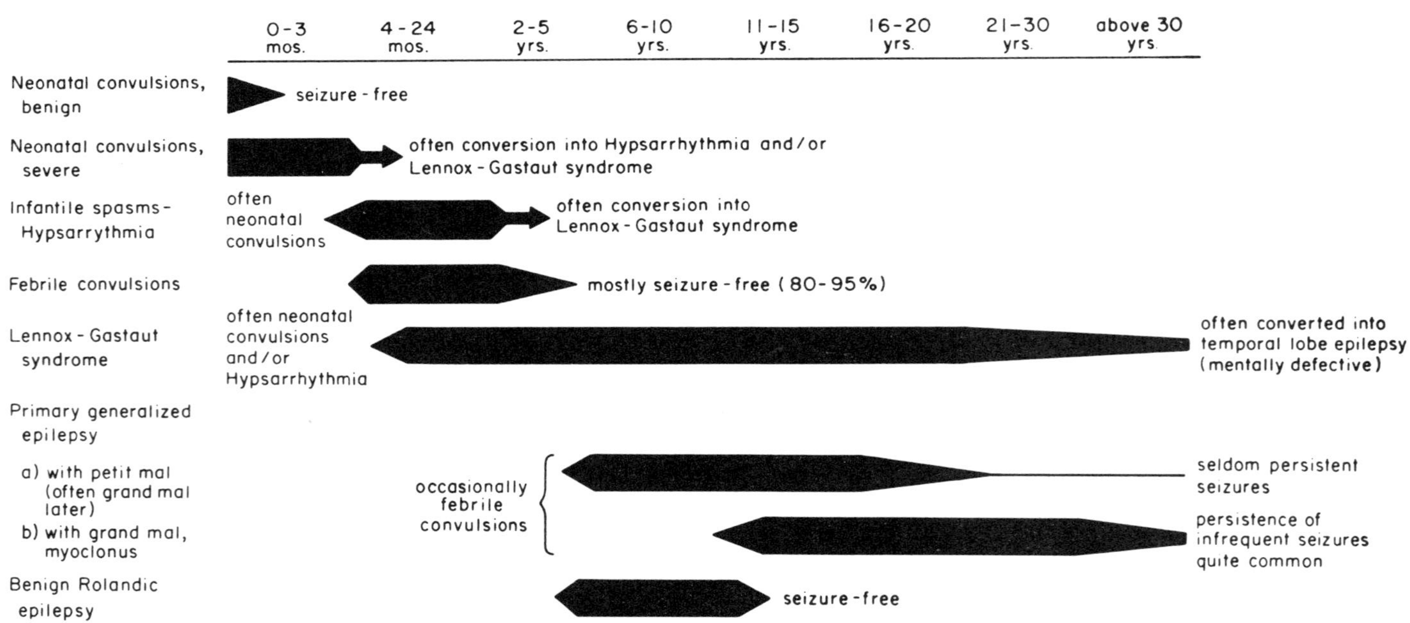

FIGURE 2. The course of age-determined epileptic conditions in longitudinal view. (From Niedermeyer [26], reprinted with permission.)

Infantile Spasms (Hypsarrhythmia)

Infantile spasms occur between 4 months and 2.5 years of age. Typical seizures and EEG abnormalities [the hypsarrhythmic pattern (48)] evolve. The most common seizure is the "jackknifing" form of flexor spasm, which has been known since an early observation of West (49), but there are also mixed or chiefly myoclonic types (50). With the occurrence of these seizures and the concomitant hypsarrhythmic EEG changes, the psychomotor development of the child slows, even to the degree of arrest.

There are cryptogenic or idiopathic forms of infantile spasms without any evidence of an underlying brain disease, evolving after a period of normal psychomotor development at around age 6 months. Symptomatic forms caused by existing brain damage are slightly more common. Many of these children have a history of neonatal convulsions. This shows the transition from one age-determined epileptic conditon to another. The prognostic outlook is guarded in the cryptogenic and poor in the symptomatic forms. Prior to the introduction of adrenocorticotropin treatment (51), the prognosis was almost uniformly poor. It is most interesting to note that infantile spasms respond chiefly to hormonal treatment (rather than to anticonvulsants). The reason for this peculiarity has been widely debated (52).

Febrile Convulsions

Febrile convulsions are probably the most common form of epileptic seizure disorder; they may occur in 3–4 percent of all healthy children (53). The age range extends from 6 months to 5 years, but the vast majority of these attacks occur between the ages of 6 months and 2 years.

Febrile convulsions are of the grand mal type. Of course, the tonic-clonic convulsion is mitigated by the small bulk of musculature at this early age. The attacks are triggered by a febrile disease, most commonly by a trivial upper respiratory tract infection. A sudden, steep rise of temperature apparently precipitates the seizure.

Although the seizures themselves are of epileptic character (from the neurophysiological viewpoint), the vast majority of these children will never have any further epileptic manifestations during the rest of their lives. Therefore, the prognosis is excellent in 90–95 percent while a minority will have further (afebrile) seizures in the future. The EEG is normal in the interictal interval in most cases.

Febrile convulsions are presumably based on a certain genetic predisposition. This benign seizure disorder must be differentiated from seizures occurring in acute febrile CNS infections (mostly hemiconvulsions); with the latter, the children are seriously ill and likely to develop a seizure disorder in the future (along with mental impairment in most cases). Some cases with protracted febrile convulsions may, however, gradually evolve into temporal lobe epilepsy.

Lennox-Gastaut Syndrome

Lennox-Gastaut syndrome has been outlined in the last few decades. It usually begins between 1 and 10 years of age. It is a severe and, in most cases, prognostically unfavorable epileptic condition characterized by a variety of seizure types. Most of these seizures are short and of rather "minor" character (tonic, atonic, clonic, myoclonic, atypical absences); there may be also psychomotor automatisms and focal motor, adversive, and grand mal attacks. Most typical is the atonic drop attack, which results in a sudden fall that often causes injuries. These falls necessitate the use of helmetlike protective headgear.

Approximately 50 percent of these patients have early infantile residual brain damage. The etiology includes various forms of cerebral palsy, CNS malformation (porencephaly, etc.), tuberous sclerosis, and progressive degenerative CNS diseases. These patients show considerable neurologic deficits. In the remaining 50 percent there is no evidence of underlying brain disease, and the seizures start without any preceding CNS disorder. These children usually have normal CT scans.

Mental retardation may be profound. The earlier the onset of seizures, the worse the intellectual deficit. Onset past the age of 10 years has been observed, and in such cases there is usually no mental retardation.

The diagnosis of Lennox-Gastaut syndrome depends heavily on the EEG finding and the type of seizures. The presence of slow (1–2.5/s) spike-wave complexes in the EEG is highly indicative; this is also true for "runs of rapid spikes." Gibbs et al. (54) first noted the association of slow spike-waves and mental deficits. However, the work of Lennox (55) and Gastaut et al. (56) was instrumental in delineating the syndrome.

The prevalence of Lennox-Gastaut syndrome has been cited at about 5 percent (all epilepsies) and 10 percent (epilepsies in patients below the age of 15 years), but these were reported by a large epilepsy center (57) and hence may be unrealistically high. These figures definitely exceed those for infantile spasms. Approximately 10–20 percent of children with Lennox-Gastaut syndrome passed through a period of infantile spasms (before age 2–3 years).

The poor prognosis is essentially due to the lack of responsiveness to anticonvulsive medication. Benzodiazepines (especially clonazepam) are at least temporarily helpful, and in children ketogenic diet may provide some improvement. Many children have to be institutionalized. In adulthood the EEG and ictal characteristics may undergo some changes with increasing signs of temporal lobe epilepsy (secondary temporalization). These patients eventually exhibit signs of a deteriorated temporal lobe epileptic.

Primary Generalized Epilepsy

Primary generalized epilepsy may be regarded as truly "idiopathic;" i.e., there is no evidence of structural CNS lesions, focal neurologic deficits, or localized EEG abnormalities. It is characterized by generalized synchronous paroxysmal EEG abnormalities, such as the 3/s spike-wave discharge with a maximum over the frontal midline. A deep thalamic midline origin [centrencephalic epilepsy (58)] has been theorized but never demonstrated; cortical and deep levels have been thought to be involved [corticoreticular epilepsy (59)].

The petit mal absence is the most typical clinical ictal manifestation, with an onset at about 4–5 or 8–10 years About 30–50 percent of these children will have a few grand mal attacks after the age of 14 years, often preceded by myoclonus. Most of these grand mal attacks occur in the morning after a night of poor sleep [awakening epilepsy (60)]. Occasionally these patients may have a history of febrile convulsions in early childhood, and a few develop petit mal absence status.

This disorder appears to be based on genetic predisposition, but the nature of the underlying genes is still enigmatic. Arousing stimuli in periods of drowsiness are capable of triggering paroxysmal bursts and clinical seizures. This renders the patients more vulnerable after a night of poor sleep. Other patients with primary generalized epilepsy are sensitive to flickering light. In this latter group, myoclonus and grand mal are the most common seizure manifestations, whereas petit mal absences are more seldom noted.

Patients with primary generalized epilepsy are usually of average intelligence, but certain psychopathic personality traits are not uncommon. They may misuse their medication and experiment with street drugs, unlike patients with other forms of epileptic seizure disorders.

The prognosis is good in the majority of the cases. Most of the patients become seizurefree in the third decade. However, in some the condition persists into later adulthood.

In adult seizure clinics one usually finds a sizable percentage of patients with primary generalized epilepsy between the ages of 20 and 30 years. At this age myoclonus and grand mal are the only major problems; petit mal absences are quite rare.

What is primary generalized epilepsy? It is presumably a genetically determined state of hyperexcitability of a system that expresses its dysfunction with generalized synchronous seizure discharges in the EEG, with or without the clinical manifestations of petit mal absence, myoclonus, or grand mal. The cue to these abnormal discharges comes from arousing stimuli [dyshormia (61)] and/or flickering light. This state of abnormal hyperexcitability is usually most pronounced between ages 4 and 16 years. The most actively involved cerebral regions (acting in bilateral synchrony) are the frontal lobes and especially the supplementary motor areas close to the interhemispheric fissure. Occasionally the differentiation of primary generalized epilepsy from focal epilepsies is rendered difficult by phenomena such as secondary bilateral synchrony and secondary temporalization. Such coexistence of focal and generalized EEG discharges is not very common (61).

Benign Rolandic Epilepsy

Found in 3- to 12-year-old patients, benign Rolandic epilepsy is essentially of neuropediatric interest. These children show copious spike activity over the central and adjacent midtemporal region in the EEG. Their seizures are either of the focal motor or the grand mal type and tend to occur during sleep (62).

This seizure disorder is also based on a dysfunction, i.e., hyperexcitability of the Rolandic cortex; there are no structural lesions and no neurologic deficits. The prognosis is excellent, and the seizures disappear at around 10–12 years of age.

Benign Rolandic epilepsy, primary generalized epilepsy, and febrile convulsions are all based on dysfunction rather than on structural pathology.

FOCAL ASPECTS

The site of an epileptogenic focus strongly determines the seizure manifestations. In other words, epileptic seizures may reflect the functional anatomy of the cortex. This was first demonstrated by the observations of Fritsch and Hitzig (63). Investigations on cortical excitability and its focal epileptic phenomena culminated with the work of Penfield and Jasper (64).

There is no "democratic equality" among the lobes of the cerebrum; some of them are more epileptogenic than others. The highest degree of epileptogenicity is found in the temporal lobe.

Temporal Lobe Epilepsy

More than 50 percent of focal epilepsies originate in the temporal lobe. Thus, a large percentage (usually between 40 percent and 60 percent) of the patients treated in adult seizure clinics consists of temporal lobe epileptics. Many, if not most, of these patients are not fully controlled, even with optimal anticonvulsive therapy, because temporal lobe epilepsy is a rather serious seizure disorder.

The cause is multifold, but most patients suffer from residual pathology such as discrete focal lesions or hippocampal sclerosis (pararhinal sclerosis, mesiotemporal sclerosis) or have areas of cortical neuronal loss with gliosis. The number of brain tumors, however, must not be underrated [12.2 percent (65)]. This is particularly true for patients with onset of seizures in adult life.

Psychomotor seizures are the classic type in temporal lobe epilepsy. Automatisms usually indicate a more serious seizure disorder than experienced psychomotor attack (see Types of Epileptic Seizures). Most temporal lobe epileptics suffer from frequent psychomotor (complex partial) seizures and occasional grand mal, but even the most recalcitrant cases may suffer from psychomotor attacks only. Such patients may have several psychomotor automatisms per day and perhaps a larger number of experienced attacks that may be "flashlike," i.e., of very short duration.

The EEG is very helpful in these cases. The typical finding is an anterior temporal spike or sharp wave focus, either unilateral or bilateral (with synchronous or independent firing), usually spreading into the frontopolar and midtemporal region. Sleep records are often more informative than waking records There are also some limitations to the use of EEG. The electroencephalographer is often perplexed by normal EEG findings that stubbornly remain normal with repeated tests. Patience usually pays off, and there may be cycles of demonstrable anterior temporal spike activity with silent and eloquent periods. Thus, the clinician must be guided by both clinical (seizure type, etc.) and EEG considerations, but in some cases the EEG evidence may be marginal or absent. Even the use of nasopharyngeal electrodes does not yield much additional information; sphenoidal electrodes are more informative but their insertion is an invasive procedure. There are patients with negative surface recordings yet with almost constant firing in limbic and neocortical temporal lobe structures when the recording is obtained from inserted depth leads. Depth recording, however, is an invasive procedure with a certain complication rate and must be reserved for patients who are potential candidates for surgical treatment of their epilepsy.

The neurologic examination is usually unremarkable unless there is gross CNS pathology. Mild weakness of the seventh nerve (upper motor neuron type) is at times found contralateral to the focus. The mental and emotional changes observed in temporal lobe epilepsy are discussed extensively in other chapters of this book.

Temporal lobe epilepsy with psychomotor (complex partial) seizures may occur any time from early childhood to old age, but it is most often found (and usually most active) in early and mid-adulthood. In most cases the therapy requires the use of anticonvulsants with special effects against psychomotor seizures (primidone, carbamazepine). Drug-resistant cases stand a good chance to benefit from temporal lobectomy provided that the affected temporal region is unilateral or predominantly unilateral. In general, the prognosis is guarded and in some cases rather poor.

What causes the temporal lobe's special proneness to epileptic seizures? The limbic structures (amygdala and hippocampus) are highly epileptogenic (low threshold areas), either generating epileptic activity or amplifying the epileptic activity originating from neocortical portions. Furthermore, the hippocampus is very vulnerable to ischemic or hypoxic damage because of its rather parsimonious blood supply.

Cortical Regions Other Than the Temporal Lobe

Frontal lobe epilepsy is much less common than temporal lobe epilepsy. Its ictal manifestations depend a great deal on the location of the epileptogenic zone within the frontal lobe. Many frontal lobe attacks lead to immediate generalization with grand mal. Frequently, there is first adversion of head and eyes to the opposite side; this may or may not be followed by a grand mal. Adversive seizures are associated with loss of consciousness if the focus lies in the intermediate frontal region. Tonic elevation of the contralateral arm and adversion of head and eyes to the opposite side are typical in seizures arising from the supplementary motor cortex (superior frontal region, vicinity of the interhemispheric fissure). There are also attacks imitating petit mal absences (even with 3/s spike-wave complexes) and sudden changes of thought processes with "forced thinking."

The EEG shows a wide variety of patterns in frontal lobe epilepsy. Neurological and mental changes depend on the extension and region of the underlying process. There may be "frontal lobish" behavior with lack of foresight and initiative, shallow euphoria, or facetiousness ("Witzelsucht").

Tumors and trauma are the most common etiologies. Frontal lobe epilepsies are most often found in early adulthood. The prognosis is guarded. Anticonvulsive therapy or partial frontal lobectomies may or may not be effective. Frontal lobe epilepsy fairly often causes status epilepticus.

Epilepsy of the motor cortex is about as common as frontal lobe epilepsy. Focal motor seizures (sometimes proceeding to a grand mal) are the classic ictal symptomatology. The EEG findings are disappointing at times. Neurologic deficits with contralateral monoparesis or hemiparesis (monoplegia or hemiplegia) are common. From the etiologic viewpoint, gross pathology is quite often present. Tumors (especially parasagittal meningioma), brain abscess, granulomas, arteriovenous malformation, chronic subdural hematoma, and acute CNS infections are notorious causes of recurrent focal motor seizures. Focal motor status may evolve in such cases (epilepsia partialis continua).

Occipital lobe epilepsy is less common than frontal and motor cortex epilepsies and is more likely to occur in acute conditions such as encephalitis rather than in chronic conditions. The ictal manifestations are either visual (elementary visual hallucinations) or motor with oculoclonic attacks [also called "epileptic nystagmus" (66, 67)]. The clinical and EEG features of "benign occipital lobe epilepsy" have been recently described by Gastaut (68).

Parietal lobe epilepsy is the least common cortical epileptic seizure disorder, encompassing a variety of somatosensory and visual phenomena.

Epilepsies Arising from Deep CNS Structures

The basal ganglia and the thalamus are most unlikely seats of epileptogenic foci. The concept of a "centrencephalic epilepsy" (58) with its seat in thalamic regions had to be abandoned. There is also no convincing evidence of a hypothalamic epilepsy.

Deep structures may fire in an epileptic manner but do not represent primary foci with secondary propagations. In trigeminal neuralgia (tic douloureux) there is good reason to presume "epileptic" firing of trigeminal nuclei (hence, the good response to certain anticonvulsants), but it would be unrealistic to term these attacks of excruciating pain "epileptic" since the element of epileptic spread is completely absent. Even the spinal cord is capable of producing epileptic phenomena, expressed as "segmental myoclonus."

UNUSUAL TRIGGER MECHANISMS OF EPILEPTIC SEIZURES

Visually Induced Epilepsies

Epileptic seizures induced by flickering light may be caused by strobe flashes used as an activation in the EEG laboratory or under natural conditions such as sunlight falling through moving foliage. Grand mal seizures and myoclonus are most common, though petit mal absences may also be triggered. More information is found in the work of Newmark and Penry (69). Patients with "natural" visual seizure precipitation do not necessarily show massive photoconvulsive responses in the EEG laboratory.

Most patients with flicker sensitivity have primary generalized epilepsy. Flicker sensitivity may also occur in other epilepsies with mental retardation; some of these patients apparently derive pleasure (even sexual pleasure) from self-induced attacks, e.g., with hand waving (70).

Paroxysmal responses may be elicited by eye closure (71). Television-induced seizures (usually grand mal) have become progressively rare with improved television sets. Visual exploration may lead to seizures (e.g., myoclonus elicited by looking at a colored scarf). A rare form of seizure induction by the viewing of geometric patterns has been described (72). Vertical black-and-white stripes are the most potent precipitating stimulus.

Reading Epilepsy

The precipitation of epileptic seizures by reading is very rare, first reported by Bickford (73). The mechanism is poorly understood. Hypermotility of the jaw and "jaw clicking" often precede the first paroxysmal EEG discharges. The attacks consist of widespread clonic and tonic movements that tend to progress to a grand mal. This seizure induction was thought to represent a form of "communication-evoked epilepsy" or "language epilepsy" (74).

Other Rare Mechanisms

Language-induced epilepsy, a rare type of precipitation, was first described by Geschwind and Sherwin (75).

Decision making-induced epilepsy is a most unusual type. It encompasses arithmetic-induced seizures and seizures caused by playing chess.

Musicogenic epilepsy was first described by Critchley (76). While myoclonus and/or grand mal is usually precipitated by the above-mentioned mechanisms, psychomotor attacks with bilateral anterior temporal spikes in the EEG are the most common in musicogenic epilepsy. Music of all styles has proved to be potentially epileptogenic in these cases. The attacks are not consistently reproducible.

Eating (77), movement-induced (78), and tapping (79) epilepsies have been described. Movement-induced epilepsy is also found in paroxysmal choreoathetosis. Widespread myoclonus is noted during examination of the tendon reflexes in tapping epilepsy.

Pure auditory precipitation of seizures (repetitive clicks, etc.) is common in certain strains of rodents. In humans auditory seizure induction must be associated with startle. Startle-induced epilepsies are found in infants with Tay-Sachs disease and also in adolescents and adults with residual hemiparetic cerebral palsy.

With the exception of flicker sensitivity and seizures induced by eye closure, all of the previously mentioned mechanisms of seizure induction are very rare. Ingenious, custom-tailored methods of seizure prevention by means of deconditioning methods have been designed (74), but anticonvulsive medication remains the basic treatment.

STATUS EPILEPTICUS

Status epilepticus denotes an epileptic seizure that is so prolonged or so frequently repeated as to create a fixed or lasting epileptic condition. A patient is considered to be in status epilepticus when a seizure state has persisted for 30 min to 1 h.

There are convulsive and nonconvulsive forms of status epilepticus. The convulsive forms comprise grand mal status, tonic status, myoclonus status, adversive status, hemiconvulsive status, and hemiclonic status. The nonconvulsive forms consist of petit mal absence status and psychomotor status. Whereas the former may progress to dangerous and life-threatening conditions, the latter are of particular interest for the psychiatrist because they present as abrupt behavioral changes.

Status Epilepticus Grand Mal (Tonic-Clonic Status)

A grand mal status must be distinguished from simple clusters of seizures. A true status grand mal is a very serious condition; until recently, its mortality was very high (up to 50 percent). In this condition the seizures repeat themselves in rapid succession (intervals of a few minutes only) while the patient remains in coma between the attacks. Central hyperthermia is common, often in association with blood leukocytosis and albuminuria. The dangers and pathophysiologic problems in status epilepticus have been discussed elsewhere (26).

A grand mal status is more common in focal (partial) forms of seizure disorder than in primary generalized epilepsy. Frontal lobe epilepsy shows a special propensity toward evolution into grand mal status. Brain tumor, craniocerebral trauma, and cerebral arteriosclerosis are the most common causes of this serious event. Grand mal status was noted in up to 50 percent of patients with no previous history of epileptic seizure disorder.

Other Convulsive Forms Of Status Epilepticus

Tonic status occurs almost exclusively in children and adolescents with Lennox-Gastaut syndrome. Myoclonic status is rare; this condition must be distinguished from progressive myoclonus epilepsy (Lafora-Unverricht) and dyssynergia cerebellaris myoclonica (Ramsay Hunt). Prolonged myoclonus in profound coma is rather common in acute cerebral anoxia following cardiorespiratory arrest and resuscitation. Hemiconvulsive and hemiclonic status usually occur in childhood; adversive status is more common among the elderly.

Focal motor status is also known as epilepsia partialis continua or Koshevnikoff's syndrome. In such cases localized muscle twitching may persist for weeks, months, or years. The most prolonged and stubbornly persistent forms are caused by the Siberian spring-summer encephalitis. The focal motor status represents a post-encephalitic sequela in these cases. Further information can be found in the study of Thomas et al. (80).

Petit Mal Absence Status

The term "petit mal absence status" (81) refers to a series of petit mal absences occurring in very rapid succession or, more often, a prolonged state of impaired consciousness with sluggish mentation or stuporous behavior (characterized by petit mal-like EEG activity, i.e., generalized 3–4/s spike-wave discharges with minor or major modifications). This latter condition is of considerable interest since it may be masked as a psychiatric episode with predominant stuporous behavior. Problems of differential diagnosis are demonstrated in Table 4.

The petit mal absence is not always a nonconvulsive form of status. Myoclonic twitching of extremities or orofacial muscles may be a prominent feature; a grand mal attack may evolve during the episode.

The duration of a petit mal absence status usually ranges from

TABLE 4. *Prolonged episodes of confusion or stupor*

Epileptic ictal episodes
Petit mal absence status
In a patient with a history of primary generalized eilepsy
In a patient with no previous history
In a patient with a history of focal seizures
In a patient with a frontal lobe focus (unilateral)
Psychomotor status
Epileptic nonictal episodes
Postconvulsive confusion or delirium after grand mal
Epileptic psychosis, subacute
Chronic psychosis (mostly schizophreniform) in epileptics, mostly in temporal lobe epilepsy
Nonepileptic episodes
Hypoglycemic episodes
Amnestic episodes (transient global amnesia)
Psychogenic episodes (hysterical stupor, dissociative states)

From Niedermeyer (26), reprinted with permission.

6 to 48 h, but there are occasionally much shorter episodes of 30 min or so. The intravenous administration of benzodiazepines (diazepam, clonazepam) usually terminates the status almost immediately. A much less responsive form of petit mal absence status may occur in children with Lennox-Gastaut syndrome.

Petit mal absence status falls into the category of primary generalized epilepsy This condition is usually most active between the ages of 4 and 20 years. Petit mal absence status, however, seems to occupy an exceptional position within the frame of primary generalized epilepsy. Onset in adulthood and even in old age is not uncommon, even in septuagenarians and octogenarians without a good history of earlier epileptic manifestations. This is an enigmatic feature of petit mal absence status.

In problems of differential diagnosis (see Table 4) the EEG will provide an answer, with the demonstration of massive and almost constant generalized paroxysmal activity that does not have to be of the spike-wave type; bursts of polyspikes or almost spikefree, rhythmic 3–4/s activity of very high voltage may be found instead. The prompt response to intravenous benzodiazepines is also an important differential diagnostic criterion.

Petit mal absence status is a rare but not extremely rare condition. In a major medical institution, one can expect one case per year.

Psychomotor (Complex Partial) Status

A status of psychomotor (complex partial) automatism is extremely rare and much less common than a petit mal absence status. This status is discontinuous and consists of a succession of automatisms and postictal confusional states, but the possibility of a continuous psychomotor status cannot be ruled out with absolute certainty.

From the clinical-behavioral viewpoint, there is a wide variety of clinical pictures ranging from distinct automatisms to twilight states with or without psychotic appearance (82).

CLINICAL EVALUATION OF THE EPILEPTIC PATIENT

In the case of a presumed seizure disorder, the following questions ought to be answered: (a) Are the reported episodes epileptic or nonepileptic in character? (b) If epileptic: What type of seizure? Is there any evidence of an age-determined epileptic condition? Is there any evidence of an epileptogenic focus? What is the cause (underlying pathology) of the attacks? Is there any evidence of a special triggering mechanism?

Table 5 schematically demonstrates the diagnostic process. In spite of the availability of highly modernized diagnostic equipment, history taking is of paramount importance. This must be followed by a thorough general physical and neurological examination. Neuropsychological studies may be very helpful. A variety of blood tests will be necessary, selected according to the general diagnostic impression of the physician.

The EEG is uniquely contributory in the differential diagnosis (as a function-oriented test). Without adequate training, however, an electroencephalographer could do more harm than good. The interpretation of interictal paroxysmal discharges must be judicious; spikes or spike-wave discharges may have a different meaning in various clinical contexts. Even negative (normal) EEG findings may be diagnostically very informative, e.g., the usual normal interval EEG findings in patients with alcohol withdrawal seizures.

As previously mentioned (with regard to temporal lobe epilepsy), some cases may be most puzzling by the lack of convincing EEG abnormalities. The EEG provides a window for data collection within a limited period of time (30–60 min, sometimes longer) under rather favorable laboratory conditions with the availability

TABLE 5. *Diagnostic evaluation of the adult epileptic*

Clarify problem:

Acute versus chronic epileptic seizure disorder
Acute cases: emergency room, on the ward
  Cause of acute condition:
    Metabolic, cerebrovascular disease, CNS infection, CNS trauma, CNS poisoning, CNS anoxia after cardiopulmonary arrest? Status epilepticus in a chronic seizure disorder? Acute exacerbation of brain tumor or neglected subdural hematoma?

After elimination of acute cases:
  One recent seizure, first in life, or chronically recurrent seizures, thus far untreated or treated without success.

Step 1: Rule out chronic alcoholism.
  If patient is a chronic alcoholic, differentiate between:
    A chronic epileptic who happened to become an alcoholic (mostly abnormal EEG)
    Seizure types: grand mal, psychomotor,or focal

    A chronic alcoholic with epileptic seizures in alcohol withdrawal (EEG mostly within normal limits of variability)
    Seizure type: grand mal only

  Send patients with withdrawal seizures into special treatment program for alcoholics; do not start anticonvulsive treatment (seizure disorder being "self-inflicted").

Step 2: Carefully establish type of seizure. At this point make every effort to eliminate possibility of a nonepileptic seizure type.
  Consider:
    Hypoglycemic (confusional states with sweating, tremor, also grand mal)

    Syncope (special problem: convulsive syncope)

    Drop attack syncope (older persons with vertebrobasilar artery insufficiency)

    Attacks related to sleep disorder

    Migrainous episodes

    Hyperventilation syndrome

    Psychogenic attacks

    Malingered attacks

TABLE 5. *(Continued)*

Step 3: You are confident that nonepileptic seizures can be eliminated—try to define the type of seizures.

Distinction between petit mal absence and psychomotor (complex partial) seizures may be difficult.

Consider age:

Petit mal absences rarely start in adulthood.

Psychomotor seizures are much more common, especially in adulthood.

Tongue biting is highly indicative of grand mal. In case of grand mal, is there any aura?

Step 4: Try to determine under which circumstances (or in which setting) the seizures occur.

Irrespective of time of the day—

In most forms of seizures due to cerebral pathology, especially in temporal and frontal lobe epilepsy

Mainly in sleep—

Not very helpful in adults—once more, try to rule out sleep disorders such as nocturnal terror

Mainly in the morning—

And especially after a night of poor sleep: myoclonic jerking and/or grand mal—highly indicative of primary generalized epilepsy

Mainly or exclusively with flickering light—

Light falling through moving foliage, etc.—indicative of photosensitivity occurring chiefly in primary generalized epilepsy

While closing eyes, watching television, reading, listening to music, etc.—think about rare triggering factors (see text)

Step 5: Integrate your seizure-related diagnostic impressions into the general diagnostic impression—Think about ongoing disease as a possible cause.

Any smoldering illness?

[Think about vasculitis due to subacute lupus erythematosus; in older persons, think about signs of cerebrovascular disorder (arteriosclerosis, enhanced by diabetes mellitus, hypertension, massive tobacco consumption).]

Prominent headache?

What type? Any relationship to migraine?

Chronic dull headache—any signs of intracranial hypertension? (brain tumor, subdural hematoma)

Any signs of chronic CNS infection?

(syphilis, sarcoid, fungi, certain viral infections, etc.)

TABLE 5. *(Continued)*

Any signs of chronic CNS poisoning? (heavy metals, etc.)

Any signs of a chronic degenerative-metabolic process such as essential myoclonus epilepsy (Lafora-Unverricht disease with mycolonus, ataxia, dementia, grand mal)? Think of other degenerative diseases.

Is there marked mental retardation since infancy?
Again think about degenerative-metabolic diseases; also about tuberous sclerosis.

Is there any evidence of dementia of late onset?
Think about brain tumor, chronic CNS infection, other degenerative CNS diseases.

Step 6: Look for residual brain disease or dysfunction.
A search for ongoing CNS disease has been thus far fruitless. (Remember: a brain tumor cannot be ruled out even in an alert adult with recent seizure onset.) Search for diagnostic clues from the history:

Fetal life (was mother's pregnancy uneventful?)

Birth (any asphyxia, trauma, or other suggestions of perinatal brain damage?)

CNS infection in infancy, childhood, adolescence?

Any history of process that required CNS surgery?
(for arteriovenous malformation, intracranial aneurysm, abscess, tumor, subdural or epidural hematoma, etc.).

Any significant intracranial trauma?
Remember: Posttraumatic epilepsy usually arises from cerebral lacerations.

The latency of the seizure onset usually lies between 3 and 24 months but may be longer.

Significant CNS trauma does not necessarily have to imply loss of consciousness.

With all this information collected, perform a general physical and neurological examination.

The general physical examination must not be lackadaisical or limited to vital signs. Search for degenerative stigmata (certain malformations) and vascular problems (neck vessels, heart, blood pressure).

Do not forget about thyroid function—Dysthyroid conditions may promote epileptic seizures if there is some predisposition.

Look for possible neurocutaneous syndrome (phacomatoses).

A complete neurological evaluation is a must although there will be normal findings in most of your patients.

TABLE 5. *(Continued)*

Search for remainders of cerebral palsy or suggestions of ongoing CNS disease. In patients with temporal lobe epilepsy: look for upper motor type seventh nerve weakness (contralateral to focus) and a positive hyperextensibility test.

In a patient who is already under anticonvulsive treatment, check carefully for signs of early or advanced CNS toxicity or changes outside the CNS (see text).

You may carry out a hyperventilation test at this point, but it is preferable to have this done under EEG control.

With all this information from history and physical examination, you will need laboratory data.

Blood chemistry

Urinalysis and glucose tolerance test if diabetes and/or hypoglycemia may play a role.

Blood work to rule out syphilis, other infections, subacute lupus, thyroid dysfunction.

Skull X-ray

(Still helpful in spite of CT scan availability—especially to demonstrate early meningiomatous bone change or intra- and parasellar problems.)

EEG

An absolute must, although its value depends a lot on the experience and caliber of the electroencephalographer. Resting-walking record, hyperventilation, intermittent photic stimulation, and sleep (unsedated or sedated) are part of a satisfactory evaluation.

Added nasopharyngeal leads provide very limited extra diagnostic information.

In certain focal (partial) forms, the search may be difficult and two or three tracings may be needed.

Most abnormalities are detectable in the interictal interval. Sometimes it is worthwhile to record a seizure (cautious reduction of medication may be helpful).

Sleep-deprived EEGs may or may not be informative.

CT scan

Virtually a must in every case unless there is overwhelming evidence of an old residual type of seizure disorder.

The informative value of CT scan in cases with structural lesions cannot be overrated. Do not expect CT scan clarification in primary generalized epilepsy, and expect 50 percent normal findings in Lennox-Gastaut syndrome and also in may cases of temporal lobe and other focal epilepsies.

TABLE 5. *(Continued)*

After a negative CT scan with high resolution and enhancement, you may lay to rest most of your worries about underlying tumor, abscess, subdural hematoma, arteriovenous malformation, and massive residual CNS impairment.
Nevertheless, small arteriovenous malformations cannot be ruled out without arteriography.
With unsatisfactory EEG findings after several repeat tests, advanced monitoring of EEG may be needed.
Cassette recording, 24-h EEG
EEG—biotelemetry
To observe possibly ictal behavior and concomitant EEG changes (the latter being considerably reduced—mostly four channels).

From Niedermeyer (26), reprinted with permission.

of a large number of channels. A more prolonged type of EEG monitoring can be done in special cases with special monitoring equipment with a limited number of channels. This can be combined with visual observation of the patient's behavior. In EEG biotelemetry with video monitoring, the patient is not wired to the apparatus. EEG long-term cassette monitoring is carried out in the freely moving patient for $\geq$12 h. The visual analysis of these data, however, is very laborious and time consuming. Polysomnography in a sleep laboratory can provide further information in the case of nocturnal seizures.

The use of special electrodes (nasopharyngeal, sphenoidal) was mentioned before (see Temporal Lobe Epilepsy). Depth EEG with neurosurgically implanted electrodes is reserved for potential candidates for seizure surgery.

Radiologic studies may be extremely important. Among the structure-oriented tests, the CT scan is most informative since it is capable of providing an elegant demonstration of structural brain lesions. In >50 percent of epileptic patients, a normal CT scan can be expected.

Arteriography is seldom needed these days, but the introduction of computer-assisted digital subtraction methods with the intravenous injection of the contrast has markedly reduced its risks.

Radionuclear brain scans are often very helpful. The use of positron emission computed tomography shows changes of local cerebral glucose utilization. In epileptic patients both hypo- and hypermetabolic zones have been demonstrated (83, 84). This test provides fascinating images of cerebral metabolic activity, but its true significance for epileptologic diagnosis is still unclear.

The evaluation of the patient with seizures must be guided by clinical acumen and common sense. Indiscriminate use of large numbers of expensive tests usually leads nowhere. There is no substitute for clinical experience and logical thinking. These ingredients are crucial in the diagnosis and differential diagnosis of epileptic conditions.

DIFFERENTIAL DIAGNOSIS

The differential diagnosis of the epilepsies ought to be broken down into: differentiation of epileptic seizures from nonepileptic attacks of organic origin; differentiation of epileptic seizures from nonepileptic attacks of psychogenic (hysterical) and feigned (malingering) characters.

Migrainous States and Phenomena

The relationship between epilepsy and migraine has been the topic of numerous discussions. There is now general consensus that this relationship is more distant than had been assumed in the past. Epileptic and migrainous phenomena are basically different, but there are occasional areas of overlap. Under certain unusual conditions, a massive attack of migraine may show epileptic features in the EEG as well as clinically; even a grand mal attack may occur.

This is particularly true for the special form of basilar artery migraine (85). This variant is most common in young females between 15 and 30 years of age. The classic symptoms of migraine with scintillation (teichopsia) followed by unilateral headache, nausea, vomiting, and photophobia are sometimes overshadowed by syncope (without or with convulsing movements) and full-blown grand mal. In some cases grand mal attacks are directly preceded by a very short visual aura (flashes). In these patients the interictal EEG may be stubbornly normal, awake and asleep, with repeated studies. Other patients may show occipital spiking or excessive slowing.

The failure of anticonvulsive therapy supports the diagnosis. These patients benefit from antimigrainous medication such as propranolol and particularly from ergoloid mesylate (Hydergine), preferably in combination with anticonvulsive drugs.

Syncope

A syncopal or fainting attack is caused by transient generalized cerebral ischemia due to acute circulatory insufficiency. There are various causes of syncopal attacks. Most common are those caused by peripheral circulatory inadequacy such as vasodepressor (vasovagal) syncope and postural hypotension (the Shy-Drager syndrome representing a special form). Cardiac disorders are another important causative factor; most of these attacks are arrhythmia-induced (especially the Stokes-Adams syndrome). Respiratory and pulmonary disorders may also give rise to syncope: Valsalva's phenomenon, laryngeal syncope, cough (tussive) syncope, hyperventilation, breath holding, etc. Psychogenic causes will be discussed below.

In very abrupt cerebral circulatory insufficiency, the resulting syncope may be associated with tonic or clonic convulsive phenomena (convulsive syncope). An orderly sequence of a tonic and clonic stage (as in grand mal) does not occur, and the convulsive manifestations last for only a few seconds. These intervening epileptic mechanisms are secondary and must not be used as evidence of an underlying epileptic seizure disorder.

A special form of syncope occurs in male patients during nocturnal urination (micturition syncope). Sudden drop attacks of syncopal character are found in older adults, particularly females, with vertebrobasilar artery insufficiency.

The hyperventilation syndrome is closely related to free-floating anxieties, reinforcing an abnormal breathing pattern.

Sudden Changes in Blood Chemistry

Hypoglycemia leads to profuse perspiration, imperative hunger, tremulousness, irritability, mental fatigue, muscular weakness, and occasionally headache, nausea, and vomiting. These attacks may proceed to confusion, impairment of consciousness, or even coma. In deep coma, myoclonus is very common. Grand mal seizures may be superimposed on hypoglycemic comatose or precomatose states. Hyperinsulinism may be due to a dysfunction or tumor of the pancreatic islet cells.

Hypocalcemia leads to tetanic manifestations (carpopedal spasms) that are due to peripheral mechanisms. True epileptic seizures (grand mal) may also materialize.

Episodic Cerebrovascular Changes

Transient ischemic attacks and cerebrovascular accidents must be separated from epileptic manifestations. In cerebrovascular accidents, epileptic seizures may precede, accompany, or follow the stroke.

Transient global amnesia is essentially of a nonepileptic nature.

It is based on cerebrovascular problems, interfering with memory mechanisms.

Motor Disorders (Basal Ganglia Diseases)

The motor disturbances found in basal ganglia diseases are nonepileptic. Their chronic character will hardly raise problems of differential diagnosis. In episodic disturbances, however, such problems could arise. Paroxysmal choreoathetosis (86) is characterized by paroxysms of tonic, clonic, choreic,and athetoid motions, sometimes triggered by certain active or passive movements. The EEG is usually normal. The differentiation from epileptic seizures is difficult. Some patients may even have true epileptic seizures, in addition to a motor disorder.

Sleep Disorders

The narcolepsy-cataplexy-sleep paralysis complex has a nonepileptic character. In cases of nocturnal terror or sleep apnea, the differential diagnosis should be clarified by a nocturnal polygraphic sleep study in a special sleep laboratory.

Psychogenic Seizures (Hysterical Seizures, Pseudoseizures)

The differentiation between epileptic, organic nonepileptic, and psychogenic events is a rather difficult task for the neurologist. Even if psychogenic elements are very obvious, the neurologist may be tempted to remain uncommitted. A wrong diagnosis of hysteria or psychogenic seizures in an ultimately organic case may be a hard blow to the neurologist's ego and prestige.

EEG findings must be interpreted with great caution. In dramatic psychogenic manifestations, the EEG is often obscured by movement artefacts. Normal stretches between storms of movements (with alpha rhythm as a sign of normal vigilance) are certainly very helpful and strongly support psychogenesis. Combined video and EEG documentation are particularly instructive. The EEG diagnosis in psychogenic stupor, i.e., in patients who lie calmly in a poorly defined state of consciousness, is much easier because the EEG clearly demonstrates the absence of ictal activity. The absence of postictal changes in the EEG also lends support to a psychic origin of the attack.

Can epileptic seizures occur in association with a completely normal EEG during the ictal phase? The answer is affirmative. Ictal epileptic manifestations may remain limited to deep structures, especially limbic regions, while the scalp EEG remains normal. Such cases, however, are very rare. Animal experiments have provided a good model with the local application of kainic acid, resulting in isolated ictal spiking in the amygdala (87).

Interictal EEG records also must be interpreted with great caution. In patients with indubitable psychogenic seizures, there may be mild or moderate paroxysmal EEG abnormalities such as minor temporal sharp activity or flicker sensitivity.

Thus, clinical observation of the patient still occupies an important place in the differential diagnosis. Pendular head movements strongly favor a psychogenic origin. The patient's complexion changes profoundly in a grand mal (ashen or cyanotic discoloration caused by temporary apnea) and little in a psychogenic attack. Of course, arching and rhythmic pelvic movements strongly indicate psychogenesis.

Dissociative states based on neurotic mechanisms must be carefully distinguished from epileptic states (especially petit mal absence status) and other organic conditions. The EEG provides invaluable assistance in such cases.

The occurrence of epileptic and psychogenic seizures in the same patient must be considered. This combination is not rare: Rabe (88) reported 41 observations. In some epileptics large dosages of anticonvulsants leading to CNS toxicity may facilitate psychogenic seizures (89). These patients may become unable to cope with ordinary stress and fall into archaic patterns of uncontrolled behavior (90).

Feigned Seizures (Malingering)

Feigned seizures are consciously intended and usually consist of a more or less skilled imitation of whatever the "patient" considers to be a seizure. Grand mal attacks are most commonly imitated, and even tongue bites may be found in experienced malingerers.

The ictal EEG shows massive movement artefact during the storm of motions, but there is usually good evidence of a perfectly normal stretch with alpha rhythm just before the movements start. There is also a complete lack of postictal changes.

EPILOGUE

Epileptic phenomena arise from the brain as the result of numerous diseases and dysfunctions. A disease named "epilepsy" does not exist; there are copious etiologies and various epileptic conditions. Many patients with epileptic seizures do not show any signs of intellectual impairment, and their mental capacities may reach to the lofty heights of a genius. Accompanying mental retardation or decline is attributable in most cases to the underlying brain disease rather than to seizures. Such considerations cast grave doubts on the "disease character" of epilepsy.

This sets the epilepsy patient material apart from other neurologic patient populations. Let us try to visualize the patients in the waiting room of a special clinic for a disease like multiple sclerosis or myasthenia gravis at a major medical center. The patients afflicted with such a neurologic disease resemble brothers and sisters suffering from the same disorder, some of them at an earlier, others at a more advanced stage. What is the common denominator in a group of epileptic patients in the waiting room of a seizure clinic? Fear of seizures? Some of them may be mentally too blunted and impaired to experience such fears, whereas others may be tormented by the thought of suddenly having a seizure. In other words, a very heterogeneous group of patients is found in a seizure clinic.

The neurophysiologic epileptogenic mechanisms at the neuronal level may be the same in each form of epileptic activity, but the underlying conditions are manifold. Thus, for a severely brain-damaged patient (e.g., residual state after massive cerebral palsy), the occurrence of seizures is just an extra burden on top of a serious neurologic and intellectual handicap. In others the severe character of an age-determined epileptic condition (e.g., Lennox-Gastaut syndrome) results in more or less pronounced mental decline. Some patients suffer from basically mild forms of epileptic seizure disorder (e.g., benign Rolandic epilepsy of childhood; primary generalized epilepsy of childhood, adolescence, or early adulthood); their intellectual capacity is likely to be unimpaired (unless iatrogenically depressed by overmedication), and seizure freedom may be achieved in a short time. Others have mixed or poorly defined forms of seizure disorder, each case requiring individual consideration. There is also the numerically strong group with temporal lobe epilepsy and its special problems of coexisting personality change and frank psychotic features.

These differences are obvious reasons to discourage questions such as "What is the prognosis of epilepsy?" Instead, seizure types, etiologies, and certain specific epileptic conditions must be differentiated; and then, the prognostic criteria for each subgroup can be determined. This approach requires clinical acumen and EEG expertise but will prove to be most rewarding for both patient and physician. Eventually, it will shed more light on the complexities of clinical epileptology.

REFERENCES

1. Jackson JH: Clinical remarks on the occasional occurrence of subjective sensations of smell in patients who are liable to epileptiform seizures or who have symptoms of mental derangement and in others. *Lancet* 1:659–660, 1866
2. Jackson JH, Beevor CE: Case of tumour of the right temporal-sphenoidal lobe bearing on the localization of the sense of smell and on the interpretation of a particular variety of epilepsy. *Brain* 12:346–347, 1889
3. Jackson JH, Stewart P: Epileptic attacks with a warning of a crude sensation of smell and with the intellectual aura (dreamy state) in a patient who had symptoms pointing to gross organic disease of the right temporo-sphenoidal lobe. *Brain* 22:543–549, 1899
4. Kraepelin E: *Einführung in die Psychiatrische Klinik*. 4th edition. Leipzig, Barth, 1921
5. Lange J: *Lehrbuch der Psychiatrie*. Leipzig, Thieme, 1936
6. Bumke O: *Lehrbuch der Geisteskrankheiten*. 2nd edition. Munich, Bergmann, 1942
7. Lewandowsky M (ed): *Handbuch der Neurologie*. 5 vols. Berlin, Springer, 1910–1914
8. Oppenheim H (ed): *Lehrbuch der Nervenkrankheiten*. 2 vols. Berlin, Karger, 1923
9. Ewald G: *Lehrbuch der Neurologie und Psychiatrie*. Berlin, Urban & Schwarzenberg, 1948
10. Berger H: Über das Elektroenzephalogramm des Menschen. *Arch Psychiatr Nervenkr* 87:527–570, 1929
11. Gibbs FA, Davis H, Lennox WG: The electroencephalogram in epilepsy and in conditions of impaired consciousness. *Arch Neurol Psychiatry (Chicago)* 34:1133–1148, 1935
12. Gibbs FA, Lennox WG, Gibbs EL: The electroencephalogram in diagnosis and in localization of epileptic seizures. *Arch Neurol Psychiatry (Chicago)* 36:1225–1235, 1936
13. Ward AA Jr: The epileptic neuron. *Epilepsia* 2:70–80, 1961
14. Westerum LE, White LE Jr, Ward AA Jr: Morphology of the experimental epileptic focus. *J Neurosurg* 21:1033–1046, 1964
15. Schmidt RP, Wilder BJ: *Epilepsy*. Philadelphia, FA Davis, 1968
16. Matsumoto H, Ajmone Marsan C: Cortical cellular phenomena in experimental epilepsy. Ictal manifestations. *Exp Neurol* 9:305–326, 1964
17. Schwartzkroin PA, Prince DA: Penicillin-induced epileptiform activity in the hippocampal in vitro preparations. *Ann Neurol* 1:463–469, 1977

18. Schwartzkroin PA, Wyler AR: Mechanisms underlying epileptiform burst discharges. *Ann Neurol* 7:95–107, 1980

19. Schwartzkroin PA: Ionic and synaptic determinants of burst generation, in *Epilepsy. A Window to Brain Mechanisms.* Edited by Lockard JS, Ward AA Jr. New York, Raven Press 1980, pp 83–95

20. Wyler AR, Ward AA Jr: Epileptic neurons, in *Epilepsy. A Window to Brain Mechanisms.* Edited by Lockard JS, Ward AA Jr. New York, Raven Press, 1980, pp 51–68

21. Calvin WH: Normal repetitive firing and its pathophysiology, in *Epilepsy. A Window to Brain Mechanisms.* Edited by Lockard JS, Ward AA Jr. New York, Raven Press, 1980, pp 97–121

22. Speckman E-J, Caspers H: Cortical field potentials in relation to neuronal activities in seizure conditions, in *Origin of Cerebral Field Potentials.* Edited by Speckman E-J, Caspers H. Stuttgart, Thieme, 1979, pp 205–213

23. Elger CE, Speckman E-J: Focal interictal epileptiform discharges (FIED) in the epicortical EEG and their relations to spinal field potentials in the rat. *Electroencephalogr Clin Neurophysiol* 48:447–460, 1980

24. Eccles JC: *The Inhibitory Pathways of the Central Nervous System.* Springfield, Charles C Thomas, 1966

25. Gastaut H, Broughton R: *Epileptic Seizures.* Springfield, Charles C Thomas, 1972

26. Niedermeyer E: *Epilepsy Guide. Diagnosis and Treatment of Epileptic Seizure Disorders.* Baltimore, Urban & Schwarzenberg, 1983

27. Dreifuss F: Commission on Classification and Terminology of the International League Against Epilepsy, 1981. Proposal for revised clinical and electroencephalographic classification of epileptic seizures. *Epilepsia* 22:489–501, 1981

28. Gastaut H: Clinical and electroencephalographic classification of epileptic seizures. *Epilepsia* 11:102–113, 1970

29. Macrae D: Isolated fear: a temporal lobe aura. *Neurology (Minneap)* 4:479–505, 1954

30. Williams D: The structure of emotions reflected in epileptic experiences. *Brain* 79:29–67, 1956

31. Daly DD: Ictal clinical manifestations of complex partial seizures, in *Complex Partial Seizures and Their Treatment.* Edited by Penry JK, Daly DD. New York, Raven Press, 1975, pp 57–82

32. Strauss E, Risser A, Jones MW: Fear responses in patients with epilepsy. *Arch Neurol* 39:626–630, 1982

33. Halgren E, Walter RD, Cherlow DG, et al: Mental phenomena evoked by electrical stimulation of the human hippocampal formation and amygdala. *Brain* 101:83–117, 1978

34. Gloor P, Olivier A, Quesney LF, et al: The role of the limbic system in experiential phenomena of temporal lobe epilepsy. *Ann Neurol* 12:129–144, 1982

35. Stevens JR: Interictal clinical manifestations of complex partial seizures, in *Complex Partial Seizures and Their Treatment.* Edited by Penry JK, Daly DD. New York, Raven Press, 1975, pp 85–107

36. Rodin EA: Psychomotor epilepsy and aggressive behavior. *Arch Gen Psychiatry* 28:210–213, 1973

37. Rodin EA: Aggression and epilepsy, in *Pseudoseizures.* Edited by Riley TL, Roy A. Baltimore, Williams & Wilkins, 1982, pp 185–212

38. Riley TL, Niedermeyer E: Rage attacks and episodic violent behavior: electroencephalographic findings and general considerations. *Clin Electroencephalogr* 9:131–139, 1978

39. Gibbs EL, Fuster B, Gibbs FA: Peculiar low temporal localization of sleep induced seizure discharges of psychomotor epilepsy. *Arch Neurol Psychiatry (Chicago)* 60:95–97, 1948

40. Klass DW: Electroencephalographic mechanisms of complex partial seizures, in *Complex Partial Seizures and Their Treatment.* Edited by Penry JK, Daly DD. New York, Raven Press, 1975, pp 113–140

41. Perlstein MA, Gibbs FA: Clinical significance of electroencephalography in cases of cerebral paralysis. *Arch Neurol Psychiatry (Chicago)* 62:682–685, 1949

42. Victor M, Brausch J: The role of abstinence in the genesis of alcohol epilepsy. *Epilepsia* 8:1–20, 1967

43. Hess R: Die epileptogenen Hirntumoren, in *Epilepsy. Recent Views on Theory, Diagnosis and Therapy of Epilepsy.* Edited by Niedermeyer E. Basel, Karger, 1970, pp 200–231

44. Barolin GS, Scherzer E, Schnaberth G: *Die zerebro-vaskulär bedingten Anfälle.* Bern, Huber, 1975

45. Locke J, Merrill JP, Tyler HR: Neurologic complications of acute uremia. *Arch Intern Med* 108:519–530, 1961

46. Glaser GH: Brain dysfunction in uremia, in *Brain Dysfunction in Metabolic Disorders.* Edited by Plum F. New York, Raven Press, 1974, pp 173–197

47. Lombroso CT: Neonatal electroencephalography, in *Electroencephalography.* Edited by Niedermeyer E, Lopes da Silva F. Baltimore, Urban & Shwarzenberg, 1982, pp 599–637

48. Gibbs, FA, Gibbs EL: *Atlas of Electroencephalography, Vol 2.* 2nd edition. Cambridge, Addison-Wesley, 1952

49. West WJ: On a peculiar form of infantile convulsion. *Lancet* 1:724, 1841

50. Lombroso CT: A prospective study of infantile spasms: clinical and therapeutic correlations. *Epilepsia* 24:135–158, 1983

51. Sorel L, Dusaucy-Bauloye A: A propos de 21 cas d'hypsarrhythmie de Gibbs, son traitement spectaculaire par l'ACTH. *Rev Neurol* 99:136–138, 1958

52. Riikonen R: Infantile spasms: Some new theoretical aspects. *Epilepsia* 24:159–168, 1983

53. Lennox-Buchtal MA: *Febrile convulsions. A Reappraisal.* Amsterdam, Elsevier, 1973

54. Gibbs FA, Gibbs EL, Lennox WG: The influence of the blood sugar level on the wave and spike formation in petit mal epilepsy. *Arch Neurol Psychiatry (Chicago)* 47:1111–1116, 1939

55. Lennox WG: *Epilepsy and Related Disorders.* Boston, Little, Brown, 1960

56. Gastaut H, Roger J, Soulayrol R, et al: Childhood epileptic encephalopathy with diffuse slow spike-waves (otherwise known as "petit mal variant") or Lennox syndrome. *Epilepsia* 7:139–179, 1966

57. Gastaut H, Gastaut JL, Goncalves E. Silva GE, et al: Relative frequency of different types of epilepsy: a study employing the classification by the International League Against Epilepsy. *Epilepsia* 16:457–461, 1975

58. Penfield W: Epileptic automatism and the centrencephalic integrating system. *Publ Assoc Res New Ment Dis* 30:513–528, 1952

59. Gloor P: Generalized cortico-reticular epilepsies. Some considerations on the pathophysiology of generalized-bilaterally synchronous spike and wave discharge. *Epilepsia* 9:249–263, 1968

60. Janz D: Aufwach-Epilepsien. *Arch Psychiatr Nervenk* 191:73–98, 1953

61. Niedermeyer E: *The Generalized Epilepsies.* Springfield, Charles C Thomas, 1972

62. Loiseau P, Beaussart M: The seizures of benign childhood epilepsy with Rolandic paroxysmal discharges. *Epilepsia* 14:381–389, 1973

63. Fritsch G, Hitzig E: Über die elektrische Erregbarkeit des Grosshirns. *Arch Anat Physiol* 37:300–332, 1870

64. Penfield W, Jasper HH: *Epilepsy and the Functional Anatomy of the Human Brain.* Boston, Little, Brown, 1954

65. Mathieson G: Pathology of temporal lobe foci, in *Complex Partial Seizures and Their Treatment.* Edited by Penry JK, Daly DD. New York, Raven Press, 1975, pp 163–181

66. Huott AD, Madison DS, Niedermeyer E: Occipital lobe epilepsy. A clinical and electroencephalographic study. *Eur Neurol* 9:133–156, 1974

67. Ludwig BI, Ajmone Marsan C: Clinical ictal patterns in epileptic patients with occipital electroencephalographic foci. *Neurology (Minneap)* 25:463–471, 1975

68. Gastaut H: A new type of epilepsy: benign partial epilepsy of childhood with occipital spike-waves. *Clin Electroencephalogr* 13:13–22, 1982

69. Newmark ME, Penry JK: *Photosensitivity and Epilepsy: A Review*. New York, Raven Press, 1979

70. Ehret R, Schneider E: Photogene Epilepsie mit suchtartiger Selbstauslösung kleiner Anfälle und wiederholten Sexualdelikten. *Arch Psychiatr Nervenkr* 202:75–94, 1961

71. Vignaendra V, Ghee LT, Lee TC, et al: Epileptic discharges triggered by blinking and eye closure. *Electroencephalogr Clin Neurophysiol* 40:491–498, 1976

72. Bickford RG, Daly DD, Keith H: Convulsion effects of light stimulation in children. *Am J Dis Child* 86:170, 1953

73. Bickford RG: Sensory precipitation of seizures. *J Mich Med Soc* 53:1018–1021, 1954

74. Forster FM: *Reflex Epilepsy, Behavioral Therapy and Conditional Reflexes*. Springfield, Charles C Thomas, 1977

75. Geschwind N, Sherwin I: Language-induced epilepsy. *Arch Neurol* 16:25–31, 1967

76. Critchley M: Musicogenic epilepsy. *Brain* 60:13–27, 1937

77. Binnie CD, Rowan AJ, Van Wieringen A: Eating epilepsy: report of 4 cases with review of the literature [abstract]. *Electroencephalogr Clin Neurophysiol* 53:47P, 1980

78. Burger LJ, Lopez RI, Elliott FA: Tonic seizures induced by movement. *Neurology (Minneap)* 22:656–659, 1972

79. Dawson GD: Investigations on a patient subject to myoclonic seizures after sensory stimulation. *J Neurol Neurosurg Psychiatry* 10:141–162, 1947

80. Thomas JE, Reagan TJ, Klass DW: Epilepsia partialis continua. A review of 32 cases. *Arch Neurol* 34;266–275, 1977

81. Lennox WG: The petit mal epilepsies; their treatment with Tridione. *JAMA* 129:1069–1074, 1945

82. Karbowski K: Status psychomotoricus. Klinische und elektroenzephalographische Aspekte, in *Status Psychomotoricus*. Edited by Karbowski K. Bern, Huber, 1980, pp 39–71

83. Kuhl DE, Engel JE Jr, Phelps ME, et al: Epileptic patterns of local cerebral metabolism and perfusion in humans determined by positron emission computed tomography of ^{18}FDG and ^{13}NH. *Ann Neurol* 8:348–360, 1980

84. Engel J Jr., Rausch R, Lieb JP, et al: Correlation of criteria used for localizing epileptic foci in patients considered for surgical treatment of epilepsy. *Ann Neurol* 9:215–224, 1981

85. Bickerstaff ER: Basilar artery migraines. *Lancet* 1:15–17, 1961

86. Mount LA, Reback S: Familial paroxysmal choreoathetosis. *Arch Neurol Psychiatry (Chicago)* 44:841–847, 1940

87. Menini C, Meldrum BS, Riche D, et al: Sustained limbic seizures induced by intra-amygdaloid kainic acid in the baboon: symptomatology and neuropathological consequences. *Ann Neurol* 8:501–509, 1980

88. Rabe F: *Die Kombination Hysterischer und Epileptischer Anfälle.* Berlin, Springer, 1970

89. Niedermeyer E, Blumer D, Hoscher E, et al: Classical hysterical seizures facilitated by anticonvulsant toxicity. *Psychiatr Clin (Basel)* 3:71–84, 1970

90. Krumholz A, Niedermeyer E: Psychogenic seizures: a clinical study with follow-up data. *Neurology (New York)* 33:498–502, 1983

4

Medical Treatment Of Epileptic Patients

Ernst Rodin, M.D.

The medical treatment of epileptic patients has changed considerably during the last decade. As a result of the widespread availability of anticonvulsant blood level determinations, drug regimens can be simplified, and patient compliance can be monitored. Under these circumstances, usually it is possible to avoid polypharmacy with the resultant unpredictable drug intake and drug interactions. The most common pitfalls encountered in the medical management of epileptic patients are: inadequate use of anticonvulsant levels; inadequate drug dosage, when used either singly or in combination; complex medication regimens with frequently repeated doses at differing intervals, resulting in poor compliance; wrong type of drug for given seizure type; and infrequent follow-up visits.

In the practice of psychiatry, an additional problem is likely to occur because there may be two physicians involved with a patient—the neurologist, internist, or family practitioner who treats the seizure disorder, and the psychiatrist who treats the emotional disturbances. This can place both physicians at a disadvantage, because the anticonvulsant regimen may increase psychiatric symptomatology, on the one hand, and, owing to interactions of the two types of drugs, psychotropic medications may exacerbate seizures if anticonvulsant levels drop, on the other. Furthermore, the patient's seizures may also increase if therapy causes an acute stress reaction. In addition, when stressed, some patients may report uncontrollable seizures that are, however, not necessarily epileptic in nature, as is discussed in the following chapter. These admittedly confusing situations are handled better if psychiatrists, who see the patients at more frequent intervals than their medical colleagues, are fully informed about what constitutes an adequate medication regimen.

Although it will be impossible to cover all contingencies, the following guidelines may be useful for the majority of patients. The psychiatrist is well advised to use mainly those anticonvulsant drugs for which blood level determinations are readily available. This reduces the armamentarium to the six most effective ones, allows greater familiarity with their potential side effects, and permits periodic checks on compliance. These drugs are phenytoin (Dilantin), phenobarbital, primidone (Mysoline), carbamazepine (Tegretol), ethosuximide (Zarontin), and sodium valproate (Depakene). They are effective either singly or in combination in the great majority of epileptic patients.

For tonic-clonic seizures (grand mal), the initial drug of choice is either phenytoin or valproate if the seizures are of the nonfocal variety (i.e., primary generalized) and phenytoin or carbamazepine if they have focal components (i.e., secondarily generalized). Phenobarbital and primidone (which is metabolized in part into phenobarbital) are secondary drugs because of sedative properties that can influence the patient's job performance. For partial seizures the drugs of choice, in order of preference, are carbamazepine, phenytoin, phenobarbital, and primidone. Petit mal absences are treated best with valproate; if this drug is ineffective or cannot be tolerated by the patient, ethosuximide is preferred.

It is recommended that the patient be started on one drug rather than two even though more than one seizure type is present, because the spectrum of effectiveness of a given drug overlaps seizure types. If a drug clearly proves ineffective, it should be exchanged rather than supplemented by another. What is more commonly the case, that the drug has proven moderately effective in the presence of clearly "therapeutic" levels, may justify the addition of a second drug. If seizures stop under these circumstances, the first drug may be discontinued if the patient is willing to risk a recurrence of attacks. The addition of a third anticonvulsant rarely results in further significant improvement, and patients who require three anticonvulsants usually suffer from chronic epilepsy for which the prognosis for seizure cessation is relatively poor.

The need to keep anticonvulsants to a minimum is even greater in patients with psychiatric complications, because it is likely that at least one psychotropic drug will have to be added to the regimen, with the concomitant danger of creating complex regimens with unpredictable interactions.

The next section discusses specific aspects of pharmacology, dosage and schedule of administration, side effects, and drug interactions for the six most effective anticonvulsants.

PHENYTOIN (DILANTIN)

Pharmacology

Phenytoin is a relatively insoluble weak acid. Its bioavailability depends on particle size; therefore, it presents the possibility of generic inequivalence. The drug is poorly absorbed from the stomach because of its low pH, and absorption is further decreased if an antacid is taken at the same time. The main absorption takes place in the duodenum. There is no absorption from the rectum.

After oral administration of a single dose, peak blood levels are usually reached between 4 and 8 h after administration, although they may occur as early as 3 and as late as 12 h after ingestion of the drug. The time of peak effect seems to be independent of the dose, and levels may remain at peak levels for 24 h. The plasma half-life after oral administration varies widely, and extremes of 7–42 h have been reported, with an average of about 22 h.

Phenytoin is about 90 percent bound to plasma protein, especially albumin. There is good correspondence between the free fractions in plasma, CSF, saliva, and tears (1). The drug crosses the placenta and is metabolized rapidly by the neonate exposed to the compound in utero. It is also excreted in breast milk with a milk-to-serum ratio of 0.2. Although the total serum level is relatively low, the free fraction in the neonate is about 40 percent higher than in the adult, which may be due to a displacement of the drug from its binding sites by bilirubin (2). Phenytoin has also been recovered from semen at a rate 0.17 times that of the level in plasma.

The major breakdown product is 5-(*p*-hydroxyphenyl)-5-phenylhydantoin (HPPH), which has no proven anticonvulsant activity. It is conjugated and rapidly excreted, but may accumulate with impaired renal function. Normally HPPH levels are one-tenth to one-fifth of the phenytoin level, and it is 60–65 percent protein bound (3). At higher plasma concentrations of phenytoin, the metabolism for HPPH saturates and plasma half-life lengthens (4).

Dosage and Administration

The usually effective dose of phenytoin tends to be about 5 mg/kg, but since great individual variations exist, it is advisable to obtain a blood level about 3 weeks after initiation of therapy. The dose then can be adjusted according to the laboratory results, provided the patient is compliant.

Because of its relatively long half-life, the drug can be given in one single dose, but if the patient forgets to take it, a precipitous drop in level is likely to occur, which may be accompanied by seizures. We therefore recommend two divided doses, to be taken at breakfast and dinner time. If the doses cannot be evenly divided, i.e., 300 or 500 mg, we give the higher dose in the evening.

It must be remembered that the correlation between dose and serum level is curvilinear, and small increments in doses may produce disproportionate increases in serum concentration. When the total plasma level is >10 μg/ml, it is advisable to increase doses by 25, 30, or 50 mg.

With a dose of 300–400 mg/day, therapeutic levels are usually reached within 7–10 days. With a loading dose of 1,000 mg, therapeutic levels can be reached in 8–24 hrs (5). Complications from intravenous administration consist of cardiac arrhythmias, drops in blood pressure, and respiratory arrest. Therefore, phenytoin should not be given more rapidly than 50 mg/min. When the drug is given intravenously, it can precipitate in the commonly used solutions, and its crystallization is pH dependent. Phenytoin should therefore either be used from the original ampule or given in an alkaline medium. Oral absorption of the drug is reduced by concomitant administration of oxacillin, magnesium trisilicate, or aluminum oxide, but not by calcium carbonate. Intramuscular or rectal administration is relatively ineffective because of poor absorption.

Side Effects

The side effects of phenytoin can be divided into dose related and idiosyncratic. The therapeutic range, in general, is regarded as 10–20 μg/ml for total plasma level and 1.0–2.2 μg/ml for free levels. Toxic signs are rare with a total level of <15 μg/ml. The literature states that nystagmus usually occurs at 20 μg/ml, ataxia at 25–30 μg/ml, and mental slowing at >40 μg/ml (6). At levels of >25 μg/ml, one can also find a paradoxical reaction of increased seizure frequency. In our experience, we frequently have encountered unsteadiness in walking prior to the presence of nystagmus; at times this has been mistaken for a psychogenic reaction when, in fact, the symptom promptly disappeared after the phenytoin dosage was reduced. Levels of >20–25 μg/ml may inhibit insulin release and result in hyperglycemia.

A morbilliform rash may be either dose dependent or idiosyncratic, and the same is true of gingival hypertrophy. The most important cutaneous idiosyncratic side effects are Stevens-Johnson syndrome (erythema multiforme involving skin, eyes, oropharynx, and genitalia) and exfoliative dermatitis.

As far as the immune system is concerned, there can be suppression of cellular as well as humoral immune systems with phenytoin. Decreases of lymphocytes, immunoglobulin (Ig) A, and IgG have been observed at times. This may be associated with general lymphadenopathy, malignant lymphoma, or lupus erythematosus (7, 8). The effects of phenytoin on blood are megaloblastosis and macrocytosis; these are not necessarily related to folate deficiency, which also has been attributed to the drug. Folate levels, in general, are slightly decreased, but not to the extent of causing clinically significant folate deficiency.

A relationship of folate deficiency to gingival hyperplasia has been postulated but not established (9). However, mean salivary IgA has been found to be significantly reduced in epileptic children. It was normal in untreated patients but fell during phenytoin administration. Gingival inflammation was associated with an increase in salivary IgG and serum-derived IgA (10). The severity of gingival overgrowth was related to phenytoin levels but also to the smaller root-to-crown ratio in mentally retarded children (11). Hypertrophy of masticatory mucosa was observed once in an edentulous patient (12).

Calcium and phosphorus metabolism may be disturbed with phenytoin, but this is more common in pediatric patients where ossification may also be impaired, leading to metaphyseal osteodystrophy. Generalized osteoporosis and vitamin D-responsive rickets have also been reported (13), but usually the decalcification remains within normal limits although some pathologic fractures have occurred. Chromosome studies from bone marrow and lymphocytes showed no damage when phenytoin was given alone.

CNS Effects

In response to phenytoin, movement disorders have been increasingly reported over the last few years in the forms of choreoathetosis (14), orofacial dyskinesias, limb chorea, and, in intoxicated patients, dystonia. Asterixis similar to the side effect of neuroleptic drugs has also been observed (15). In the mentally retarded population and in patients who have had previous episodes of phenytoin intoxication, one can see cerebellar and/or brainstem atrophy, which leads to permanent ataxia (16). It also has been shown that cerebellar atrophy may be asymptomatic and discernible initially only on computed tomographic scan (17). On occasion, a complex picture can be seen, consisting of psychomotor deterioration, choreiform hyperkinesia, and a dementia that is partially reversible on withdrawal of phenytoin (18).

As far as peripheral nerves are concerned, neuropathy is rarely symptomatic and consists mainly of lower extremity areflexia, sensory deficits, and reduced conduction velocity. This tends to be related to higher serum levels and to drug treatment extending for >5 years. Ocular symptoms have been reported mainly as a result of toxicity, namely, external ophthalmoplegia (19) at levels of 36–55 μg/ml; episodic convergence spasm coupled by ptosis and miosis was also seen with toxic levels (20).

Single case reports exist of interstitial nephritis (21) and acute renal failure (22). Hepatic necrosis (23) with fatal outcome in a single case was also associated with exfoliative dermatitis.

Thyroid functions may also be affected by phenytoin. A decrease in thyroxine and an increase in free thyroxine (but not triiodothyronine) have been reported. Phenytoin displaces thyroxine and, to a lesser extent, triiodothyronine from protein binding sites in serum, and increases the peripheral clearance of thyroid hormones. However, the values usually remain in the euthyroid range (24). The suggestion was made that the reduced T_4 levels were due not only to diminished protein binding but also to enhanced degradation (25). Two patients were reported to have been clinically hypothyroid; one was on phenytoin and carbamazepine, the other on carbamazepine only. These patients became euthyroid when anticonvulsants were withdrawn (26). On rare occasions a myasthenic reaction has been observed (27).

Teratogenicity

The fetal hydantoin syndrome has been reported with an incidence of 6–11 percent, but in the experience of this author, these figures appear to be rather high, and other factors apart from phenytoin administration may well play a role. In our own patient population, we have not seen significant congenital malformations (i.e., cleft lip, cleft palate, congenital heart defect) in marked excess of what might occur in the general population, especially when one considers the fact that epileptic patients have somewhat increased histories of congenital malformations in their families. The report by Bustamante and Stumpff (28) is of great interest in this respect, because it deals with the occurrence of fetal hydantoin syndrome in triplets but with different expressivity in each of the three babies. Triplet A had a low bridge of the nose, ocular hypertelorism, elevated and bifid xyphoid, as well as nail hypoplasia. Triplet B had ocular hypertelorism, undescended testes, digitalization of the right thumb, and partial fusion of the sagittal suture. The most severely affected Triplet C showed ocular hypertelorism, low bridge of the nose, bilateral cleft lip, cleft palate, large anterior fontanel, and nail hypoplasia.

Interactions

Phenytoin and phenobarbital in combination show both enzyme induction and inhibition. The phenobarbital clearance is reduced (by 20 percent) in the presence of phenytoin, whereas phenytoin clearance is not affected by the presence of phenobarbital (29). Since the interaction with phenobarbital is variable, there is, in some instances, a decline of the phenytoin level, in others no change, and in still others a rise of the level. The higher the starting plasma level of phenytoin or the higher the phenobarbital dose, the more likely is a decline of the phenytoin plasma level. Shortening of the apparent plasma half-life of Dilantin by phenobarbital has also been observed in some patients (30). Phenytoin raises the phenobarbital level whether it is derived from phenobarbital itself or from primidone. Phenytoin also raises levels of phenylethylmalonamide (PEMA; the other main metabolite of primidone).

The effects of salicylates appear to be variable: One report cites a decrease in serum phenytoin level (31, 32), but another recent study showed that on continued treatment with the phenytoin dosage held constant, the phenytoin level increased above control and became toxic (33). Isoniazid can impair phenytoin metabolism, leading to toxic levels (34, 35); one death has resulted from this interaction (36).

Bishydroxycoumarin and phenprocoumon increase the mean half-life of phenytoin and may also lead to toxic levels (37). Sulfonamides inhibit the hepatic metabolism of phenytoin, leading to an increased half-life and decreased metabolic clearance. Specific drugs reported are sulfaphenazole, sulfadiazine, sulfamethizole, and sulfamethoxazole-trimethoprim (38). Chloramphenicol likewise inhibits phenytoin metabolism with a subsequent increase in level (39, 40). Nitrofurantoin, on the other hand, can accelerate phenytoin metabolism with a resultant drop in level and the occurrence of seizures (41). The same applies to oxacillin (42). Medications that may lead to a rise in levels are disulfiram (7), methylphenidate, phenothiazines, tricyclics, antihistamines, as well as monoamine oxidase inhibitors (43). The effect appears to be variable because the opposite may also occur at times. Medications whose effectiveness has been reported to be reduced by phenytoin are steroids (cortisone, ovulation blockers), digitoxin, coumarin, antibiotics (especially tetracycline and doxycycline), tolbutamide, and L-Dopa. In the neonate, phenytoin may lead to a depression of vitamin K-dependent coagulation factors and thus to cerebral hemorrhage within the first 24 h, but this appears to occur very rarely.

The interaction of phenytoin with carbamazepine is discussed below.

Psychotropic Properties

The role of phenytoin in nonepileptic psychiatric disorders is controversial. Excellent results have been reported for a variety of conditions (44), but the review by Parnas et al. (45) has been less encouraging. Several different populations were explored, namely, male delinquents and patients with anxiety neuroses, neurotic depressions, psychoneuroses, and minimal brain dysfunctions. The results were either equivocal or negative.

PHENOBARBITAL

Pharmacology

Phenobarbital, 5-ethyl-5-phenyl barbituric acid, is a white crystalline substance with a somewhat bitter taste. The substance is quite stable in aqueous solution of low pH. Phenobarbital clearance is higher when the urine is alkaline (46). This is important for the treatment of intoxication.

In epileptic patients, peak plasma levels have been observed 1–3 h after intramuscular administration. Oral doses produce variable results, namely, 1–3 vs 2–8 h (47). In fatal poisoning, crystals have been observed in the stomach up to 12 h after ingestion. The drug is absorbed from the stomach but mostly from the small intestine. It enters the brain later than other organs, but gray matter more rapidly than white. Later, during steady state, it is found in nearly equal concentrations in all tissues of the body.

The maximum protein binding of phenobarbital, mainly to albumin at pH 7.6, is 46 percent. Binding is decreased, therefore, when albumin is decreased. The drug disappears from the plasma at a rate of 11–27 percent a day. The mean half-life in adults tends to be 96 h, the longest among anticonvulsants. From 11 to 48 percent (average 24 percent) of daily intake is excreted as unchanged drug. The main metabolite, *p*-hydroxyphenobarbital, seems devoid of hypnotic activity. Although phenobarbital is a powerful enzyme inducer, it has little effect on its own metabolism. Liver cirrhosis impairs phenobarbital metabolism, and average blood half-lives have been observed to increase up to 130 h in liver disease (48).

Dosage and Administration

Phenobarbital levels in the "therapeutic range" of 10–20 μg/ml are provided by 1.5–2 mg/kg. Since the drug has an unusually long half-life, it can be given safely as a single dose in the evening. Under these circumstances patients sometimes complain of sleepiness in the morning; if this occurs, b.i.d. administration is useful. It should be remembered that phenobarbital is a potential drug of abuse and can lead to successful suicide attempts. It is advisable, therefore, to limit prescriptions to a 1-month supply at a time.

Ever since the classic study by Buchthal and Svensmark (49), there has been practically unanimous agreement that in active seizure patients, relapses can be expected if levels drop below 10 or 15 μg/ml. There are no reports of increased effectiveness with levels of >40 μg/ml.

Side Effects

Although tolerance to drowsiness tends to develop with phenobarbital administration, this is the most significant side effect apart from an occasional rash. The latter is maculopapular, morbilliform, or scarlatiniform in nature and stops when medication is discontinued. The incidence is 1–3 percent. One case of exfoliative dermatitis has been reported. These reactions usually occur within the first 1–5 weeks. Corticosteroids may help. Systemic lupus erythematosus is an exceedingly rare complication that requires discontinuation of the drug. Impairment of cognitive and adaptive ability in proportion to phenobarbital levels has been shown, and sedation may sometimes occur at levels as low as 5 μg/ml. There is great individual variability in susceptibility, and higher levels appear to be tolerated better when the phenobarbital level is derived from primidone rather than from phenobarbital itself. At levels exceeding 40 μg/ml, dysarthria, uncoordination, ataxia, and nystagmus have been reported, but these may be complications of concomitant phenytoin administration. Levels of ≥70 μg/ml can be expected to lead to stupor or coma even in a habituated individual.

Children and the elderly may become hyperkinetic with phenobarbital. Distraction, short attention span, mood fluctuation, and aggressive outbursts are not related to blood levels but appear to be idiosyncratic in nature. The mood may become depressed, and memory as well as learning may be impaired (50–53). Reynolds and Travers (54) reported that patients with levels around 19 μg/ml showed psychomotor slowing, some intellectual deterioration, and personality changes. This did not occur with levels around 13 μg/ml. The substitution of carbamazepine for phenobarbital in children has led to better classroom performance. Depression of the critical flicker fusion rate and short-term memory impairment have also been reported.

Phenobarbital produces physical dependence, and the withdrawal symptoms consist of anxiety, emotional lability, insomnia, tremor, diaphoresis, confusion, and seizures. Since the drug crosses the placenta, fetal withdrawal symptoms may occur, but permanent sequelae have not been reported. Another side effect, which must be kept in mind especially for male patients, is sexual impotence. Still other side effects include liver dysfunction, megaloblastic anemia, macrocytosis, and low folate levels. Mattson et al. (55) found an inverse relationship between folate and phenobarbital levels in serum and CSF, but no change in CSF folate levels on folate treatment. Phenobarbital stimulates the rate of T_4 and T_3 clearance. It increases the rate of T_4 removal, which is countered by an increase in the thyroid secretion of T_4, so that serum levels stay constant in euthyroid individuals. The extent of the conversion of T_4 to T_3 is probably not significantly altered by phenobarbital.

The concurrent use of alcohol and phenobarbital can cause respiratory depression, leading to unsuspected and unintended suicide. Heroin deacetylation can be increased. Oral contraception breakthrough bleeding was reported in >50 percent of 52 females and was positively correlated with phenobarbital dosage; bleeding occurred in 4 percent of the control population (56). The drug enhances bilirubin elimination and is thus used to treat hyperbilirubinemia in infants, reducing the need for exchange transfusion. In toxicity, elimination can be increased by alkalinization with ammonium chloride and induction of forced diuresis.

Teratogenicity

No single malformation has been definitely attributed to phenobarbital as monotherapy.

Interactions

The phenytoin-phenobarbital interaction is variable. There is some evidence that phenobarbital levels rise with phenytoin administration, but this is rarely of significant magnitude. There is also a suggestion that phenytoin prolongs the phenobarbital half-life. Valproate increases phenobarbital levels, but with great individual variability. This also occurs when phenobarbital comes from primidone, but the reaction is not quite as predictable. A ketogenic diet may likewise cause an increase of phenobarbital levels similar to that seen with valproate.

Other drugs that raise phenobarbital levels are furosemide, acetazolamide, pheneturide, chloramphenicol, and propoxyphene. Folic acid, pyridoxine, dicumarol, and phenylbutazone have been reported to lower phenobarbital levels. In the presence of phenobarbital, carbamazepine levels drop while the level of its metabolite epoxide remains unchanged or declines only a small extent. A drop in the levels of chlorpromazine, desipramine, and nortriptyline has also been reported (30).

PRIMIDONE (MYSOLINE)

Pharmacology

Primidone is a weakly acidic cyclic amide and was first described as having clinical anticonvulsant properties by Bogue and Carrington in 1953 (57). The major metabolites are PEMA and phenobarbital. In epileptic patients the main peak absorption time is 3.2 h, with a range of 0.5–9.0 h. In another single-dose study, the average peak level occurred in 2.7 h, with a range of 0.5–7 h. The half-life for primidone itself in epileptic patients has been reported as 7.2 ± 1.5 h, with a range 3.3–12.5 h. But there is great individual variability, and comedication may play a significant role. In patients on monotherapy, the average half-life was 14.4 h compared with 7.3 h for patients on polypharmacy.

Primidone is poorly bound to protein. The free fraction is 76 ± 11.9 percent, and the free phenobarbital derived from primidone is 45 ± 11.2 percent of the total level. Principal excretion is in the kidney, mainly as unconjugated primidone. A comparable amount is excreted as unconjugated PEMA and the least amount as phenobarbital and conjugates. Biotransformation occurs in the liver. The drug passes through the placenta and is also excreted in breast milk (58).

Dosage and Administration

An effective dosage range for primidone tends to be between 500 and 750 mg; because of its relatively short half-life, the drug is given in two or three divided doses. The effective range of drug levels is regarded as 6–15 μg/ml, but the high end may not be attained in some cases because of concomitant excessive phenobarbital rise.

Side Effects

In some patients an initial toxic reaction may occur 0.5 h after the first dose and may last up to 48 h. It consists of dizziness, drowsiness, gastrointestinal distress, and, rarely, hallucinations. This reaction is more common when patients are not already on anticonvulsants, especially phenobarbital. Treatment should therefore be started with 125 or even 50 mg at bedtime.

Symptoms of overdose include somnolence, lethargy, ataxia, dysarthria, nystagmus, nausea and vomiting, depression of deep tendon reflexes, and flaccidity. These may be due to primidone itself rather than to phenobarbital or PEMA, because the latter levels may go up as the patient improves (59).

Idiosyncratic side effects include personality changes, paranoid reactions, confusion, a schizophreniform psychosis, decreased libido, difficulties with memory and concentration, as well as lack of energy. Three cases of partial or total external ophthalmoplegia have also been reported. Twenty-two grams of the drug has been ingested in a suicidal attempt without permanent sequelae. Crystalluria is a prominent factor of overdose and should raise suspicion of primidone or phenobarbital intoxication. Isolated reports exist also of megaloblastic anemia, thrombocytopenia, thrombocytopenic purpura, leukopenia, and lymphadenopathy. On rare occasions edema has been observed with no renal or hepatic involvement.

Cutaneous rashes are rare; they usually occur at the onset of therapy and may disappear spontaneously or when the drug is stopped. At times the drug can be reintroduced without recurrence of the rash. Systemic lupus erythematosus has been reported once. There are too few instances of monotherapy to allow statements with regard to teratogenicity (59).

Interactions

There is considerable variability, but when phenytoin is used, the phenobarbital level derived from primidone increases. A decrease in phenytoin level was seen in children when primidone was given as comedication. No significant interaction has been reported with ethosuximide. Carbamazepine may increase the metabolism of primidone to its metabolites, but an increase of primidone levels as a result of carbamazepine has been reported also. Isoniazid can increase primidone levels; in one report it nearly doubled the primidone plasma half-life, but aspirin was also given in that instance. Valproate initially increased primidone levels, but they returned to the original values within 1–3 months. Another report showed no change at steady state (60).

SODIUM VALPROATE (DEPAKENE)

Pharmacology

First synthesized in 1882, valproic acid could be regarded as the oldest of the modern anticonvulsant drugs. Its anticonvulsant properties, however, were not appreciated until 1963, and the first clinical trials were reported in 1964. The drug is highly water soluble and completely absorbed throughout the intestinal tract. Peak concentrations in plasma are dependent upon food intake. With immediate-release formulations, peak concentrations are obtained in the fasting state within 2 h and after a meal within 3–8 h. This is important with regard to dosage regimens, which will be discussed below. On whole-body autoradiography, the majority of the drug can be found in the blood, liver, kidneys, and intestines. It passes through the placenta and enters the fetus with similar distribution. In the brain, labeled material was found initially more in white than in gray matter (especially in the cerebellar fiber tracts), but later on radioactivity was more prominent in gray matter. Valproate penetrates breast milk in about 2 percent of the serum concentration. CSF concentrations are about 10 percent of those in serum.

Valproic acid is bound extensively to plasma protein, mainly albumin. The free fraction amount is nonlinear with respect to total plasma. It ranges from 5 to 13 percent and increases as total plasma sodium valproate increases. The mean half-life in normal volunteers ranged from 9.5 to 17.7 h. In epileptic patients the mean half-life was about 9 h, which may well be related to comedications. Its rapid absorption, short half-life, and saturable plasma binding result in extensive variations in serum levels during chronic therapy (61).

Sodium valproate undergoes various oxidative processes, but the most important urinary metabolite is the glucuronide that is formed in the liver. It accounts for about 20–40 percent of the urinary excretion. Some of the metabolites have anticonvulsant properties (especially alpha-, beta-, and unsaturated valproate), which may explain in part the lack of a direct relationship between plasma valproate concentrations and seizure control (62).

Dosage and Administration

The minimum effective dosage of sodium valproate tends to be between 15 and 30 mg/kg. The drug can be given as a single dose in spite of its relatively short half-life because of the anticonvulsant properties of its metabolites. Until recently this was usually not feasible, because in the United States the compound was available only in 250-mg capsules, and thus a rather large amount of medication had to be taken at one time, which could also lead to increased gastric complaints. An enteric-coated 500-mg preparation has just been marketed, and this may make once-daily regimens feasible. Currently we give the drug in two divided doses, similar to phenytoin. In order to avoid initial toxicity, the drug is introduced very gradually, in increments of one capsule every 3 days, with the first dose taken in the evening. Gastric discomfort can also be minimized by giving the drug at mealtime or at least with a glass of milk. There is also a suggestion that an uneven dosage regimen, i.e., two-thirds in the evening and one-third in the morning, leads to more stable free levels of the bound and free fractions, thus reducing the marked diurnal fluctuations that are otherwise found (63).

When given as the sole drug, sodium valproate has a slower clearance and longer half-life, thus leading to higher levels for a given dose. The low levels in the presence of comedication may even prevent optimal therapeutic results. The generally accepted therapeutic range is from 50 to 100 μg/ml, and the lowest effective level appears to be about 40–50 μg/ml. The relationship between the mg/kg dose and levels is linear, unless comedication is used. If treatment begins with combination therapy and other anticonvulsants are discontinued, valproate levels rise, and the sodium valproate dose can be decreased. In adults doses of >2,500 mg are not recommended (64).

Side Effects

The most common side effects with sodium valproate are gastrointestinal complaints, especially anorexia, indigestion, nausea, and occasional vomiting. These can be minimized by a gradual introduction of the drug and an associated food intake. Appetite may increase, leading to weight gain. This can be a serious problem because females tend to be more affected, and a 1,000-cal diet may have to be prescribed. If, under those circumstances, weight gain persists, the drug may have to be discontinued and another anticonvulsant introduced. Drowsiness is rare and occurs in only 0.2 percent on monotherapy; it can become a problem, however, because of the interaction with other anticonvulsants.

Increased hair loss occurs in 2.6–12 percent; although very frightening, especially to females, it is temporary in nearly all instances. Only reassurance is required. Tremor, another of the slightly more common side effects, may be improved by a decrease in dosage or the administration of propranolol. Occasionally, irregular menses and secondary amenorrhea have been observed. Among the more serious side reactions are hepatitis, pancreatitis, and blood dyscrasias. The latter are rare, but transient or persistent neutropenias have been observed, as well as thrombocytopenia and occasional coagulation defects. This is most likely when dosages exceed 50 mg/kg. Elevations in serum glutamic-oxaloacetic and pyruvic transaminases are usually asymptomatic and may respond to dose reduction. Hepatotoxicity is unrelated to dosage or levels, and occurs mostly in infants and children on multiple therapy. Hyperammonemia may occur especially when comedications are used, and this might be considered as another sign of liver failure.

Deaths resulting from hepatic involvement, as reported by Jeavons (64), were idiosyncratic, and it is not clear that sodium valproate was the sole responsible agent. Jeavons reviewed these cases carefully and found that toxic hepatitis and pancreatitis, if present, occurred most commonly within 3 months of the initiation of treatment, rarely in <1 month, but in all before 6 months. The mean onset was 62 days. In all but five cases, there was comedication, particularly phenytoin. Most of the serious problems occurred in children with mental retardation and intractable epilepsy. Prodromal symptoms consisted of loss of seizure control, lethargy, drowsiness, weakness, vomiting, anorexia, and jaundice. Dosages and levels were in the therapeutic range. Jeavons felt that clinical monitoring was more important than laboratory testing; for the first 2 months, patients should be reviewed every 2 weeks, and then every month for the next 4 months. No serious side effects were observed with doses of <30 mg/kg. Pancreatitis should be suspected if vomiting occurs after 5–6 weeks of treatment and if there is marked abdominal pain. Serum amylase determination is indicated.

Accidental or purposeful suicide attempts with valproic acid have been reported in 23 cases. Of these 22 recovered and 1 died; the serum level in the latter case was 197 μg/ml.

Teratogenicity

There have been recent reports of the increased incidence of spina bifida with the administration of sodium valproate. The U.S. Centers for Disease Control have estimated the risk for neural tube defects at 1.2 percent.

Interactions

Because of high protein binding, sodium valproate has several interactions with anticonvulsants as well as with other drugs. Serum phenobarbital levels rise with valproate; this increase may be from 25 to 200 percent, with a usual range of 15–70 percent. This does not occur in all patients, but it is sufficiently common to be of considerable clinical significance. Sodium valproate probably inhibits the biotransformation and hydroxylation of phenobarbital and increases its elimination half-life, resulting in the elevation of the serum phenobarbital levels. Phenytoin tends to be displaced from its binding sites, with a resultant drop in the total plasma level and an increase in the free level, leading at times to clinical intoxication in the presence of average therapeutic phenytoin levels.

An effect on ethosuximide levels is less frequent, although a report exists of increased ethosuximide levels as a result of valproate (65). The potential interaction with carbamazepine is more important because that drug is 75 percent protein bound. A rise in the free level of carbamazepine induced by sodium valproate may result in intermittent toxic symptoms that cannot be explained by carbamazepine total plasma levels, similar to those occurring with phenytoin. In the presence of suspected toxicity, it is valuable to monitor both the free and total level of the drugs. Another important finding, the mechanism of which is still unknown, is reported with benzodiazepines, especially clonazepam. The free fraction of sodium valproate may rise two- to threefold in the presence of clonazepam so that at times the clonazepam must be discontinued.

Salicylates, especially aspirin, can displace valproate from protein, thus resulting in high free levels of the drug. This is less common with phenylbutazone, and no interaction with warfarin has been demonstrated. Lowered total valproate in the presence of high free drug occurs also in disease states associated with lowered serum albumin, e.g., malnutrition, hepatic, renal, and gastrointestinal disease, malignancy, and protein loss secondary to burns (66).

ETHOSUXIMIDE (ZARONTIN)

Pharmacology

Ethosuximide was first reported as an effective agent against petit mal seizures in 1958. The compound, 2-ethyl-2-methylsuccinimide, is highly water soluble (67). Its main metabolite, 2-(1-hydroxyethyl)-2-methylsuccinimide, is formed by hydroxylation of the carbon atom next to the ring on the ethyl side chain. Ethosuximide is present in two isomers that are partly conjugated with glucuronic acid and excreted in the urine (68). The plasma half-life ranges from 15 to 68 h, with a mean of 36–39 h. Absorption is rapid, and peak levels have been observed in adults within 3 h after administration. Plasma levels have been reported to rise more sharply with increasing doses in females. Even in males the dose-plasma level relationship may not be linear. Equal increments of doses may give progressively steeper levels. In pregnant women the levels may increase after delivery in spite of the same dose. Ethosuximide passes through the placenta, and the neonatal half-life was reported as 41.3 h.

The drug is poorly bound to protein and appears rapidly in CSF, milk, and saliva (69). A dosage of 20 mg/kg in children younger than 11 years gives levels of about 50 μg/ml, whereas only 15 mg/kg will give similar results in older children (70).

Dosage

An optimum daily dose of ethosuximide tends to be around 20 mg/kg, which can be given b.i.d. With levels of 40–100 μg/ml, 60 percent of petit mal absence patients can be expected to become seizurefree, and another 20 percent can expect a substantial reduction in seizures (70).

Side Effects

Side effects of ethosuximide consist mainly of nausea, abdominal discomfort, drowsiness, anorexia, hiccups, and headache. All of these are dose related, except headache. Reports exist of an increase in other seizure types, but these are not well documented.

Occasionally there are behavioral problems including psychotic episodes with visual or auditory hallucinations and ideas of persecution. These are idiosyncratic and not dose related. Other idiosyncratic reactions are rash, Stevens-Johnson syndrome, erythema multiforme, lupus erythematosus, and scleroderma. Blood dyscrasias, especially leukopenia, thrombocytopenia, pancytopenia, and bone marrow depression, are the most serious potential problems (71). Most fatalities have occurred within the first year of treatment. Granulocytopenia may be dose related, and if it is the only abnormality, reduction in the total daily dosage can be tried while the patient is closely supervised with frequent hemograms.

There is little information available on teratogenicity because the drug is used rarely in adults. It is probably clinically insignificant.

Interactions

No consistent significant drug interactions with ethosuximide have been established. Because, however, the drug can affect the hematopoietic system, it should not be combined with other agents that tend to produce blood dyscrasias, e.g., carbamazepine and mephenytoin (Mesantoin).

CARBAMAZEPINE (TEGRETOL)

Pharmacology

Carbamazepine, 5-carbamyl-5*H*-dibenz[*b,f*]azepine-5-carboxamide, is a derivative of iminostilbene and is chemically related to the tricyclic antidepressants, especially imipramine. Carbamazepine is a white crystalline compound that is poorly soluble in water but readily soluble in ethanol, acetone, and propylene glycol (72). Its poor water solubility may be clinically important, because part of the compound is excreted unchanged in feces. Its solubility can be enhanced by taking the drug with meals, thereby increasing gastrointestinal secretions. Peak plasma levels are reached from 4 to 8 h after an oral dose, but individual variability is seen beyond this range (73).

Carbamazepine is about 70–80 percent protein bound in plasma. Whether it binds mainly to albumin is still under investigation. The drug passes through the placental barrier, and it can also be passed on through breastfeeding to the baby. The half-life on chronic therapy ranges between 10 and 30 h for adults and 8 and 20 h for children. No difference in the half-life between newborns and adults has been found (74). The main breakdown product of carbamazepine is its 10,11-epoxide, which is further metabolized mostly to the 10,11-dihydroxide. Two-thirds of the 10,11-dihydroxide is eliminated in free form in the urine, and the rest is conjugated with glucuronic acid. Iminostilbene can also be recovered in the urine as a further minor metabolite (75).

Dosage and Administration

Early reports indicated that the therapeutic plasma levels of carbamazepine ranged from 4 to 7 μg/ml. This estimate has been revised upward to 6–12 μg/ml (76). Levels of >10 μg/ml need not be alarming if they are not accompanied by side effects. Plasma levels frequently do not correspond exactly to mg/kg intake, even in hospitalized patients in whom compliance is not a factor (77). Virtually all investigators of the pharmacokinetics of carbamazepine have noted not only considerable interindividual differences but also intraindividual differences in absorption and breakdown. Nevertheless, it is agreed that the highest levels and longest half-lives with the least amount of drug are achieved when the drug is used alone (78).

When carbamazepine is given as monotherapy, 600–800 mg tends to produce satisfactory blood levels; this amount can be given b.i.d. In the presence of other anticonvulsants, the total daily dosage frequently may have to be increased to 1,200 or even 1,400 mg, and under these circumstances it is better to adopt a t.i.d. regimen. If satisfactory levels are not obtainable with 1,400 mg, increasing the dose further is not likely to be useful, and if carbamazepine is indeed regarded as the drug of choice, comedications would have to be discontinued. This problem arises mainly in brain-damaged patients with severe intractable seizure disorders.

Side Effects

Dose-related symptoms and signs of carbamazepine consist of dizziness, drowsiness, ataxia, diplopia or blurring of vision, nystagmus, and possible irritability or hyperactivity. Less common are orofacial dyskinesias, dystonia, and oculogyric crises. The lowest level at which diplopia, ataxia, and nystagmus were reported was 7.6 μg/ml (79). The usual levels for these symptoms are 10.2–12.5 μg/ml. At 13.5 μg/ml sleepiness, restlessness, and disorientation can be expected, and at 22.0 μg/ml general apathy. The average level for side effects is 11.6 ± 4.3 μg/ml. The anticipated threshold for side effects is about 8.9 μg/ml. The carbamazepine levels fluctuate throughout the day and so may the side effects. Intermittent symptoms of diplopia, drowsiness, and headache did not correlate with morning levels, but there was a rapid rise in levels observed by the afternoon, which was accompanied by side effects (80). Fewer symptoms occur with carbamazepine monotherapy. When a t.i.d. regimen is used, the noon dose should be relatively small. On monotherapy the fluctuation of levels ranged from 27 to 38 percent, with a mean of 32.5 percent, throughout the day; on polypharmacy from 41 to 84 percent, with a mean of 61 percent.

Decreased plasma sodium concentration, decreased plasma osmolality, and decreased ability to tolerate a water load occur in a small minority of patients taking carbamazepine. Clinical water intoxication has occurred rarely (81, 82). This phenomenon varies directly with the carbamazepine plasma concentration. Hyponatremia is more likely to occur in patients taking carbamazepine alone than in those taking carbamazepine and phenytoin in combination because the latter drug lowers the former's plasma concentrations (83).

Idiosyncratic reactions include exfoliative dermatitis, jaundice, lymphatic hyperplasia, lenticular opacities, aplastic anemia, thrombocytopenia, and pancytopenia. Urticarial-type rash and depression of one or more values of cellular or humoral immune responses may occur; these can be dose related or idiosyncratic. Several early reports of serious bone marrow depression in association with carbamazepine therapy led to a special bold-print warning on the package insert and the recommendation that frequent blood cell counts be obtained.

Recent comprehensive reviews of all available data indicate that the hematopoietic toxicity of carbamazepine is much less than originally feared (84, 85). Hart and Easton (84) tabulated the prevalence of carbamazepine-hematologic toxicity as follows: aplastic anemia, $<1/50{,}000$ (a total of 20 cases); transient leukopenia, 10 percent; persistent leukopenia, 2 percent; thrombocytopenia, 2 percent; and anemia, <5 percent. Pisciotta (85) calculated similar risks and pointed out that in many of the reported cases of carbamazepine-hematopoietic toxicity, the patient was taking other drugs that either have hematopoietic side effects of their own or may potentiate latent ones.

Teratogenicity

When carbamazepine monotherapy is used, teratogenicity does not appear to be a major problem. There is only one report of a decrease in head circumference of neonates born to mothers on phenytoin or phenobarbital monotherapy (86).

Interactions

Serum levels drop when carbamazepine is administered in combination with phenytoin, phenobarbital, or primidone (87). The addition of carbamazepine decreases the clearance and increases the plasma concentration of phenytoin (88), but does not appear to change the plasma concentration of phenobarbital, although carbamazepine may cause an increase in the plasma concentration of phenobarbital derived from primidone. It increases the clearance of ethosuximide and valproic acid. A reduction in the plasma concentration and elimination half-life of clonazepam has also been observed (87). Carbamazepine may accelerate the metabolism of warfarin as well as tetracycline, and may also increase or induce bradycardia resulting from digitalis. On theoretical grounds an interaction would be expected to occur between carbamazepine and monoamine oxidase inhibitors, but no cases have been reported so far. Propoxyphene may increase carbamazepine levels to toxicity but without change in the epoxide.

Psychotropic Effects

The psychotropic effects of carbamazepine in epileptic patients are still somewhat controversial. Since most reports deal with the subjective impressions of a relatively few patients who tend to be on complex medication regimens, caution is indicated in interpretating the results.

Our own acute, double-blind study (89) failed to demonstrate a psychotropic effect when a large variety of behavioral and neuropsychologic scales was used, but the study had two potential drawbacks. One was that it lasted for only 3 weeks, which may have been an inadequate amount of time in which to demonstrate significant objective behavioral changes. The other was that carbamazepine was merely added to phenytoin and phenobarbital; a better method would have been the simultaneous withdrawal of one of the other two compounds. Although statistical evaluation did not bear out the presence of psychotropic effects, several patients were improved emotionally on carbamazepine.

The statistical results from other double-blind studies are somewhat more encouraging. When the effectiveness of carbamazepine versus primidone was investigated, it was found that patients scored higher on the psychopathic deviate scale of the Minnesota Multiphasic Personality Inventory while taking primidone than while taking carbamazepine ($p < 0.01$). There was also a significantly greater impairment in repeatable cognitive perceptual motor tests with primidone than with carbamazepine (90). Troupin et al. (91) reported fewer errors on tasks requiring attention and problem solving when patients were taking carbamazepine rather than phenytoin. Patients scored slightly better on all MMPI scales when they were using carbamazepine, but only the F scale was affected to a statistically significant degree. A study of children using carbamazepine by Groh (92) showed an increase in drive level and mood improvement.

Evidence is accumulating that carbamazepine may have greater promise as a psychotropic agent in nonepileptic patients than epileptologists have been able to prove in the past. This may be due to the fact that neurologists have used carbamazepine mainly in combination with other anticonvulsants. This practice may mask its psychotropic properties because of the sedative effects of comedications and the fact that maximum therapeutic levels of carbamazepine may not be attainable. If carbamazepine is given as a single drug, therapeutic levels of 7–10 μg/ml can readily be obtained in the vast majority of patients with 600–800 mg/day, but in the presence of one and especially two anticonvulsants, this goal may not be attainable at all. It is therefore recommended that, whenever possible, carbamazepine be given as a single drug.

BENZODIAZEPINES

The benzodiazepines occupy an intermediate position between anticonvulsants and psychotropic drugs. Diazepam, chlordiazepoxide, clorazepate, as well as oxazepam have some anticonvulsant properties but are more effective as anxiolytic agents. Clonazepam has no appreciable psychotropic properties and is used exclusively as an anticonvulsant. Because of frequent undesirable side effects, limited efficacy, interaction with other anticonvulsants, and the fact that blood level determinations require electron capture techniques that are not available in all laboratories, the clinical usefulness of clonazepam tends to be limited to otherwise intractable patients.

Diazepam has received widespread acceptance as an anticonvulsant mainly because of the work of Gastaut et al. (93), which demonstrated its usefulness in the termination of status epilepticus. It has become the drug of first choice for this condition, and is given slowly in a 10- to 20-mg intravenous dose. Since it has a half-life of <1 h, seizures tend to recur within 0.5–1 h if the patient has even moderately severe status epilepticus. Therefore, additional anticonvulsant medications in the form of either intravenous phenytoin (18 mg/kg) or sodium amytal (500 mg) should be given. Orally, diazepam is rapidly absorbed, and peak blood levels are reached within 30–90 min. Rectal absorption is even more rapid: A 0.5- or 1-mg/kg dose via rectal tube resulted in peak plasma concentrations of 300–800 ng/ml within 4–5 min or of 600–1,400 ng/ml within 10–60 min. In infants and children under 11 years of age, administration of 1 mg/kg gives plasma levels of about 500 ng/ml, consistent with acute seizure control, within 10 min. Suppositories are not useful because of delayed peak and low plasma levels.

The drug is metabolized in the liver, mainly to *N*-desmethyldiazepam and *N*-methyloxazepam (94). *N*-Desmethyldiazepam has significant anticonvulsant, sedative, as well as anxiolytic properties, and clorazepate's effectiveness may be entirely due to that compound. Diazepam is highly protein bound to albumin (96–97 percent), but apparently does not displace phenytoin from its binding sites. Hypoalbuminemia may be associated with toxic symptoms resulting from relatively small doses (95). It has no effect on the plasma levels of warfarin, tricyclic antidepressants, or ethanol, but its absorption is enhanced in the presence of ethanol. The relationship between dose and plasma level, especially for oral ingestion, is quite poor, and it is not possible to make accurate predictions. The recommended dose for long-term treatment for adult patients is 0.2–0.4 mg/kg.

It needs to be emphasized that diazepam is not a primary anticonvulsant, and significant seizure control cannot be expected at these doses. Its main usefulness resides in its anxiolytic properties, but since tolerance appears to develop, it is best to limit its administration to acute stress reactions. Long-term treatment over several years is rarely indicated in epileptic patients.

The side effects from oral administration are usually minor and consist of drowsiness, dizziness, and ataxia. Ataxia may be due, however, to an interaction with other anticonvulsants, especially phenytoin. In children, irritability, inattention, and hypotonia have been reported with diazepam. Other side effects are quite rare, and teratogenicity has not been proven.

On intravenous administration of diazepam, the most serious side effects are apnea, hypotension, and cardiac arrest. It is therefore essential that the drug not be given as a bolus, but at an injection rate not exceeding 5 mg/min. Even under these circumstances, it is advisable to have equipment and personnel available for cardiopulmonary resuscitation if necessary. When injected into a small vein, or as a result of precipitates developing when the compound is mixed with saline solution, thrombophlebitis may occur. Accidental intraarterial administration must be avoided since it can lead to extensive tissue necrosis.

Whereas diazepam and chlorazepate are used mainly in primary generalized seizures (especially myoclonic attacks and absences), chlordiazepoxide in doses between 20 and 75 mg seems to be more useful at times as an adjunct in the treatment of partial complex (temporal lobe or psychomotor) seizures. An occasional side effect, which may limit its use in patients who have a tendency toward acting out, is increased aggressivity, and the drug may have to be discontinued under these circumstances.

OTHER PSYCHOTROPIC AGENTS

Antipsychotic agents can be used safely when needed in epileptic patients, provided anticonvulsant levels are maintained in the therapeutic range. This author has used mainly trifluoperazine and haloperidol with considerable success, especially in the interictal or postictal psychoses that occur at times in patients with complex partial seizures. The duration of the psychosis can be dramatically shortened to a few days, but it is important that the initial doses be given parenterally. These psychoses frequently have a paranoid character, and patients may refuse oral medications or pretend to take it but subsequently remove it when no longer observed. This can have dangerous consequences because anticonvulsant medications are not taken under these circumstances either, and recurrent seizures, possibly even status epilepticus, may appear. Five milligrams of haloperidol intramuscularly, repeated if needed at 4- to 8-h intervals for the first 24 h, is usually sufficient to break through the initial agitation and combativeness. The patient then can be maintained on oral medications for another 7–10 days. By that time an interictal or postictal psychosis usually has subsided sufficiently that antipsychotic medication can be either discontinued altogether or markedly reduced.

It is important to know the patient's history in detail so that an idiosyncratic reaction to certain anticonvulsant drugs can be excluded. This would merely be masked by the antipsychotic agent and would persist as long as the offending drug is given. Idiosyncratic psychotic reactions tend to occur within the first 3–6 months after that particular anticonvulsant has been prescribed. They are unlikely to be due to drug reaction if the patient has been on this medication regimen for 6 months to 1 year.

The single most psychotogenic drug on the market for seizure disorders is phenacemide. Although it is very effective at times in patients with complex partial seizures, it produced, in the author's personal experience, psychoses with such regularity that its use has been practically abandoned. Methsuximide, ethosuximide, and primidone may also cause psychoses, but this side effect as a result of phenytoin, phenobarbital, carbamazepine, or valproate has not been encountered by this author.

The antidepressant drugs can also be used safely, provided that anticonvulsant levels are carefully supervised and not allowed to drop below the middle therapeutic range. This applies to monoamine oxidase inhibitors as well as the tricyclics. Although the literature contains several references to the convulsant properties of imipramine especially (96–99), its use does not tend to be a problem in the treatment of epileptic patients unless the dose is suddenly raised sharply or anticonvulsant levels are allowed to drop. There is some suggestion from the work of Fromm et al. (100) that imipramine may have a diphasic action. At doses of 0.7–3.5 mg/kg and resultant levels of 40–120 μg/ml, it was found to have anticonvulsant properties in patients with absence and myoclonic-astatic seizures.

The use of lithium in patients with known seizure disorders is controversial at this time and requires further controlled studies. The literature gives evidence for the aggravation (101–103) as well as the improvement (104,105) of behavior and/or seizures. At the present time, psychiatrists would be well advised to use lithium with caution in patients who have moderately severe to severe epilepsy. Therapy should be initiated in the hospital with careful supervision of anticonvulsant levels, lithium levels, and the EEG. Deterioration of the EEG can occur in the presence of therapeutic lithium levels and outlast the discontinuation of the drug by several weeks.

Thioridazine in doses up to 200 mg is beneficial at times, especially because it has mild anticonvulsant properties as well. On rare occasions idiosyncrasy may lead to the precipitation of seizures. (In two of our cases, seizures occurred within 3–4 h of the first dose after several months of seizure freedom; this may, of course, have been mere coincidence.) This is so rare that it should not lead to the avoidance or discontinuation of the use of the drug. Although we have seen EEG and clinical seizure deterioration that mandated the discontinuation of lithium, this has not occurred with thioridazine. The most problematic side effects of the latter are drowsiness and lethargy, which limit its usefulness in outpatient treatment by interfering with either school or employment.

Aggressive acting-out behavior can be a serious problem, especially in adolescents and young adults. Antipsychotic drugs as well as lithium may be effective. However, this behavior tends to be difficult to treat medically, because social factors in the home situation frequently also are responsible in part, and these may not be rectifiable. Under these circumstances it is important that the anticonvulsant regimen be such that it does not contribute to an individual's aggressiveness. Phenobarbital, primidone, as well as chlordiazepoxide should therefore be avoided.

FOLATE AND PSYCHIATRIC DISORDERS

The role of folate in the genesis of psychiatric problems in epileptic patients is also still somewhat controversial. In the past two decades, many papers have been published that link folate deficiency to chronic anticonvulsant intake and psychiatric symptoms, especially depression. This has been disputed, and the book by Botez and Reynolds (106) provides an up-to-date, state-of-the-art report.

We have studied the question in 140 patients hospitalized for seizures with or without associated mental changes and have found, in agreement with Reynolds et al. (107), that lower folate levels are more common in epileptic patients than in the general population, and that levels of <3 ng/ml are associated with a statistically significant degree with depression as seen on psychological tests. There was no relationship to other psychiatric findings in this sample of patients.

It is advisable, therefore, to keep the possible contribution of folate deficiency, especially to depressive symptomatology, in mind, and to obtain plasma and red blood cell folate levels in these patients. Folate and B_{12} levels are not significantly correlated. It appears that folate deficiency, when symptomatic at all, may show itself mainly in mental changes, whereas pure B_{12} deficiency tends to result more commonly in spinal cord pathology. In spite of some suggestions in the literature that folate supplements may cause an increase in seizures (108, 109), it has been the experience of the author that these can be given safely in doses of 1–5 mg/day provided that anticonvulsant levels are kept stable.

PROBLEMS OF CHILDBEARING

The psychiatrist may be asked by female patients or relatives about the advisability of having children and the teratogenic effects of anticonvulsant medications. These questions have to be answered on an individual basis. The risk of having an epileptic child for a parent with epilepsy is increased 3.2 times over that for the general population (110). The risk increases further when both parents have epilepsy. On the other hand, if there is only a hereditary trait without associated cerebral injury, the seizure disorders tend to be relatively easily controllable, especially when the patients are treated immediately after the first seizure. If the problem is compounded by pre- or perinatal CNS damage or cerebral infection (especially in childhood), the result may be an individual who has a very serious, lifelong illness that may be uncontrollable. The prospective parents should know about these risks and make every effort to ensure excellent pre-, peri-, and postnatal care.

Great individual variability exists in regard to seizure frequency during pregnancy. Progesterone has anticonvulsant properties, and some prospective mothers are seizurefree during their pregnancies on amounts of anticonvulsant medication that had not been fully effective before or after the pregnancy. In case of a multipara, one can be guided by the history. Anticonvulsant levels tend to drop in most instances because the drugs are in part siphoned off into the baby and because there may also be changes in protein binding. Under ordinary circumstances it is not necessary to "treat the level"; it is essential, however, that the regimen that had been initiated prior to pregnancy be adjusted if either toxic symptoms or excess of seizures occurs. In the author's personal practice, the patient is merely followed at regular intervals throughout the pregnancy with anticonvulsant level determinations and no changes are made unless dictated by clinical necessity. At the time of delivery, the patient must continue with her anticonvulsant regimen, and "NPO" orders should not apply to anticonvulsants when given with one sip of water. This principle is also important when patients go to surgery for any other reason.

The risk of congenital malformation has already been discussed under the individual drugs, but it is, in all probability, somewhat enhanced if there is a family history of congenital malformations. This is part of the information the physician should have available during the counseling of individual patients. On the other hand, if a woman has already given birth to a healthy child, chances that subsequent children will be deformed as a result of the same anticonvulsant she had taken previously are, in all probability, considerably lessened. Fortunately, the malformations reported in association with the various anticonvulsants tended to be relatively mild and surgically correctable, if they occurred in otherwise healthy families.

CONCLUSION

Psychiatrists intermittently have to treat patients with seizure disorders and should therefore be familiar with the principles of anticonvulsant therapy. Unfortunately, many patients are still not cared for according to current standards of modern anticonvulsant treatment.

The most important principle is that the anticonvulsant regimen be kept as simple as possible, with one or maximally two drugs, supervised by anticonvulsant level determinations, and one psychotropic agent when needed. Under these circumstances, interactions and toxicity can be minimized, and psychotherapy can be carried out most successfully.

REFERENCES

1. Morselli PL, Franco-Morselli R: Clinical pharmacokinetics of antiepileptic drugs in adults. *Pharmacol Ther* 10:65–101, 1980
2. Richens A: Clinical pharmacokinetics of phenytoin. *Clin Pharmacokinet* 4:153–169, 1979
3. Chang T, Glazko AJ: Phenytoin. Biotransformation, in *Antiepileptic Drugs*. Edited by Woodbury DM, Penry JK, Pippenger CE. New York, Raven Press, 1982, pp 209–226
4. Woodbury DM: Phenytoin. Absorption, distribution, and excretion, in *Antiepileptic Drugs*. Edited by Woodbury DM, Penry JK, Pippenger CE. New York, Raven Press, 1982, pp 191–207
5. Wilder BJ, Serrano EE, Ramsay RE: Plasma diphenylhydantoin levels after loading and maintenance doses. *Clin Pharmacol Ther* 14:797–801, 1973
6. Kutt H, Winters W, Kokenge R, et al: Diphenylhydantoin metabolism, blood levels and toxicity. *Arch Neurol* 11:642–648, 1964
7. Kaspar U: Diphenylhydantoin [German]. *Schweiz Rundsch Med Prax* 69:795–802, 1980
8. Jungi WF, Senn HJ, Stanisic M, et al: Malignant lymphoma following years of hydantoin treatment for epilepsy [German]. *Schweiz Med Wochenschr* 105:1735–1737, 1975
9. Vogel RI: Gingival hyperplasia and folic acid deficiency from anticonvulsive drug therapy: a theoretical relationship. *J Theor Biol* 67:269–278, 1977
10. Aarli JA: Phenytoin-induced depression of salivary IgA and gingival hyperplasia. *Epilepsia* 17:283–291, 1976
11. Girgis SS, Staple PH, Miller WA, et al: Dental root abnormalities and gingival overgrowth in epileptic patients receiving anticonvulsant therapy. *J Periodontol* 51:474–482, 1980
12. Dreyer WP, Thomas CJ: Diphenylhydantoinate-induced hyperplasia of the masticatory mucosa in an edentulous epileptic patient. *Oral Surg* 45:701–706, 1978
13. Stogmann W: Disturbances of calcium-phosphate-metabolism by anticonvulsant drugs in relation to their serum concentration [German]. *Paediatr Pathol* 14:89–95, 1979
14. Rasmussen S, Kristensen M: Choreoathetosis during phenytoin treatment. *Acta Med Scand* 201:239–241, 1977
15. Chadwick D, Reynolds EH, Marsden CD: Anticonvulsant-induced dyskinesias: a comparison with dyskinesias induced by neuroleptics. *J Neurol Neurosurg Psychiatry* 39:1210–1218, 1976
16. Iivanainen M, Viukar M, Helle EP: Cerebellar atrophy in phenytoin-treated mentally retarded epileptics. *Epilepsia* 18:375–386, 1977

17. Koller WC, Glatt SL, Fox JH: Phenytoin-induced cerebellar degeneration. *Ann Neurol* 8:203–204, 1980

18. Meistrup-Larsen KI, Hermann S, Permin H: Chronic diphenylhydantoin encephalopathy in mentally retarded children and adolescents with severe epilepsy. *Acta Neurol Scand* 60:50–55, 1979

19. Spector RH, Davidoff RA, Schwartzman RJ: Phenytoin-induced ophthalmoplegia. *Neurology (New York)* 26:1031–1034, 1976

20. Guiloff RJ, Whiteley A, Kelly RE: Organic convergence spasm. *Acta Neurol Scand* 61:252–259, 1980

21. Sheth KJ, Casper JT, Good TA: Interstitial nephritis due to phenytoin hypersensitivity. *J Pediatr* 91:438–441, 1977

22. Agarwal BN, Cabebe FG, Hoffman BI: Diphenylhydantoin-induced acute renal failure. *Nephron* 18:249–251, 1977

23. Lee TJ, Carney CN, Lapis JL, et al: Diphenylhydantoin-induced hepatic necrosis. A case study. *Gastroenterology* 70:422–424, 1976

24. Finucane JF, Griffiths RS: Effect of phenytoin therapy on thyroid function. *Br J Clin Pharmacol* 3:1041–1044, 1976

25. Heyma P, Larkins RG, Perry-Keene D, et al: Thyroid hormone levels and protein binding in patients on long-term diphenylhydantoin treatment. *Clin Endocrinol (Oxf)* 6:369–376, 1977

26. Aanderud S, Strandjord RE: Hypothyroidism induced by antiepileptic therapy. *Acta Neurol Scand* 61:330–332, 1980

27. Kaspar U: Diphenylhydantoin [German]. *Schweiz Rundsch Med Prax* 69:795–802, 1980

28. Bustamante SA, Stumpff LC: Fetal hydantoin syndrome in triplets. A unique experiment of nature. *Am J Dis Child* 132:978–979, 1978

29. Vree TB, Henderson PT, van der Kleijn E, et al: Drug interactions at the metabolic level: a reality in drug treatment of epilepsy, in *Clinical Pharmacology of Antiepileptic Drugs*. Edited by Schneider H, Janz D, Gardner-Thorpe C, et al. Berlin, Springer-Verlag, 1975, pp 34–42

30. Kutt H, Paris-Kutt H: Phenobarbital. Interactions with other drugs, in *Antiepileptic Drugs*. Edited by Woodbury DM, Penry JK, Pippenger CE. New York, Raven Press, 1982, pp 329–340

31. Neuvonen PF, Lehtovaara R, Bardy A, et al: Antipyretic analgesics in patients on antiepileptic drug therapy. *Eur J Clin Pharmacol* 15:263–268, 1979

32. Olanow CW, Fin AL, Prussak C: The effect of salicylate on the pharmacokinetics of phenytoin. *Neurology (New York)* 31:341–342, 1981

33. Inoue F, Walsh RJ: Folate supplements and phenytoin-salicylate interaction. *Neurology (New York)* 33:115–116, 1983

34. Miller RR, Porter J, Greenblatt DJ: Clinical importance of the interaction of phenytoin and isoniazid. *Chest* 75:356–358, 1979

35. Geering JM, Ruch W, Dettli L: Diphenylhydantoin poisoning due to diphenylhydantoin-isoniazid interaction [German]. *Schweiz Med Wochenschr* 104:1224–1228, 1974

36. Johnson J, Freeman HL: Death due to isoniazid (INH) and phenytoin. *Br J Psychiatry* 129:511, 1976

37. Skovsted L, Kristensen M, Hansen JM, et al: The effect of different oral anticoagulants on diphenylhydantoin (DPH) and tolbutamide metabolism. *Acta Med Scand* 199:513–515, 1976

38. Hansen JM, Kampmann JP, Siersbaek-Nielsen K, et al: The effect of different sulfonamides on phenytoin metabolism in man. *Acta Med Scand (Suppl)* 624:106–110, 1979

39. Koup JR, Gibalki M, McNamara P, et al: Interaction of chloramphenicol with phenytoin and phenobarbital. *Clin Pharmacol Ther* 24:571–575, 1978

40. Rose JQ, Choi HK, Schentag JJ, et al: Intoxication caused by interaction of chloramphenicol and phenytoin. *JAMA* 237:2630-2631, 1977

41. Heipertz R, Pilz H: Interaction of nitrofurantoin with diphenylhydantoin. *J Neurol* 218:297–301, 1978

42. Fincham RW, Wiley DE, Schottelius DD: Use of phenytoin serum levels in a case of status epilepticus. *Neurology (Minneap)* 26:879–881, 1976

43. Pippenger CE, Siris JH, Werner WL, et al: The effects of psychotropic drugs on serum antiepileptic levels in psychiatric patients with seizure disorders, in *Clinical Pharmacology of Antiepileptic Drugs*. Edited by Schneider H, Janz D, Gardner-Thorpe C, et al. Berlin, Springer-Verlag, 1975, pp 135–144

44. Dreyfus J. *A Remarkable Medicine Has Been Overlooked*. New York, Simon & Schuster, 1981

45. Parnas J, Flachs H, Gram L: Psychotropic effect of antiepileptic drugs. *Acta Neurol Scand* 60:329–343, 1979

46. Maynert EW: Phenobarbital. Absorption, distribution, and excretion, in *Antiepileptic Drugs*. Edited by Woodbury DM, Penry JK, Pippenger CE. New York, Raven Press, 1982, pp 309–317

47. Booker HE: Phenobarbital. Relation of plasma concentration to seizure control, in *Antiepileptic Drugs*. Edited by Woodbury DM, Penry JK, Pippenger CE. New York, Raven Press, 1982, pp 341–350

48. Maynert EW: Phenobarbital. Biotransformation, in *Antiepileptic Drugs*. Edited by Woodbury DM, Penry JK, Pippenger CE. New York, Raven Press, 1982, pp 319–327

49. Buchthal F, Svensmark O: Serum phenobarbital and phenytoin as related to EEG findings and anticonvulsant effects. *Acta Psychiatr Neurol Scand* 36 (suppl 150):208–210, 1961

50. Mattson RH, Cramer JA: Phenobarbital. Toxicity, in *Antiepileptic*

Drugs. Edited by Woodbury DM, Penry JK, Pippenger CE. New York, Raven Press, 1982, pp 351–362

51. Camfield CS, Chaplin S, Doyle AB, et al: Side effects of phenobarbital in toddlers: behavioral and cognitive aspects. *J Pediatr* 95:361–365, 1979
52. MacLeod CM, Dekaban AS, Hung E: Memory impairment in epileptic patients: selective effects of phenobarbital concentration. *Science* 202:1102–1103, 1978
53. Cordes CK: Chronic drug intoxication causing pseudoretardation in a young child. *J Am Acad Child Psychiatry* 12:215–222, 1973
54. Reynolds EH, Travers RD: Serum anticonvulsant concentrations in epileptic patients with mental symptoms: a preliminary report. *Br J Psychiatry* 124:440–445, 1974
55. Mattson RH, Gallagher BB, Reynolds EG, et al: Folate therapy in epilepsy: a controlled study. *Arch Neurol* 29:78–81, 1973
56. Hempel E, Klinger W: Drug stimulated biotransformation of hormonal steroid contraceptives: clinical implications. *Drugs* 12:442–448, 1976
57. Bogue JY, Carrington HC: The evaluation of "Mysoline"—a new anticonvulsant drug. *Br J Pharmacol* 8:230–236, 1953
58. Schottelius DD: Primidone. Absorption, distribution, and excretion, in *Antiepileptic Drugs*. Edited by Woodbury DM, Penry JK, Pippenger CE. New York, Raven Press, 1982, pp 405–413
59. Leppik IE, Cloyd JC: Primidone. Toxicity, in *Antiepileptic Drugs*. Edited by Woodbury DM, Penry JK, Pippenger CE. New York, Raven Press, 1982, pp 441–447
60. Fincham RW, Schottelius DD: Primidone. Interactions with other drugs, in *Antiepileptic Drugs*. Edited by Woodbury DM, Penry JK, Pippenger CE. New York, Raven Press, 1982, pp 421–427
61. Levy RH, Lai AA: Valproate. Absorption, distribution, and excretion, in *Antiepileptic Drugs*. Edited by Woodbury DM, Penry JK, Pippenger CE. New York, Raven Press, 1982, pp 555–578
62. Schobben F, van der Kleijn E: Valproate. Biotransformation, in *Antiepileptic Drugs*. Edited by Woodbury DM, Penry JK, Pippenger CE. New York, Raven Press, 1982, pp 567–578
63. Haidukewych D, Rodin EA: Monitoring free valproic acid in epilepsy patients medicated with coanticonvulsants. *Ther Drug Monit* 4:209–212, 1982
64. Jeavons PM: Valproate. Toxicity, in *Antiepileptic Drugs*. Edited by Woodbury DM, Penry JK, Pippenger CE. New York, Raven Press, 1982, pp 601–610
65. Mattson RH, Cramer JA: Valproic acid and ethosuximide interaction. *Ann Neurol* 7:583–584, 1980

66. Mattson RH: Valproate. Interactions with other drugs, in *Antiepileptic Drugs*. Edited by Woodbury DM, Penry JK, Pippenger CE. New York, Raven Press, 1982, pp 579–589

67. Glazko AJ: Ethosuximide. Chemistry and methods of determination, in *Antiepileptic Drugs*. Edited by Woodbury DM, Penry JK, Pippenger CE. New York, Raven Press, 1982, pp 617–622

68. Chang T, Glazko AJ: Ethosuximide. Biotransformation, in *Antiepileptic Drugs*. Edited by Woodbury DM, Penry JK, Pippenger CE. New York, Raven Press, 1982, pp 631–635

69. Glazko AJ, Chang T: Ethosuximide. Absorption, distribution, and excretion, in *Antiepileptic Drugs*. Edited by Woodbury DM, Penry JK, Pippenger CE. New York, Raven Press, 1982, pp 623–629

70. Sherwin AL: Ethosuximide. Relation of plasma concentration to seizure control, in *Antiepileptic Drugs*. Edited by Woodbury DM, Penry JK, Pippenger CE. New York, Raven Press, 1982, pp 637–645

71. Dreifuss FE: Ethosuximide. Toxicity, in *Antiepileptic Drugs*. Edited by Woodbury DM, Penry JK, Pippenger CE. New York, Raven Press, 1982, pp 647–651

72. Kutt H, Paris-Kutt H: Carbamazepine. Chemistry and methods of determination, in *Antiepileptic Drugs*. Edited by Woodbury DM, Penry JK, Pippenger CE. New York, Raven Press, 1982, pp 453–463

73. Morselli PL, Bossi L: Carbamazepine. Absorption, distribution, and excretion, in *Antiepileptic Drugs*. Edited by Woodbury DM, Penry JK, Pippenger CE. New York, Raven Press, 1982, pp 465–482

74. Morselli PL: Clinical pharmacokinetics in neonates. *Clin Pharmacokinet* 1:81–98, 1976

75. Faigle JW, Feldmann KF: Carbamazepine. Biotransformation, in *Antiepileptic Drugs*. Edited by Woodbury DM, Penry JK, Pippenger CE, New York, Raven Press, 1982, pp 483–495

76. Cereghino JJ: Carbamazepine. Relation of plasma concentration to seizure control, in *Antiepileptic Drugs*. Edited by Woodbury DM, Penry JK, Pippenger CE. New York, Raven Press, 1982, pp 507–519

77. Johannessen SI, Strandjord RF: Concentration of carbamazepine (Tegretol) in serum and in cerebrospinal fluid in patients with epilepsy. *Epilepsia* 14:373–379, 1973

78. Strandjord RE, Johannessen SI: Single drug therapy with carbamazepine in patients with epilepsy: serum levels and clinical effect. *Epilepsia* 21:655–662, 1980

79. Schneider H: Carbamazepine: an attempt to correlate serum levels with antiepileptic and side effects, in *Clinical Pharmacology of Antiepileptic Drugs*. Edited by Schneider H, Janz D, Gardner-Thorpe C, et al. New York, Springer-Verlag, 1975, pp 151–158

80. Hoppener RJ, Kuyer A, Meijer JWA, et al: Correlation between daily fluctuations of carbamazepine serum levels and intermittent side effects. *Epilepsia* 21:341–350, 1980

81. Stephens WP, Epsir MLE, Tattersall RB, et al: Water intoxication due to carbamazepine. *Br Med J* 1:754–755, 1977

82. Ashton MG, Ball SG, Thomas TH, et al: Water intoxication associated with carbamazepine treatment. *Br Med J* 1:1134–1135, 1977

83. Perucca E, Richens A: Water intoxication produced by carbamazepine and its reversal by phenytoin. *Br J Clin Pharmacol* 9:302P, 1980

84. Hart RG, Easton JD: Carbamazepine and hematological monitoring. *Ann Neurol* 11:309–311, 1982

85. Pisciotta AV: Carbamazepine. Hematological toxicity, in *Antiepileptic Drugs*. Edited by Woodbury DM, Penry JK, Pippenger CE. New York, Raven Press, 1982, pp 533–541

86. Iivanainen M: Effect of antiepileptic drugs on human body maturation, in *Antiepileptic Drug Therapy in Pediatrics*. Edited by Morselli PL, Penry JK, Pippenger CE. New York, Raven Press, 1983, pp 65–73

87. Levy RH, Pitlick WH: Carbamazepine. Interactions with other drugs, in *Antiepileptic Drugs*. Edited by Woodbury DM, Penry JK, Pippenger CE. New York, Raven Press, 1982, pp 497–505

88. Gratz ES, Theodore WH, Newmark ME, et al: Effect of carbamazepine on phenytoin clearance in patients with complex partial seizures. *Neurology (New York)* 32 (part 2):A223, 1982

89. Rodin EA, Rim CS, Rennick PM: The effect of carbamazepine on patients with psychomotor epilepsy: results of a double-blind study. *Epilepsia* 15:547–561, 1974

90. Rodin EA, Rim CS, Kitano H, et al: A comparison of the effectiveness of primidone versus carbamazepine in epileptic outpatients. *J Nerv Ment Dis* 163:41–46, 1976

91. Troupin A, Ojemann LM, Halpern L, et al: Carbamazepine—a double-blind comparison with phenytoin. *Neurology (Minneap)* 27:511–519, 1977

92. Groh C: The psychotropic effect of Tegretol in non-epileptic children with particular reference to the drug's indications, in *Epileptic Seizures—Behaviour—Pain*. Edited by Birkmayer W. Berne, Hans Huber, 1976, pp 259–263

93. Gastaut H, Naquet R, Poire R, et al: Treatment of status epilepticus with diazepam. *Epilepsia* 6:167–182, 1965

94. Schmidt D: Benzodiazepines. Diazepam, in *Antiepileptic Drugs*. Edited by Woodbury DM, Penry JK, Pippenger CE. New York, Raven Press, 1982, pp 711–735

95. Greenblatt DJ, Koch-Weser J: Clinical toxicity of chlordiazepoxide and diazepam in relation to serum albumin concentration: a report from the Boston Collaborative Drug Surveillance Program. *Eur J Clin Pharmacol* 7:259–262, 1974

96. Trimble M: Non-monoamine oxidase inhibitor antidepressants and epilepsy: a review. *Epilepsia* 19:241–250, 1978

97. Petti TA, Campbell M: Imipramine and seizures. *Am J Psychiatry* 132:539–540, 1975

98. Legg NF, Swash M: Clinical note: seizures and EEG activation after trimipramine. *Epilepsia* 15:131–135, 1974

99. Schulze B: Problem of drug-induced cerebral reactions—a case of myoclonic state under treatment with tricyclic antidepressive agents [German]. *Nervenarzt* 43:332–336, 1972

100. Fromm GH, Wessel HB, Glass JD, et al: Imipramine in absence and myoclonic-astatic seizures. *Neurology (Minneap)* 28:953–957, 1978

101. Lauter H. Middelhoff HD: Epilepsy caused by lithium therapy [German]. *Nervenarzt* 40:549–551, 1969

102. Demers R, Lukesh R, Prichard J: Convulsion during lithium therapy. *Lancet* 2:315, 1970

103. Jus A, Villeneuve A, Gautier J, et al: Some remarks on the influence of lithium carbonate on patients with temporal epilepsy. *Int J Clin Pharmacol* 7:67–74, 1973

104. Erwin CW, Gerber CJ, Morrison DS, et al: Lithium carbonate and convulsive disorders. *Arch Gen Psychiatry* 28:646–648, 1973

105. Kavallinis GP: Lithium in epilepsy. *Clin Electroencephalogr* 8:51–56, 1977

106. Botez MI, Reynolds EH (eds): *Folic Acid in Neurology, Psychiatry, and Internal Medicine*. New York, Raven Press, 1979

107. Reynolds EH, Chanarin I, Milner G, et al: Anticonvulsant therapy, folic acid and vitamin B_{12} metabolism and mental symptoms. *Epilepsia* 7:261–270, 1966

108. Reynolds EH: Effects of folic acid on the mental state and fit-frequency of drug-treated epileptic patients. *Lancet* 1:1086–1088, 1967

109. Chanarin I, Laidlaw J, Loughridge LW, et al: Megaloblastic anaemia due to phenobarbitone. The convulsant action of therapeutic doses of folic acid. *Br Med J* 1:1099–1102, 1960

110. Annegers JF, Hauser WA: The risk of seizure disorders among relatives of patients with epilepsy, in *Epilepsy, Pregnancy, and the Child*, Edited by Janz D, Dam M, Richens A. New York, Raven Press, 1982, pp 509–520

5

Epileptic and Pseudoepileptic Seizures: Differential Diagnostic Considerations

Ernst Rodin, M.D.

The differential diagnosis of epileptic from other forms of short-lived episodic behavioral derangements has been discussed extensively in various recent publications (1–3). This chapter, therefore, will rely mainly on the personal experience of the author.

In order to diagnose epilepsy, as well as the type or types of epileptic seizures a patient is having, the physician must have an accurate history by a reliable observer and must also be thoroughly familiar with the pathophysiologic mechanisms that operate in the most common seizure types discussed below. Since the days of Charcot, it has been well known that "hysteria" can mimic organic disease. Unless one has some understanding of functional neurophysiology, it can become very difficult to distinguish between attacks that result from excessive neuronal firing in the brain, i.e., epileptic seizures, and those in which other mechanisms are operative, especially those of a psychogenic nature.

The problem is compounded further by the fact that a number of patients with proven epileptic seizures also have psychogenic attacks that mimic organic ones. These are due to acute stress reactions, attention-getting mechanisms, or the need of the patient for invalidism. The precise processes underlying hysteria as opposed to outright malingering are still poorly understood. Emotional factors are paramount; however, symptom choice (namely, attacks versus paralysis, anesthesia, etc.) may well depend on constitutional factors in the sense of Adler's organ inferiority concept. Slater's follow-up study (4) of patients who had been diagnosed as hysteric is quite sobering, because in at least one-third the hysterical symptom was merely the initial expression of an organic process. Instead of the prevailing trend to dichotomize disorders as either "organic" or "psychogenic," it is much more useful to think in terms of the relative contributions of organic pathology and psychogenic elements to a given symptom at a given time.

Neurologists currently do not agree on a uniform term to denote attacks that appear to be epileptic but are not. The terms "hysterical," "psychogenic," and "pseudoseizures" are most commonly used. The first is pejorative, and the last, although currently in vogue, is not accurate because the patient is having a seizure that is not epileptic. The term "psychogenic" focuses on etiology, and has been objected to because, on occasion, genuine epileptic attacks can be precipitated by emotional stress. Fenton (5) has therefore used the term "pseudoepileptic seizure" for attacks that are clinically similar to epileptic seizures but are not due to cerebral epileptic mechanisms.

Since the attacks are also influenced by sociocultural factors, we no longer see the typical "grande hystérie" as described by Charcot, and since pseudoepileptic seizures are protean in their manifestations, even in the same patient, it is not useful to describe everything that could happen during an attack. It is therefore better to acquaint the psychiatrist in some detail with the clinical features of epileptic seizures, using mainly the terms of the International Classification of Epileptic Seizures (6).

GENERALIZED CONVULSIVE SEIZURES (GRAND MAL)

Nonfocal grand mal has been reclassified as primary generalized, and focal onset grand mal as secondary generalized tonic-clonic seizures. Before entering into the fine distinctions, which are open to dispute at times, the common features and typical sequence of events during a tonic-clonic seizure need to be reemphasized.

First, there is sudden unresponsiveness and loss of consciousness associated with loss of postural tone, resulting in a hard fall unless the patient is in the prone position. The head may initially be turned to one side (not necessarily to the same side in different attacks), and there is flexion and some abduction of the upper and lower extremities. At that point the mouth is opened widely, and a cry or guttural noise may be emitted. This lasts for <10 s. The tonic phase follows, during which the mouth clenches tightly shut, and if the tongue gets caught it is severely bitten on the lateral edge. The head, if it had been turned to one side, returns to and remains rigidly fixed at the midline. The arms change from flexion and abduction to extension and adduction alongside the body, and the legs are likewise in extension. There may be spontaneous dorsiflexion of one big toe. The hands are partially flexed at the metacarpophalangeal joints with thumbs adducted but extended alongside the hand, similar to what is seen in a tetanic seizure. In secondary generalized tonic-clonic seizures, particularly those that arise from temporal lobe structures, when the arms, instead of being extended, are flexed across the chest, the hands may be fisted (7).

Constant maximal tonic firing lasts for <20 s and is followed by flexion clonus. The individual clonic jerks are symmetrical in the upper and lower extremities and last only a fraction of a second, but they repeat for about 30 s. These are not thrashing movements, but constitute intermittent inhibition of tonus. As neuronal firing decreases, the intervals between the myoclonic jerks lengthen from 1 to about 2 or 3 s, and the entire attack ends within 1 min of the onset. Bladder control tends to be lost during the tonic or clonic phase, but this appears to be dependent on the interval since the patient last voided. Bowel incontinence is quite rare. When it occurs at all, it is usually in a brain-damaged patient. Seminal emission is also exceedingly rare. Throughout the seizure the patient is apneic, and the apnea may persist for several seconds after the last clonic jerk, with resultant cyanosis.

At this point the patient is deeply comatose and areflexic, except that positive plantar signs may be elicited. The pupils are fixed and unresponsive to light. Respiration then returns with a deep inspiration frequently accompanied by a guttural sound. Initially, respirations are stertorous, and since there is frequently excessive salivation, the colloquial "frothing at the mouth" occurs at this time. This period tends to last 1 or 2 min, after which the patient either arouses spontaneously or becomes arousable, but is confused and may thrash around, especially if restrained. When left alone, the patient is likely to fall asleep for a variable period of time and subsequently awaken with amnesia for the events.

The tonic-clonic seizure is an orderly sequence of events that utilizes phylogenetically old pathways and, as such, is quite similar in rats, cats, monkeys, and humans. Only when the events as outlined above have occurred, in their proper sequence and duration, is one justified to make the diagnosis of a tonic-clonic or grand mal seizure. Although any one aspect of the tonic-clonic seizure may be retained in a pseudo-grand mal seizure, it will be out of sequence or unduly prolonged. One should mention, however, that the attack as described above occurs in this form only in patients who are intellectually intact. Patients with severe diffuse brain damage may produce more atypical attacks, but these are diagnostic problems found mainly in an institutional setting.

Typical of pseudoepileptic grand mal is the marked involvement of truncal musculature, with some opisthotonus (a complete arc de cercle is rare nowadays), pelvic thrusts, and thrashing movements in the ictal rather than postictal state. If the tongue is bitten at all, which is rare, the bite wounds are minor and occur either on the tip rather than the side of the tongue or on the lips rather than the cheeks. Loss of bladder control is uncommon, but may occur. Pupillary reaction to light is retained during the seizure, but this may be difficult to test when a patient is moving about actively. Side-to-side throwing of head and body are common but do not occur in a tonic-clonic seizure. The facial expression during a grand mal is characterized by trismus in the tonic phase and symmetrical twitching during clonus, whereas in pseudo-grand mal it reflects either repose or a variety of emotions including ecstasy. Injuries from falls are rare in pseudo-grand mal but can occur on occasion.

"Auras" may suggest pseudoepilepsy if they are highly complex, if they contain a great number of somatic or visceral sensations, and especially if they differ on different occasions. The epileptic aura signals the transition of the interictal firing of epileptogenic tissue into a continuous discharge that recruits additional neuronal circuits. Unless the patient has multifocal disease—which occurs only in cases of extensive brain damage and, as such, is diagnosable independently of epilepsy—the aura, if present at all, will be identical or at least highly similar in different attacks. Neither the presence nor absence of auras per se provides a differential diagnostic criterion, and the type of aura is also not reliable. An ascending sensation from the epigastrium was, around the turn of the century, regarded as hysterical and provided the origin of the term "globus hystericus." As now recognized, it occurs commonly in patients whose epileptic seizures originate in temporal lobe structures. Pain, on the other hand, in the body, extremities, or head, is exceedingly uncommon as an epileptic aura, and other etiologies for the attack should be sought. The only exception is provided by a seizure focus in the parietal area, but under these circumstances there is usually also numbness and additional spread to the motor cortex so that the affected extremity will show clonus.

There are also some patients who present with pseudo-status epilepticus. In organic status epilepticus, the patient does not regain consciousness in the postictal period but instead has further seizures separated by intervals of no more than 15–30 min. In the interictal state, the patient is comatose or at least stuporous. As status progresses the seizures become somewhat shorter and less vigorous, but there are never thrashing or throwing movements as commonly seen in pseudo-status epilepticus. It is most important to make the correct diagnosis immediately, because status epilepticus has to be treated vigorously to prevent possible death, whereas in pseudo-status epilepticus an opposite regimen needs to be pursued, as will be mentioned in detail later. The diagnosis should be verified by electroencephalography (EEG). There will always be seizure discharges in association with the attacks in status epilepticus, whereas pseudo-status, which may well occur in epileptic patients, shows only the individual's usual (interictal) tracing and muscle movement and electrode artefacts during the episode.

SIMPLE PARTIAL SEIZURES

In simple partial seizures, previously called "Jacksonian," consciousness is retained and the movements are clonic although not as vigorous as in the grand mal seizure. They do not consist of trembling or shaking.

The cortical motor representation shows that the face, thumb, and hand occupy the largest portion of the lateral surface of the motor strip (8). The trunk has a very small representation, and the legs are on the mesial surface. For this reason epileptic attacks originating in the motor area affect mainly the face, thumb, and hand. Jerking of the shoulder or elbow in the absence of jerking of the face and hand is therefore unlikely to be of epileptic origin. Furthermore, since in most right-handed patients and in 60 percent of left-handed individuals, speech is dependent on the function of the left hemisphere, a right-sided motor seizure is usually associated with speech arrest. If speech is preserved during a clinically right-sided seizure and the patient is not left-handed, an epileptic etiology becomes somewhat unlikely.

GENERALIZED NONCONVULSIVE SEIZURES

Petit mal absences consist merely of momentary cessation of speech and activities with a staring facial expression. Occasionally there is rhythmic blinking of the eyelids and slight rhythmic jerking of the hands. They are often confused with simple daydreaming episodes. These episodes usually last up to 10 s, but may occasionally last up to 50 or 60 s. The longer the absence attacks last, the more likely it is that some slight automatic activity will occur, but these are simple automatisms rather than the complex activity one observes in patients who have temporal or frontal pathology. These automatisms consist mainly of wetting the lips or some other slight repetitive behavior.

Patients who suffer only from petit mal absences are usually psychiatrically intact and will therefore rarely be seen by the psychiatrist except when petit mal status is misdiagnosed. Though not common, this condition occurs in adult life, at times even without prior history of absence attacks or tonic-clonic seizures. In three personally observed instances, the patients functioned normally, but for 2–3 days per month they would have, as one patient expressed it, "goofy days." She would be unable to concentrate, not know how to prepare meals, and, when unattended, simply sit or wander around in a confused state. On examination these patients do not have a typical organic mental syndrome; they are not disoriented or delirious, but have severe concentration difficulties. They are slow in their thought processes, and since they tend to be pleasant people, they may smile inappropriately to cover their deficit. If one is not aware that the condition is clearly episodic, a diagnosis of simple schizophrenia could readily be made. The concentration problem would be regarded as blocking and the smile as inappropriate affect. The correct diagnosis is immediately apparent from the EEG, which shows nearly continuous diffuse spike-wave discharges.

Tonic seizures occur mainly in brain-damaged patients and as a second or third seizure type. They therefore should not represent a significant problem for the psychiatrist. If an intellectually intact patient presents with episodic tonic manifestations as the sole attack form, nonepileptic etiologies must be looked for.

Myoclonic jerks occur mainly in patients with primary generalized tonic-clonic seizures, where they are readily treatable. They also occur in patients with Lafora's disease and Jakob-Creutzfeldt disease, which are progressive neurologic disorders with fatal outcome. Myoclonic jerking usually of the upper extremities in an otherwise healthy epileptic patient commonly begins in late adolescence or young adulthood. Isolated jerking of the upper extremities is usually noticed in the morning upon arising. The toothbrush may fly out of the hand, breakfast dishes may be thrown to the floor, and food or drink may be spilled. If these jerks come in close succession, the patient is liable to have a tonic-clonic seizure. Some patients learn to recognize this sequence of events and stay home from work or school on these days. It should be emphasized that these patients are completely healthy in all other respects and, if treated appropriately, provide the most gratifying results. This group of patients as well as those with petit mal absences may be sensitive to intermittent photic stimulation.

COMPLEX PARTIAL SEIZURES

The most problematic seizure types for the psychiatrist are the "partial seizures with complex symptomatology." In this group of patients, the disciplines of neurology and psychiatry overlap. Even epileptologists still have a problem arriving at an exact definition of terms. In order to understand the reasons for this state of the art, it is necessary to give a brief historical overview.

The seizure types that we are concerned with here were initially called "epileptic equivalents," "epileptic automatisms," or "psychomotor automatisms" (8–11). When EEG studies showed that these episodic behavioral disturbances were accompanied in the interictal tracing by spikes or sharp waves in one or both temporal areas, the term "temporal lobe seizure" became synonymous with "psychomotor automatism." The older clinical terms concentrated mainly on only one aspect of the attack, namely, automatic movements. They did not readily encompass the sensory manifestations or the aphasia that is sometimes the main symptom. The use of the term "temporal lobe seizures," on the other hand, presupposes that all of these attacks originate within temporal lobe structures. We now know that there are also frontal automatisms that can be very difficult to distinguish clinically from those of temporal origin.

The distinction between simple partial and complex partial seizures was supposed to have resolved this conflict, but that distinction rests entirely on the presence or absence of consciousness during the attack. Although all patients with clinical automatic behavior have impairment of consciousness, there are others who do not have automatisms but only visceral sensations with or without a déjà vu. These are clearly of temporal origin, but the patients maintain steadfastly that they are fully aware of their surroundings and can handle themselves appropriately during the event. Although this is not a frequent occurrence, it presents a significant problem to the patient and physician even apart from classification difficulties.

A recent patient of mine insisted that she was unjustly penalized by "the system": Had she simply ignored the episodes, she would not have received the diagnosis of epilepsy and thus would not have been prevented from driving a motor vehicle. Both the patient and her father insisted to me that a bystander would never know that she was experiencing an attack unless she mentioned it; yet she had a definite right temporal sharp wave focus and the visceral sensory symptoms were absolutely typical. Furthermore, since these brief attacks can be quite refractory to anticonvulsant medications, one cannot even hold out the hope that such a patient will ever legally obtain a driver's license under current regulations. It would seem that a person like this has really only two options, namely, either to lie or to become litigious, neither of which is desirable.

In spite of our problem with terminology, for the sake of conformity with international rules, the term "complex partial seizure" will be retained here for these seizure types. When one reads the textbook descriptions, it is readily understandable why psychiatrists who have not had many opportunities to see a great number of typical patients with complex partial seizures should be bewildered by the seemingly endless variety of symptoms the patients may present. Therefore, the most common events and their differences from pseudoepileptic "temporal lobe" seizures will be described.

The patient frequently reports an aura, but this is not invariably the case. When present, it consists of olfactory, gustatory, abdominal, or epigastric sensations, and especially a feeling of something rising from the epigastrium. It may also consist of vertigo, dizziness, auditory, or visual sensations. Any of these may be accompanied by a déjà vu sensation. In general, olfactory-gustatory sensations tend to result from a focal discharge in the uncus of the hippocampus, abdominal and epigastric sensations from the amygdala or Island of Reil, vertigo and auditory phenomena from the temporal surface (especially Heschl's gyrus), and formed visual hallucinations from the temporoparietal occipital junction. Crude visual sensations originate from the occipital lobe. At times the patient is unable to give a good description of the aura and refers to it simply as a "funny feeling." After the aura the patient's report becomes unreliable, because at that point the patient's level of consciousness is impaired; the rest of the description has to be obtained from a witness.

From the observer's point of view, the seizure begins in one of three ways: (a) There may simply be an arrest reaction where the patient stops what he or she had been doing, is unresponsive, and has a preoccupied, vacant, staring expression. (b) The patient may utter a repetitive, stereotyped phrase or question. (c) There is tonic postural flexion or extension of one arm, at times both, which may be coupled with deviation of the head to one side. Either of these is then frequently followed by chewing, smacking, or swallowing motions. The attack may cease at this point or continue with behavioral automatisms. These consist of seemingly purposeful, repetitive, stereotyped activity that is, in fact, purposeless and inappropriate to the situation of the patient. The movements are best described as "fussing" type of behavior.

The descriptions of the attacks differ widely among patients, but in a given patient tend to be consistent although variable in intensity and duration. The behavioral phenomena are understood best when one realizes that the patient has partial awareness of the environment and reacts to a variety of internal and external stimuli without having, however, moment-to-moment recall of what he or she is doing. If the patient is right-handed and the seizure originated in the right temporal lobe, the patient may utter some stereotyped, repetitive phrase during the automatism, but it will have no relevance to outside events.

In contrast to petit mal absences where the return to consciousness is quite abrupt, the patient with a complex partial seizure recovers more gradually. Although the attack itself lasts only about 1 min, the postictal state can be quite prolonged. It consists of confusion, sometimes disorientation, memory difficulties, drowsiness, and at times headaches. If the attack originated in the dominant hemisphere, there is also postictal aphasia that changes later to dysphasia, which may contribute to the patient's apparent confusion. Memory for relatively recent events may not be restored for up to about 0.5 or even 1h. If the patient has a seizure in the office and is unaccompanied, it is advisable to thoroughly check memory functions before he or she is released.

The patient's attacks may occur in various degrees of severity and intensity on different occasions, but this will be mainly a variation on the basic theme; the differential diagnosis against pseudoepileptic seizures is easier when one remembers the pathophysiologic mechanisms that are operative. As long as the patient has only an aura, there is limited spread and there are no clinical behavioral manifestations. The clinical automatism occurs when the discharge has spread to the contralateral hemisphere. At that time the hippocampal structures in both hemispheres are actively firing, and this effectively prevents memory traces from being laid down. The patient is therefore physiologically unable to carry out goal-directed, purposive activity, because this requires access to immediate, recent, and, to some extent, remote memory. Textbooks state that patients may perform bizarre acts like undressing in public, but since undressing as well as dressing require sequential thinking, it is unlikely that this has ever occurred as an ictal event.

In the postictal confusional period, it is conceivable that a male patient may respond to an urge to urinate by taking out his penis in public. The circumstances of the event would be such that a diagnosis of exhibitionism need not be entertained, because the behavior of an exhibitionist is clearly purposeful, premeditated, and not accompanied by confusion. The same applies to goal-directed violence. Ictal aggression that has produced bodily harm to another human being is extremely rare (12, 13). The reason lies again in the fact that goal-directed aggression requires memory which is simply not available during a genuine complex partial seizure associated with automatic behavior. An exception to this rule would be if the patient were to be physically restrained during the attack. Since the patient is stimulus bound, he or she might well strike out in perceived self-defense, but would not, however, go to a drawer, take out a knife or gun, and use it on some bystander.

Although there is some greater possibility of postictal violence, it again tends to be defensive rather than offensive in nature. In the author's personal experience, all patients who have shown postictal aggression have also had significant behavior problems in the interictal state. What appears to happen is that the basic personality structure of the individual is released in the postictal period. Thus, an individual without aggressive tendencies will engage in harmless, confused behavior, whereas the habitually dysphoric patient is likely to vent anger.

From a differential diagnostic viewpoint, the sequence and duration of events are again as important as in the tonic-clonic seizure and must be elicited from a witness. Any automatic behavior that lasts for more than a few minutes is not likely to be epileptic in nature. To make the diagnosis of postictal automatic behavior, which at this point is no longer simple and stereotyped but can be quite complex, one has to have a description of preceding ictal behavior that lasted for about 1 min. Differential diagnostic difficulties arise frequently when patients complain only of a variety of sensory or mental phenomena (including déjà vu) without automatic behavior, because patients with beginning schizophrenia or borderline states may also present with these symptoms. In epileptic patients symptoms are clearly limited in number as well as in time, are extremely similar on different occasions, and last for <1 min. In the schizophrenic or borderline patient they are all pervasive. These patients may have intense déjà vu at one time, marked dizziness or vertigo at another, gustatory sensations at a third, etc. It is the patterns in which the abnormal sensations occur as well as their duration that are the best diagnostic guidelines. Although some of the patients with complex partial seizures also have associated interictal symptomatology that can be regarded as schizophreniform, they have preserved affect that, as a matter of fact, is usually excessive and can at times be readily manipulated (14).

If the patient's sensory symptoms and/or purposeless confused behavior are accompanied by intense sweating, hypoglycemia must be considered. A 5-h glucose tolerance test should be obtained. If the patient were to have an attack in the physician's presence, blood for a sugar level should be drawn immediately. One should also remember that hypocalcemia may at times present with seemingly epileptic rather than tetanic seizures. This possibility should be entertained especially if the patient has had a thyroidectomy.

ATONIC SEIZURES, EPISODIC FALLING

Differential diagnostic problems can also arise in patients who simply intermittently fall to the ground and remain unresponsive for varying periods of time with no associated muscular activity. The most common organic causes are vasovagal or orthostatic syncope in younger individuals and vertebrobasilar insufficiency in older persons. Occasionally the symptom also occurs in patients who have temporal foci in the EEG. In all of these conditions, the episode lasts maximally 2–3 min, and the patient regains consciousness spontaneously. Cataplexy also leads to sudden drop attacks, but these are invariably preceded by an emotional stimulus and the patients do not lose consciousness.

Epileptic drop attacks of the astatic-myoclonic variety, on the other hand, occur without provocation. The patient loses consciousness and falls exceedingly hard, which frequently results in injuries. Attacks last for <0.5 min; the patients then collect themselves and get off the floor without assistance. These seizures typically occur only in brain-damaged individuals and seldom as the only seizure type. The patients usually also have tonic-clonic, tonic, or complex partial seizures on other occasions. Since they have serious intellectual limitations, referral to psychiatrists is rare.

This leaves a group of patients who seem to "faint" at times for no apparent reason, but remain seemingly unarousable for minutes or, when placed on a couch, for hours. In these psychogenic "faints" the patient is conscious and can hear whatever is said. Therefore, comments to nursing personnel should be such that the patient is not put on the defensive and forced to prove that the symptom is "really organic," thereby prolonging the attack. When asked to see a patient in this state, it is advisable first to check the eyes for position and the pupillary reaction. Since the lids are closed, they have to be opened; if the patient resists, it is clear that consciousness is retained. If the eyes are rolled upward, one would not be able to test pupillary reaction, but corneal sensation may be testable. Most of the time the eyes are in the midline, although they may at times oscillate from side to side, and the pupils are reactive to light. The deep tendon reflexes are preserved, and there are no pathologic reflexes. Facial color is normal or flushed. If an EEG is obtained during the episode, one sees normal waking activity. Although the patients may appear asleep, they are not, and thus there is no difficulty distinguishing this state from narcolepsy, in which the patient would be aroused by the examination.

OTHER EPISODIC ORGANIC BEHAVIORAL DISTURBANCES

Other episodic organic behavioral disturbances that can give rise to confusion with psychogenic reactions are startle- or movement-induced epilepsy, paroxysmal choreoathetosis, Kleine-Levin syndrome, and transient global amnesia.

In startle- or movement-induced seizures (15–17), the patient suddenly drops to the ground, with an associated brief loss of consciousness, as the result of a sudden startle stimulus or when suddenly getting up from the sitting position. The attack is short lived, and the patient returns to consciousness immediately. It usually results from a myoclonic jerk, and the EEG frequently shows spike-wave discharges.

Patients with paroxysmal choreoathetosis (18, 19) suffer from episodes initiated with restless movements of the upper and lower extremities that progress to typical choreiform activity. The patients remain conscious, usually do not fall, and are acutely embarrassed by the symptom so that they tend to retreat to a private facility like the bathroom. The attacks may last between 30 min and several hours. They tend to be precipitated by emotional stress, coffee, and beer, and may be aggravated by anticonvulsant medication, especially phenytoin, which is prescribed at times when a seizure disorder has been mistakenly diagnosed. Frequently there is a positive family history for this condition.

The Kleine-Levin syndrome occurs mainly in adolescent males (20). The etiology is obscure, although hypothalamic mechanisms have been suggested. Patients develop a marked behavioral change for a 2- to 3-day period per month. They become morose, irritable, and poorly responsive, eat excessively, and, if left alone, sleep excessively. The patients do not show signs of an organic mental syndrome, but could be regarded as schizophrenic during the acute episode. The author has seen only one of these patients, but the behavioral change was most dramatic. The EEG during the episode showed slight slowing of background rhythms, which disappeared as the symptoms abated.

Transient global amnesia (21, 22) differs from fugue states insofar as the patient merely continues with routine activities but fails to lay down a permanent memory trace. The etiology is not clear but since it occurs in middle-aged individuals, vascular factors have been held responsible. This author is not aware of any case on record where a patient, during an attack of transient global amnesia, has committed a criminal act.

FUGUE STATES

The conditions reviewed in the preceding section are rare. More frequently one encounters patients who perform bizarre acts with or without bodily harm to another person and subsequently claim amnesia for the attacks. Although temporal lobe disease is frequently suspected, it is rarely proven. It occurs most commonly in patients who have had a past history of mild or moderate head injury, and the acute episode tends to be precipitated by alcohol. The differential diagnosis of fugue states lasting several hours versus postictal automatic behavior rests on the absence of immediately preceding ictal activity, their long duration, and the absence of other epileptic phenomena.

The relationship of aggression to epileptic phenomena has been discussed earlier in the section on complex partial seizures and has been reviewed extensively (9).

LABORATORY DIAGNOSIS

As far as laboratory diagnostic aids are concerned, the EEG is the single most important tool. To yield definitive information, it should be obtained during the state of altered behavior, since interictal tracings may be normal or misleading by showing slight changes that have no relevance to the patient's symptoms. To solve difficult diagnostic problems, it is advisable to admit the patient to the hospital and have an EEG machine and technician available for stat recordings. If possible, prolonged video monitoring of the EEG and the patient's behavior is helpful, but this is time consuming and therefore expensive. Pharmacologic activation methods, especially pentylenetetrazol and bemegrid, are not useful because they may produce generalized tonic-clonic seizures and thus obscure the picture. We have therefore recently employed more physiologic stresses such as sleep deprivation combined with extra fluid intake and psychologic testing while the patient is video monitored.

Interictal temporal EEG abnormalities are useful in the diagnosis only if they consist of continuous, random slow wave activity or clear-cut spikes or sharp waves, as defined by international standards, located in the anterior rather than mid- or posterotemporal areas. The latter may be asymptomatic at times, especially in children. Their amplitude should be at least 75 μV.

Trimble (23) has recently demonstrated that prolactin levels rise after a tonic-clonic seizure and has shown that this may be useful in differentiating epileptic grand mal seizures from nonepileptic pseudo-grand mal. Since there is no elevation after complex partial or other types of minor seizures, the method cannot be used for distinguishing between epileptic and nonepileptic attacks in those instances.

In doubtful cases every effort should be made to reproduce, whenever possible, the precipitants of a spontaneous attack. Video monitoring is helpful because the tape can be shown to responsible relatives for confirmation that the attack is indeed the patient's habitual episode. In certain instances of pseudoepileptic seizures, we have also shown the attack to the patient as part of psychotherapy, as have Feldman et al., and this has proven helpful at times (24).

MANAGEMENT

It may be useful in conclusion to briefly cover the acute management of epileptic and pseudoepileptic seizures. In a tonic-clonic seizure, no specific measures need be taken except to prevent patients from injuring themselves during the clonic phase. Since the tongue is bitten in the beginning of the tonic phase, insertion of a mouthpiece during the attack is not useful unless one can carefully time it to the rhythmic opening of the jaws during the clonic phase. Oxygen administration in the ictal or postictal state is unnecessary because cyanosis when present is due to apnea and disappears as soon as respirations resume.

The patient with simple partial seizures needs no help, nor does the patient with petit mal absences. The patient with complex partial seizures should not be interfered with during the attack, and in the postictal state should not be restrained. Simple verbal reassurance that everything is all right is sufficient. The patient should be prevented from leaving the office, by locking the door if possible, or else one person should accompany the patient on his or her wanderings until consciousness has fully returned. This becomes problematic only if the patient has an associated personality disorder, because under these circumstances aggressive behavior can surface. If this is a habitual part of the seizure pattern, the problem must be addressed psychotherapeutically, because now one is no longer dealing with a purely epileptic process.

If one is called to see a patient who presents with pseudo-grand mal or an unresponsive state, it is best to keep conversations with bystanders to a minimum, because the patient can hear what is going on; whatever is said should be of a reassuring nature, ostensibly addressed to the nursing staff rather than the patient. This author tells the nursing staff and thus the patient that the attack is "due to nerves," is not dangerous, and will soon be over. We then place the patient in a private room and tell the nursing personnel that when the patient has recovered he or she is free to get out of bed. Nursing and physician personnel then leave, thus allowing the patient to return to normal activities without embarrassment.

The same applies to pseudo-grand mal status epilepticus. In these instances the nursing personnel are informed that the patient has had enough medications and that the intravenous drip and other measures taken such as oxygen administration can be discontinued. The patient is then left alone and will recover when there is no audience.

Although the acute management of these patients is relatively simple, the long-term treatment designed to prevent further recurrences is at times quite difficult and can be a serious challenge to the psychotherapeutic skills of the treating physician.

REFERENCES

1. Trimble MR: Hysteria and other nonepileptic convulsions, in *Epilepsy and Psychiatry*. Edited by Reynolds EH, Trimble MR. Edinburgh, Churchill Livingstone, 1981, pp 92–112
2. Riley TL, Roy A (eds): *Pseudoseizures*. Baltimore, Williams & Wilkins, 1982
3. Pond DA; The differential diagnosis of attacks and the borderlands of epilepsy, in *A Textbook of Epilepsy*. Edited by Laidlaw J, Richens A. New York, Churchill Livingstone, 1982, pp 270–274
4. Slater E: Diagnosis of 'hysteria.' *Br Med J* 1:1395–1399, 1965
5. Fenton GW: *Hysterical Alterations of Consciousness*. Edited by Roy A. New York, John Wiley & Sons, 1982, pp 229–246
6. Commission on Classification and Terminology of the International League Against Epilepsy: proposal for revised clinical and electroencephalographic classification of epileptic seizures. *Epilepsia* 22:489–501, 1981
7. Rodin E: Some relationships of induced seizure patterns to clinical findings in epileptic patients. *Epilepsia* 5:21–32, 1964
8. Penfield W, Jasper H: *Epilepsy and the Functional Anatomy of the Human Brain*. Boston, Little, Brown, 1954
9. Rodin E: Aggression and epilepsy, in *Pseudoseizures*. Edited by Riley TL, Roy A. Baltimore, Williams & Wilkins, 1982, pp 185–212
10. Jackson JH: On temporary mental disorders after epileptic paroxysms, in *Selected Writings of John Hughlings Jackson, Vol 1: On Epilepsy and Epileptiform Convulsions*. Edited by Taylor J. London, Staples Press, 1958, pp 119–134
11. Turner WA: *Epilepsy: A Study of the Idiopathic Disease*. New York, Raven Press, 1973
12. Delgado-Escueta AV, Mattson RH, King L, et al: The nature of aggression during epileptic seizures. *N Engl J Med* 305:711–716, 1981
13. Rodin E: Psychmotor epilepsy and aggressive behavior. *Arch Gen Psychiatry* 28:210–213, 1973
14. Rodin E: Psychosocial management of patients with complex partial seizures, in *Advances in Neurology, Vol 11: Complex Partial Seizures and Their Treatment*. Edited by Penry JK, Daly DD. New York, Raven Press, 1975, pp 383–414
15. Gimenez-Roldan S, Martin M: Effectiveness of clonazepam in startle-induced seizures. *Epilepsia* 20:555–561, 1979
16. Gimenez-Roldan S, Martin M: Startle epilepsy complicating Down's syndrome during adulthood. *Ann Neurol* 7:78–80, 1980
17. Baier WK: The "startle disease" in brain-damaged patients. Report of a case. *Neuropaediatrie* 11:72-75, 1980

18. Mount LA, Reback S: Familial paroxysmal choreoathetosis. *Arch Neurol Psychiatry* 44:481-487, 1940

19. Lance JW: Familial paroxysmal dystonic choreoathetosis and its differentiation from related syndromes. *Ann Neurol* 2:285-293, 1977

20. Carpenter S, Yassa R, Ochs R: A pathologic basis for Kleine-Levin syndrome. *Arch Neurol* 39:25-28, 1982

21. Jensen TS, deFine OB: Transient global amnesia as a manifestation of transient cerebral ischemia. *Acta Neurol Scand* 61:115–124, 1980

22. Shuping JR, Rollinson RD, Toole JF: Transient global amnesia. *Ann Neurol* 7:281–285, 1980

23. Trimble MR: Serum prolactin in epilepsy and hysteria. *Br Med J* 2:1682, 1978

24. Feldman RG, Paul NL, Cummins-Ducharme J: Videotape recording in epilepsy and pseudoseizures, in *Pseudoseizures.* Edited by Riley TL, Roy A. Baltimore, Williams & Wilkins, 1982, pp 122–126

6

Behavioral Alterations in Patients with Temporal Lobe Epilepsy

David Bear, M.D.
Roy Freeman, M.D.
Mark Greenberg, Ph.D.

THE NATURE OF BEHAVIORAL ALTERATIONS

The international neurologic and psychiatric literature, extending over more than a century, documents distinctive features of behavior in patients with temporal lobe epilepsy (1–4). Yet the existence of characteristic behavioral alterations associated with epileptic foci in the temporal lobe has been disputed (1, 5, 6).

The issue of behavioral change is important for at least two reasons. First, temporal lobe epilepsy is a common illness, the most frequent epilepsy in adulthood, with a prevalence of roughly 3 per 1,000. According to some estimates, 30 to 40 percent of patients experience persistent psychiatric symptoms that, more frequently than uncontrolled seizures, become the most incapacitating aspect of the illness (4, 7). Second, if behavioral changes are characteristic of some patients, temporal lobe epilepsy might serve as a valuable model illness in neuropsychiatry, allowing a

We gratefully acknowledge the secretarial assistance and infinite patience of Ms. Christine McNulty in preparation of this manuscript. As well, we are grateful to Mr. Jeffrey Saver for exceptional editorial and grammatical expertise. The Delbert Coleman Foundation, and Dr. and Mrs. Henry Murray provided financial assistance essential for our clinical studies which are summarized in this chapter.

direct correlation between localized electric dysfunction and specific features of human emotion, cognition, and personality (8).

Given the considerable practical and theoretical importance of behavioral changes in temporal lobe epilepsy, how is one to understand and clarify the debate on this topic? In this chapter we first attempt to illustrate the many features of altered behavior that have been reported by numerous authors in Europe and the United States. In our view the observations are robust and include, remarkably, parallel elements of behavior: deepened emotions, changes in sexual function, aggressivity, development of nascent religious or philosophic interests, circumstantiality, and interpersonal viscosity (1, 2, 7, 9).

It is difficult to dismiss the careful documentation of behavioral symptoms in many patients with temporal lobe epilepsy. In fact, we believe that much apparent controversy has no bearing on the reality of behavioral changes per se, but on independent, secondary, and often confounded issues: the frequency of such changes among temporal lobe epileptics, the specificity of these behavior changes to this neurologic illness, and the differentiation of particular behavioral features from those of idiopathic psychiatric syndromes.

There are additional sources of confusion regarding the behavioral observations. For example, it might be assumed that if behavior were affected by a limbic epileptic focus, the alterations would take the form of brief, episodic, paroxysmal activation of such basic drives as sex and aggression; following these ictal (seizurelike) perturbations in behavior, for which the patient would be amnesic, he or she would revert to an unremarkable interictal personality. The misunderstanding here is a confusion of ictal with interictal events. During the ictal period the limbic functions of drive activation and memory are most commonly inhibited, as suggested by the terms "absence," "automatism," and "psychoparesis" (1). By contrast, the interictal emotional state is generally characterized by an intensification of affective responses that form the basis of the majority of behavioral features to be described below (1, 9, 10).

The deepening of affect may lead to characteristic features of interictal behavior, but many of these—such as an interest in cosmologic issues and a tendency to write extensively—need not constitute psychopathology as defined by current psychiatric nomenclature. Thus, many commentaries on "interictal psychopathology" in temporal lobe epilepsy erroneously equate the observation of specific behavior patterns with the existence of psychopathology as reflected in psychometric scores or admission to psychiatric hospitals. In this chapter we hope to provide a coherent picture of interictal behavior changes without the unnecessary attribution of pathologic diagnostic labels.

For clarity of exposition, we will group these behavioral features into several categories: alterations of physiologic drives such as sexuality and aggression; intellectual and dispositional characteristics, including circumstantiality, religious or philosophic interests, interpersonal viscosity, and hypergraphia; severe syndromes including paranoid thought disorder, which has been termed "schizophreniform psychosis of epilepsy"; and the rarer phenomena of prolonged dissociative states and multiple personalities. We will also discuss cognitive impairments in temporal lobe epileptic patients, especially those affecting memory and language. Following the presentation of these clinical features, we will consider the important, incompletely resolved questions of their frequency, specificity, neural mechanism, and treatment.

ALTERATIONS IN DRIVE-RELATED BEHAVIOR

Sexuality

The importance of the temporal lobes in mediating sexual behavior has been demonstrated by numerous investigators. This observation has been derived from stimulation and ablation studies in humans and animals (11, 12). Thus, it is not surprising that a range of sexual behaviors has been described during the ictal, interictal, and postictal periods in patients with temporal lobe epilepsy. Gastaut and Collomb (13) drew attention to global hyposexuality that occurs interictally in many temporal lobe epileptics. Their observations have been repeatedly confirmed in case reports and retrospective studies. Abnormalities have been described, encompassing the spectrum of sexual behaviors, including lack of sexual interest and curiosity, absence of sexual dreams and fantasies, loss of libido, inability to experience orgasm, and diminution in frequency of sexual intercourse or masturbation (14–19).

Authors have also drawn attention to the occurrence of impotence in temporal lobe epilepsy, although most patients have developed normal secondary sexual characteristics and remain capable of complete sexual arousal (20, 21). An inverse relationship between epileptic activity in the temporal lobe and sexual behavior is suggested by the return of normal sexual behavior following control of seizures by medication or surgery (17). This observation contradicts the view that hyposexuality in epileptic patients is an adverse effect of seizure medication. The inverse relationship is further supported by the development of hypersexuality, on occasion, in the months following a temporal lobectomy and the return of hyposexuality if seizures recur (22).

The frequency of changes in sexual behavior may have been underestimated because hyposexuality in the temporal lobe epileptic, in contrast to psychogenic sexual disturbance, may be perceived as ego-syntonic (14, 17). This is often the case when the epileptic focus was present prior to the development of secondary sexual characteristics. In the interpersonal realm, altered sexuality can result in chaotic relationships, marital discord, or social isolation, and may influence mate selection (14, 16).

Temporal lobe epilepsy has also been associated with sexual deviations and perversions in numerous case studies. Observations include transvestism, transexualism, voyeurism, exhibitionism, fetishism, sadism, masochism, heterosexual and homosexual pederasty, and genital self-mutilation (15, 17, 19, 21–24). In an unselected sample, 11 of 49 male temporal lobe epileptic patients showed deviant sexual behavior. This was often associated with temporal lobe damage prior to the first year of life (15).

Case 1
Hyposexuality followed by sexual preference conflict with deepened emotions, circumstantiality, and hypergraphia

A 34-year-old man suffered febrile convulsions early in childhood. He was aware of interruptions in consciousness during elementary school, but these were attributed to daydreaming and were never evaluated medically. Only as a college freshman did he suffer a generalized tonic-clonic convulsion. The electroencephalogram (EEG) then revealed a right temporal lobe spike focus. While taking anticonvulsants he experienced complex partial seizures, heralded by an aura of dread, followed by rotation of his head to the left and lip smacking.

This man was a professional writer whose productions were marked by endless recitation of seemingly peripheral details. For his initial medical evaluation, he prepared a 20-page "essay" summarizing childhood experiences for the physician; no detail was left unexamined.

Of particular note was his sexual development. He had acquired secondary sexual characteristics early in adolescence. Yet he had "absolutely no interest" in sexual matters and virtually no knowledge of sexual anatomy until his freshman year in college. This hyposexuality was not a matter of concern, for he "preferred platonic relationships" with both men and women throughout high school. The phenomenon of dating had been a curiosity to him.

Classmates in college ridiculed him for his sexual naiveté. Thereupon, he commenced a "crash course" in sexuality, proposing liaisons with both women and men through advertisements in a local newspaper. He first consummated a relationship with a female prostitute, but subsequently had multiple sexual relations with men. Eventually he entered a continuing sexual and deeply emotional relationship with a woman 40 years his elder. Privately he also experimented with cross-dressing, followed by masturbation in front of his mirror. His mannerisms and vocal habits became effeminate.

In contrast to frequent sexual alterations occurring interictally in temporal lobe epileptics, on rare occasions the ictus will include complex motor automatisms such as masturbatory activity, pelvic thrusting, and exhibitionism for which the patient is usually amnesic (25–28). Somatosensory genital sensations as well as sexually associated emotions such as sexual arousal, erotic thoughts, and orgasm are rare ictal experiences (27, 28).

In the immediate postictal period, inappropriate sexual behavior such as exhibitionism or unseemly sexual advances may occur, perhaps owing to the lack of inhibition and judgment occurring in a setting of confusion and amnesia. Blumer (22) has also drawn attention to appropriate postictal sexual arousal in some patients. This is usually expressed with a receptive partner or through masturbation in a private environment without associated confusion or amnesia.

Anger, Irritability, and Aggression

The temporal lobe epileptic frequently experiences intensified feelings of anger or irritability. Occurring in conjunction with humorlessness and a moralistic sense of right and wrong, this personality alteration often results in sanctimonious or self-righteous behavior.

Epidemiologic studies of overt aggression among temporal lobe epileptics in the general population are hampered by semantic, reporting, and recognition difficulties. In fact, there are few issues more emotionally charged than that of the association of aggression with epilepsy (5, 29, 30). Studies of selected groups with a high incidence of violence, such as incarcerated prisoners, must control for other factors (e.g., head trauma and malnutrition) that will coincidentally increase the incidence of epilepsy. From these groups one must be cautious in drawing cause-and-effect relationships between epilepsy and violence.

The issue has been confused still further by the failure to distinguish among three clearly different patterns of aggression that may occur in the epileptic patient: ictal, postictal, and interictal aggression (29).

In a recently reported study (31), a panel of experts reviewed the histories of 5,400 epileptic patients and then examined the videotapes of 33 epileptic attacks in the 19 patients thought to display ictal violence. Using strict criteria only 13 were felt to have incontestable epilepsy; of these 7 were felt to demonstrate unequivocal violence as defined by the "directed exertion of extreme and aggressive physical force which if unrestrained would result in injury, destruction, or abuse." Three of these patients had been reported previously in the literature.

The aggressive actions included spitting, shouting, swearing, scratching, karate blows, and the destruction of property; all lasted for <1 min, with an average of 29 sec. In five cases the aggression was accompanied by an angry mood; the other two patients appeared frightened and confused. In all cases there was amnesia for the event. This study, while emphasizing the rarity of directed ictal violence, failed to address postictal or interictal aggression (29).

Postictal irritability is a well-described clinical event; in fact, in the study above (31), two patients demonstrated this phenomenon, screaming wildly as they were restrained for 3–4 min postictally. This behavior may be similar to that of the confused or concussed patient who mistakes attempts at medical assistance for threats.

It has been our clinical experience that the most frequent and potentially serious phenomena involve aggression during the interictal period. In this situation an aggressive act might be carried out for a clear motive, often following considerable planning in response to an objectively minor provocation. The patient frequently experiences moral concerns or a sense of outrage. The perpetrator does not generally claim amnesia for the event and may recall these actions with considerable regret (29).

This behavior is often associated with other features of the interictal behavior syndrome. In a recent study, psychiatrically hospitalized temporal lobe epileptics were distinguished from patients with aggressive character disorders by the presence of religiosity, interpersonal clinging, circumstantiality, bizarre humor, and philosophical interests. Contrary to the prevailing clinical dogma, the temporal lobe patient was more inclined to accept responsibility for angry outbursts and less inclined to claim amnesia for the event or to blame the actions on uncontrollable impulses (32).

Case 2
Aggressivity with hypermoralism, paranoia, and hypergraphia

This 37-year-old ambidextrous man had experienced sinking sensations in his stomach and feelings of fear followed by brief interruptions of consciousness since age 9. In subsequent years he experienced generalized tonic-clonic seizures. The most recent EEG revealed spikes and focal slowing over the right temporal area. Dilantin 300 mg daily had been prescribed for many years. General physical, neurologic, and computed tomographic (CT) examinations were unremarkable.

The patient initially minimized problems with his temper, emphasizing that he "went out of his way to avoid trouble." However, when provoked by teasing about his seizures in high school, he injured people on several occasions. He retained vivid memories of these altercations and generally felt morally justified in "fighting back." On one occasion the patient came upon a thief attempting to steal his car. Filled with indignation, he attacked the man and held him at gunpoint; subsequently, he was overcome by the thief's accomplice. He became convinced that this crime and insult would never be avenged by the authorities. Over a 6-month period, the patient constructed and allegedly executed an elaborate plan to identify the accomplice, befriend and intoxicate him, and beat him into unconsciousness.

During the interictal period the patient presented his physicians with a voluminous diary of his early experiences. He was also an avid writer of letters, many detailing minor deviations from a safety code in his place of work; this sensitivity to minor infractions eventually led to his suspension. He felt that he had been maligned and persecuted by both his employer and the union. Formerly a man of deep religious conviction, he had become disillusioned by a God who "caused my epilepsy." He sought emergency psychiatric consultation at several hospitals, where he was described as depressed, paranoid, and potentially suicidal or homicidal (29).

Interictal aggressive behavior should be contrasted with the aggression occurring in frontal lobe disease—in particular, resulting from lesions of the orbital prefrontal cortex—in which trivial stimuli elicit brief, aggressive outbursts that are usually unplanned, unsustained, ineffectual, and soon forgotten. The shallow mood and affect of the frontal lobe patient stand in sharp contrast to the deepened emotionality of patients with the interictal behavior syndrome of temporal lobe epilepsy (29).

Epilepsy has been invoked as a defense in crimes of violence with increasing frequency—in at least 12 cases of violent crime since 1977. In 1979 epilepsy was cited as a defense in five cases of murder (33). The claim most typically has been that violence occurred during a seizure. Because of the rarity of directed ictal aggression, we suspect that this defense is seldom justified.

However, interictal aggression has not, to our knowledge, been invoked as a defense in a court of law. Since this behavioral alteration occurs as a result of intrinsic brain disease, it could be considered "a mental disease or defect." Thus, it is conceivable that the interictal behavior syndrome might be raised in the future in support of a plea of diminished criminal responsibility or insanity in a patient with well-documented temporal lobe epilepsy.

ALTERATIONS IN EMOTIONAL AND INTELLECTUAL BEHAVIOR

Deepened Emotions, Viscosity, Circumstantiality, and Religiosity

In addition to alterations in biologic drives such as sexuality and aggression, the interictal behavioral changes described in temporal lobe epilepsy include a cluster of emotional and intellectual characteristics. The development of a heightened intensity of many feelings and ideas is central to this behavior pattern. In the affective sphere, this might manifest as deepened emotions; emotional lability; mood states such as depression, elation, or euphoria; or fear-related experiences such as anxiety, panic attacks, phobias, or paranoia (1, 4, 9, 10).

Intellectual features include nascent philosophic interests and metaphysical concerns, a humorless sobriety, and a sense of increased significance of both the internal and external world. These phenomena form the basis of some of the most characteristic aspects of the interictal behavior syndrome (1, 4, 9).

Interpersonal viscosity, or "clinging," is familiar to many physicians involved in the care of the temporal lobe epileptic. This trait may manifest as the inability to bring a conversation to an appropriate end, insensitivity to temporal or spatial cues regulating social interactions, or prolonged clinical interviews followed by frequent attempts to reestablish contact with phone calls, letters, notes, or messages (1, 4, 32). This interpersonal viscosity, or excessive social cohesion, is often associated with circumstantiality—a style of speaking or writing characterized by the incorporation of multiple, often peripheral details and containing excessive clarifications, qualifications, and circumlocutions (1, 4, 9, 10, 32).

Many authors have drawn attention to the increased religious and philosophic interests in the temporal lobe epileptic patient (1, 3, 4, 9, 10, 32). Patients may exhibit a profound interest in religious texts, undergo multiple conversions from one faith to another, or develop strong moral convictions or commitment to secular ideologies.

Hypergraphia

Waxman and Geschwind (34) were the first to document the occurrences of hypergraphia (a tendency to excessive and compulsive writing) in patients with temporal lobe epilepsy. Other aspects of the interictal behavior syndrome are often reflected in the contents of these writings: verbosity, circumstantiality, meticulous attention to details, and frequent religious and metaphysical allusions. This behavior may be exhibited in the writing of notes; diaries; letters to physicians, church officials, and politicians; novels; poems; hymns; and autobiographies. The form of writing often incorporates idiosyncratic stylistic devices for emphasis: parentheses, underlining, different colored inks, and the rewriting of written numbers in arabic form. We have also noted an extensive tendency to draw in several of our patients.

Case 3
Hypergraphia with emotional deepening, religious preoccupation, pansexuality, and aggressivity

This 55-year-old black woman had suffered seizures since early childhood. Originally she experienced interruptions of consciousness. She subsequently developed a prolonged aura consisting of foul odor, followed by focal movements of the left face and arm that sometimes progressed to a generalized seizure. The EEG revealed a spike focus over the right temporal lobe; spike bursts were recorded from the right amygdala with depth electrodes. A stereotactic radiofrequency lesion within the right amygdala at age 42 produced no apparent change in seizure pattern or interictal behavior.

This patient initially presented her physician with >20 spiral notebooks filled with somber personal reflections, religious exegeses, and angry diatribes against former physicians, police, and politicians. For several months she completed a 70-page notebook with new writing each week. Her writing efforts were all the more remarkable because she suffered painful and deforming rheumatoid arthritis that forced her to write with finger and wrist supports.

With her permission, we include a typical page from these diaries (Figure 1).

She also carried satchels filled with audio cassettes of her own sermons on biblical themes. Despite her unmistakable religious and moral fervor, she reported sexual activity from age 6, with bisexual preference, and prostitution beginning in adolescence.

Yet another aspect of her intense emotionality was striking. She had been prosecuted for multiple aggravated assaults including an attempt to castrate an unsatisfactory sexual partner and beating a policeman unconscious.

Case 4

Hypergraphia—poetry and painting—with deepened emotions, philosophic interests, irritability, and sexual conflict

A 29-year-old single woman experienced the onset of spells 8 years previously during which "everything appeared wavy and faces looked like caricatures." These recurrent episodes included rushing thoughts and voices and a sense of imminent disaster. At these times she was aware of people talking to her but gave inappropriate responses to their questions. The EEG revealed bilateral midtemporal sharp waves on two occasions. Neurologic examination and CT scan were normal. She had sustained a traumatic loss of consciousness at age 18 following an automobile accident.

There was a dramatic change in her affect following the onset of spells. The patient developed deepening emotions, with a marked, self-reported tendency to become angry about trivial events. In the last 2 years, even normal volume sounds led to violent outbursts in which she smashed furniture or struck her cat.

This highly intelligent woman composed music, wrote poems, and frequently combined poetic texts with elaborately detailed or vividly colored illustrations. Philosophic reflections and moral aphorisms were frequently depicted, as exemplified in Figure 2.

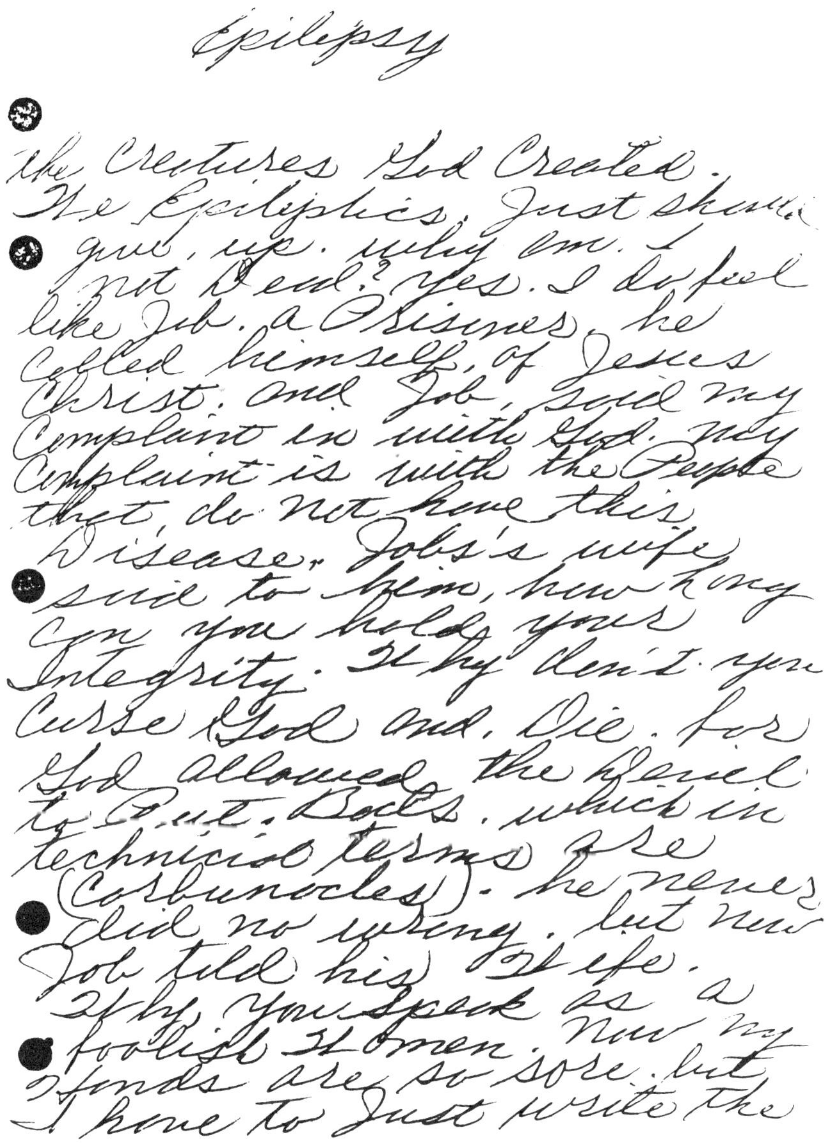

Epilepsy

the Creatures God Created.
The Epileptics, Just should
give, up. why am. I
not Dead? yes. I do feel
like Job. a Prisoner, he
called himself, of Jesus
Christ. and Job, said my
Complaint in with God. my
Complaint is with the People
that, do not have this
Disease. Jobs's wife
said to him, how long
Can you hold your
Integrity. Why don't you
Curse God and. Die. for
God allowed the Devil
to Put. Boils. which in
technical terms are
(Carbuncles). he never
did no wrong. but now
Job told his Wife.
Why You speak as a
foolish Women. now my
friends are so sore. but
I have to Just write the

FIGURE 1. *Typical page from the diary of a patient with temporal lobe epilepsy and hypergraphia*

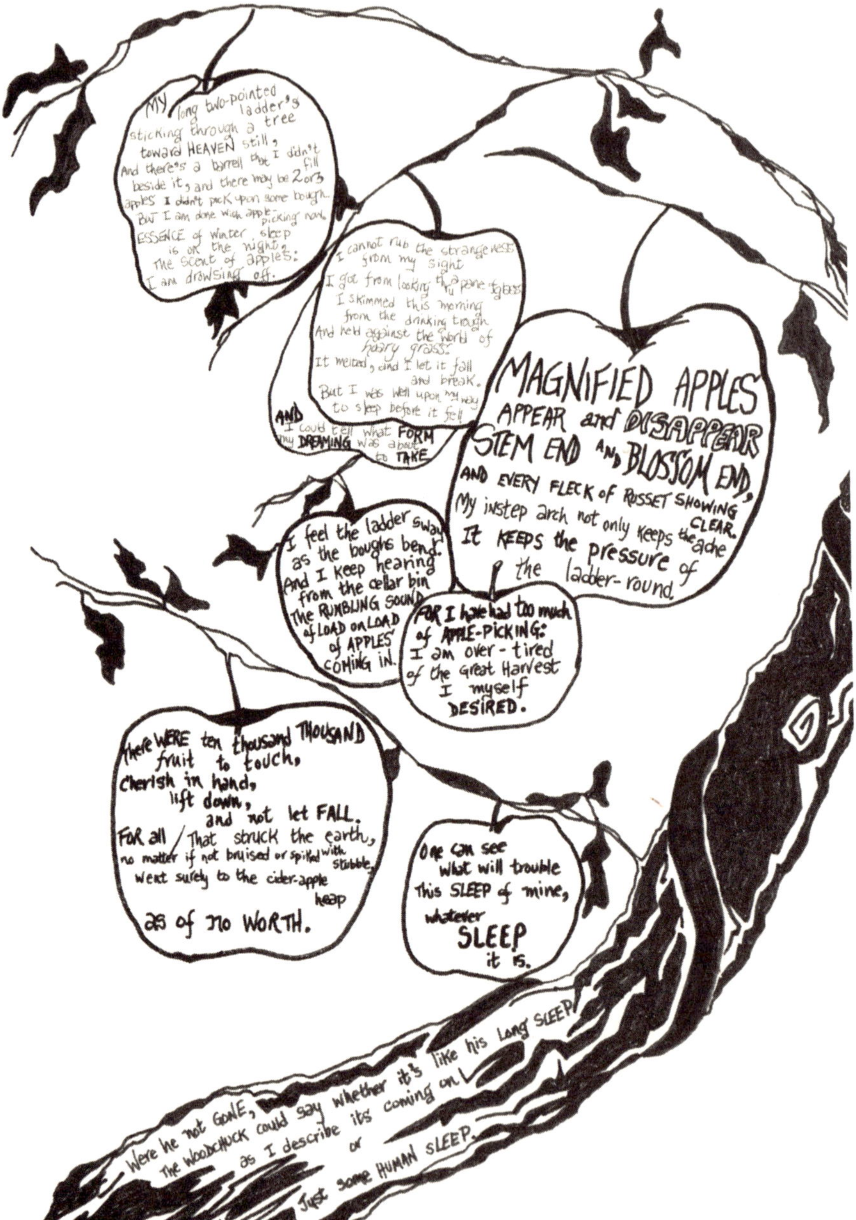

FIGURE 2. *Example of a detailed illustration drawn by a patient with temporal lobe epilepsy*

Other features of the interictal behavior syndrome were present: readily elicitable sadness with recurrent suicidal depressions, religious preoccupation leading to enrollment in a divinity school, and continuing conflict regarding sexual preference (29).

The mechanism of hypergraphia remains unresolved. Waxman and Geschwind (9), Bear (1), and Bear and Fedio (10) have suggested that hypergraphia reflects intellectualized expression of intensified emotions. In a recent retrospective review, Roberts et al. (35) noted the association of hypergraphia with right-sided or predominantly right-sided foci, and emphasized the possible contribution of an intact language-dominant hemisphere. However, other studies have not confirmed this lateralization (10, 36).

Psychoses

The association of psychotic states with epilepsy was described as early as the nineteenth century (37). More recent developments in electrophysiology have made possible the accurate localization of seizure foci as well as the differentiation of psychoses occurring ictally, interictally, and postictally (38).

Early investigators claimed an inverse relationship between seizure frequency and psychosis among epileptics (39, 40), an observation that may have led von Meduna to introduce convulsive therapy as a treatment for schizophrenia. Based on observations that the onset of psychotic behavior in epileptics occurred in the setting of diminishing seizure frequency, Gibbs (40) described the psychiatric and seizure manifestation of temporal lobe epilepsy as "physiologically antithetic." Landolt (41) commented on the diminution or absence of spike discharges (occurring spontaneously or caused by anticonvulsant therapy) in the setting of psychosis. He called this phenomenon "forced normalization" of the EEG.

A more questionable concept of antagonism was based on the observation of early epidemiologists that the combination of schizophrenia and epilepsy occurred less frequently than predicted by chance. Slater and Beard (3), on the other hand, felt that the association of epilepsy with psychosis occurred with a frequency far greater than predicted by chance. They described 69 patients referred to two London hospitals over 2 years. They argued that this number was >10 times greater than would be predicted for the entire London area. The psychosis occurred an average of 14.1 years after the onset of seizures, in patients with a mean age of 29.8 years. Over 70 percent of their patients had temporal lobe epilepsy.

Such symptoms as delusions and hallucinations (in clear consciousness), paranoid behavior, and, more rarely, thought blocking, neologisms, and catatonia were described in the interictal period of temporal lobe epilepsy. Beard and Slater emphasized that all of the cardinal symptoms of schizophrenia were manifest at some time in their patients. However, they confirmed the observation of Pond (42) that, in contrast to idiopathic schizophrenics, these patients had warm, appropriate affects and did not suffer the clinical deterioration of schizophrenia. This led to the use of the term "schizophreniform psychosis of temporal lobe epilepsy," which is not synonomous with the "Schizophreniform Disorder" defined in the third edition of the *Diagnostic and Statistical Manual of Mental Disorders* (1980).

Case 5
Paranoid psychosis with aggressivity, homosexual preoccupation, religiosity, and hypergraphia

A 38-year-old man developed paroxysmal abdominal pains at age 7. These persisted into adult life and responded to anticonvulsant medication. No gastrointestinal pathology had been identified. Although his behavior and academic records were good throughout high school, he was forced to abandon college during the freshman year because of "paranoid thoughts, dreamy states, and an urge to hit people." He then entered military service at age 18; during his first year, he assaulted a man with a razor blade. This episode and additional fights led to his arrest. At this time he described auditory hallucinations and a desire to hurt or kill people. He was diagnosed as schizophrenic, although the EEG then and subsequently documented spike activity over the right temporal lobe.

Since this incident he was chronically hospitalized and treated with neuroleptics and anticonvulsants. His birth had been complicated by a difficult delivery, requiring the use of high forceps. Neurologic abnormalities included right hemicranial and left-sided atrophy, hyperreflexia, and a left extensor plantar response.

His delusional and paranoid thoughts, tangential associations, fears of homosexuality, and auditory hallucinations led to the diagnosis of schizophrenia. However, the deepened emotionality, writing of religious poems, and marked interpersonal warmth and clinging are consistent with an alternative diagnosis. In the presence of unambiguous EEG and neurologic find-

ings, it seems most likely that this patient suffers from the "schizophreniform psychosis of temporal lobe epilepsy" (29).

Flor-Henry (43), in a retrospective study of 50 patients, pointed out a statistical association between epileptic foci in the dominant hemisphere and schizophrenialike psychotic behavior, whereas nondominant hemisphere foci were associated with manic-depressive symptoms. The latter finding has not been replicated; the former has received inconsistent support in the literature (2, 10, 44).

The development of psychosis in temporal lobe epilepsy has been linked to specific anatomic and clinical features. Taylor (44) noted the association of hamartomas (congenital dysplasias) with psychosis in temporal lobe epilepsy. Specific types of aura have also been associated by several authors with the development of psychosis. Jensen and Larsen (45) noted that psychosis occurred more commonly in patients with ictal hallucinations or complex motor automatisms than in patients with visceral auras. Herman et al. (46) described the development of psychosis in patients with ictal fear. The fact that Case 5 developed schizophreniform psychosis with a visceral aura and right-sided epileptic focus underscores the exceptions to many of these reported associations.

Dissociative States

Several authors have drawn attention to the association of temporal lobe epilepsy with dissociative states (47, 48). These include the classic multiple personality syndrome in which two or more personalities exist independently, with amnesic barriers between them. In a less dramatic form of dissociative disorder, the patient, usually female, describes herself as having more than one side to her personality, attributing different thoughts and behaviors to alternative aspects of the self. Other patients have attributed their thoughts, behavior, and emotions to benevolent or malevolent powers or spiritual entities such as demons.

Case 6
Dissociative state (possession) with aggression, deepened emotions, hypergraphia, and religiosity

The patient was a woman in her mid-twenties whose complex partial seizures included feelings of panic, depersonalization, and déjà vu, followed by interruption of consciousness, lip smacking, and rocking movements. The EEG revealed bilateral temporal lobe spiking. She had noted a definite personality change since the onset of her seizures. A previously outgoing and happy person, she had become depressed and introverted. She was extremely religious and hypergraphic. At times she believed there was a demon in her body; she sensed a presence and heard a voice urging her to perform aggressive acts. She often complied with the voice and attacked people. However, she denied feeling anger, insisting that her hostile behavior resulted from the demon. She went to a priest to be exorcised and felt that this was somewhat successful (48).

In most reported cases, the dissociative states occur as interictal events in patients who are alert, attentive, and capable of responding appropriately to the environment. It has been suggested that the intensified dysphoric affects that may develop as features of the interictal behavior syndrome predispose some individuals to dissociative reactions (48). These phenomena should be distinguished from simple automatisms, fugue states, and poriomania (4), which may occur as ictal or periictal events.

COGNITIVE IMPAIRMENTS IN TEMPORAL LOBE EPILEPSY

Clinical Presentations

Assessment of cognitive abilities is an important part of the evaluation of patients with temporal lobe epilepsy. Memory and language functions are most frequently affected (49–53).

Patients commonly complain of amnesic gaps in their experience before, during, and after seizure activity. Indeed, the absence of postictal amnesia is often used as a criterion in the identification of hysterical pseudoseizures. In addition to these ictal symptoms, we believe that interictal changes in memory function are frequent. These changes may be subtle and insidious and therefore go unreported, especially in patients whose occupation or avocation places limited demands on their memory capacity.

Adequate clinical evaluation requires comparing information from several sources: the patient's spontaneous complaint; the patient's response to direct inquiry about specific abilities (e.g., finding words, remembering appointments, faces, names, written material, landmarks, or music); reports from others—friends, family, coworkers; standardized, objective tests of cognitive function, with established norms.

By comparing data from these sources, the clinician can delineate and quantify the nature and severity of cognitive impairment.

In addition, estimates of premorbid ability or multiple samples taken over time allow for an analysis of the progressive nature of the deficits. This information can also elucidate the relation between cognitive impairment and other clinical variables such as seizure frequency and medication levels.

Some patients tend to minimize their difficulties, and when confronted with their poor test results, emphasize that they were, for example, "never good with designs." The family and coworkers of such patients are often more acutely aware of their difficulties. Other patients who are introspective and anxious may exaggerate their difficulties, claiming that they are "unable to think anymore," although objective testing reveals only minor deficits. In each case a disparity between objective findings and self-report alerts the clinician to a characteristic response bias (minimizing versus maximizing). These tendencies have important implications for the interpretation of the patient's other physical and psychologic complaints.

Approach to Neuropsychologic Testing

Because problems outside the realm of memory can cause patients to complain of trouble in remembering, an initial assessment of the patient's attention, concentration, distractibility, and level of alertness should precede inquiry into memory function. In addition, special notice should be paid to obsessional concerns or the presence of preoccupations of thought that may interfere with evaluation of memory.

There are many psychometric instruments designed to examine distinct aspects of memory function, including remote memory, episodic memory, imagery, and incidental memory (54–56). In our experience tests of new learning—which present the patient with unfamiliar material and require immediate and delayed recall—provide an efficient and sensitive index of temporal lobe pathology. Both verbal and visual new learning tasks should be administered. In the verbal realm the basic testing strategy is to expose the patient to a flood of information that is beyond his or her span of apprehension, and requires the patient to transform and reduce it to a manageable form in order to encode and ultimately recall the information (57).

The amount of information assimilated in one exposure is then quantified along with a qualitative assessment of the spontaneous strategy employed. Particular attention is devoted to determining which aspects of the original material the patient fails to recall, along with an analysis of errors of commission (perseverative versus intrusive versus confabulatory errors). Successive reexposures allow an assessment of the incremental acquisition over several trials (the learning curve) and the consistency of the strategy. Furthermore, an additional recall condition after a distraction or 20-min delay allows an evaluation of retention ability. This crucial dimension is often overlooked in bedside testing. A 15-item, 5-trial list of words to be recalled (such as the Rey Auditory Learning Test [58]) provides a precise and pragmatic test of verbal memory. Established norms allow comparison with different age and occupation groups.

In the visuospatial realm a similar basic approach is employed (57). The patient is asked to copy a complicated design that defies verbal description. The examiner notes the quality of the patient's copying strategy (systematic or haphazard, segmented or holistic, right to left, left to right, etc.). Then the patient is required to immediately redraw the figure (recall). Is the internal detail remembered at the expense of configural relationships? Is the size expanded? Are features distorted? Reduplicated? Symmetrical? Is the left side emptier than the right or vice versa? Answers to such questions reveal clues as to the quality of the deficit. Finally, a drawing is made after a 20-min delay and compared with the immediate recall. The Rey-Osterreith Complex Figure (59) is an excellent test for this purpose.

Anomia, or word-finding difficulty, is probably the most frequent language complaint of the temporal lobe epileptic. The patient generally describes the frustrating feeling of being unable to articulate the word for which he or she is looking, often settling for a poor semantic substitute. Frequent pauses and stereotypic utterances such as "umm" and "you know" tend to fill the gaps of spontaneous speech. This difficulty often is exacerbated by stress or performance anxiety. There is a theoretic debate as to whether anomia is a problem in retrieving overlearned information from semantic memory or a true language disturbance (60, 61). Two standard measures of anomia are visual confrontation naming, in which the patient is asked to provide the names of pictures of objects (The Boston Naming Test [62]), and word fluency, in which the patient is required to generate as many words as he or she can that begin with a particular letter in a specified amount of time (the Controlled Word Association Task [63]). Norms for both tests are available.

Having collected the test data, the examiner searches for patterns of deficits. One discrepancy may be between verbal and visual memory. The literature consistently documents that right temporal lobe pathology (irritative foci and/or lobectomy lesions) yields relatively greater visual than verbal memory impairment, whereas the opposite pattern is obtained with left temporal lobe damage (52, 53, 64, 65). Thus, a marked discrepancy can have localizing value. However, inferences drawn from neuropsychologic data as to the localization and lateralization of lesions are dependent on additional factors: sex, age, handedness, familial handedness, etiology, etc. Such a discrepancy may also lead to a recommendation that patients develop ways of relying on their strengths and avoiding their weaknesses.

Memory for details can be superior to memory for the overall configuration. If so, this pattern can be demonstrated to the patient, and predictions about situations in which difficulty is likely to be encountered can be made with some confidence.

A disparity between immediate and delayed recall can also have important implications. If immediate memory is relatively more impaired than delayed recall (indicating adequate retention), the patient should be encouraged to rehearse, check, and use other mnemonic devices, since information will not decay once it is successfully encoded. However, if delayed memory is relatively more impaired than immediate, the patient can be encouraged to use external aids such as tape recorders, lists, and outlines to retain important information.

Periodic retesting of these basic functions is an effective means of monitoring the severity of neurologic compromise and the adequacy of treatment. The following case illustrates many of the above points.

Case 7

Impairment in verbal memory with spared visual memory

A 42-year-old right-handed physician developed complex partial seizures at age 21. These seizures were initiated by an experience of déjà vu, followed by an interruption of consciousness and lip smacking. Occasionally, an aversive smell preceded the attacks. Repeated EEGs revealed spikes and slow waves localized to the left mesial temporal lobe. His seizure frequency of approximately five per month was reduced to fewer than four seizures per year with carbamazepine.

Before the onset of seizures, he had been a superior student, having won a highly regarded fellowship in high school. However, limitations, especially in memory, led to severe difficulty in medical school and failure to obtain advanced specialty cer-

tification. This situation resulted in professional limitation and lowered self-esteem.

Neuropsychological testing revealed mild to moderate impairment in verbal memory with considerable loss of detail, inconsistent and inadequate strategies, some intrusive errors, and a significant amount of decay after a delay.

By contrast, visual memory was superior. Thus, his immediate recall of a complex visual figure was superb, with retention of both the external outline and the internal details. There was no significant decay of visual information after a 20-min delay, indicating excellent retention. Further testing revealed a remarkable capacity to generate visual images in which many details might be encoded.

A program of utilizing cognitive imagery to enhance memory was initiated, with the goal of compensating for impaired verbal memory by exploiting his superior visual recall. After 2 months of practice in generating images, he was able (after many rehearsals) to recall a list of >150 words by linking visual images in the form of rebuses. He could recall words forward or backward at any point of the list, as well as retrieve words by their ordinal position. This encouraged him to resume advanced medical study with renewed confidence.

UNRESOLVED ISSUES CONCERNING INTERICTAL BEHAVIOR

Quantifying the Interictal Behavior Syndrome

What constitutes an appropriate measure of the interictal behavior syndrome? Standardized psychologic tests, designed to segregate patients into idiopathic psychiatric diagnostic categories, may not be appropriate. There are inherent test limitations (for example, low sensitivity and specificity for interictal changes) as well as inadequate validation and normative data on temporal lobe epileptics. In the previously cited study of Bear and Fedio (10), an inventory in which specific features ascribed to the interictal behavioral syndrome (for example, writing interests, religious concerns, changes in sexual preference) were sampled powerfully discriminated between temporal lobe epileptics and both normal controls and patients with other neurologic diseases. To our knowledge, in every study utilizing this inventory, temporal lobe epileptics have obtained higher scores than normal subjects (10, 36, 66, 67). The inventory was an attempt to sample clinical features of the interictal behavior syndromes more accurately than existing standardized tests. With the future description of presently unrecognized features of the interictal behavior syndrome, the diagnostic power of such self-report instruments will improve.

In addition, biologic markers of the interictal behavior syndrome, such as neurochemical profile, patterns of autonomic responsivity, and increased incidence of associated diseases, will add further dimensions to the current clinical picture (68).

Furthermore, the recognition of additional variables exerting influences that either promote or inhibit the development of the interictal behavior syndrome will further refine the clinical entity; for example, psychosis with left focal discharge among left-handed females (44), emotional alterations with the limbic rather than neocortical location of the epileptic focus (69), severer cognitive and emotional changes with bilateral spike discharges (70), and an increased incidence of paranoid symptoms among patients whose auras include the experience of fear (46). Moreover, elucidation of those variables that lower the probability of developing behavioral alterations will be of considerable interest.

In the absence of satisfactory measures of behavioral change, its actual frequency remains unknown. Few observers doubt an elevated incidence of psychiatric illness, suicide attempts, aggressive disturbances, and sexual dysfunction among temporal lobe epileptics (1–3, 7, 14, 17, 29). However, these overt indications of psychopathology or maladaptive behavior may substantially underestimate the number of patients with more subtle features of an interictal behavioral syndrome. For example, in a small sample of consecutively tested temporal lobe epileptics attending outpatient neurology clinics, one-third had attempted suicide and 40 percent had been psychiatrically hospitalized. Yet, based on questionnaire data sampling traits of the interictal behavioral syndrome, 90 percent of the temporal lobe epilepsy patients could be distinguished from both normal controls and other neurologic patients by a discriminant function analysis (10). These results by no means constitute an estimate of the true frequency of behavior changes, but indicate a high prevalence of such alterations in temporal lobe epilepsy.

Neurologic Specificity of the Interictal Behavior Syndrome

The observation of an "interictal behavior syndrome" associated with temporal lobe epilepsy implies that multiple features of behavior—such as deepened emotions, altered sexual behavior, and hypergraphia—appear in concert with some patients with this disorder. We wish to emphasize the evidence for such a simultaneous appearance or clustering of multiple features of behavior in individual patients (1, 9, 10, 32).

Such a behavioral syndrome has not been reported in response to the stress of general medical illnesses such as myocardial infarction, diabetes mellitus, and asthma (1, 10); patients with life-threatening or disfiguring neurologic illness did not exhibit interictal features to a greater extent than did normal controls (10). Patients with multiple sclerosis or rheumatoid arthritis exhibited patterns of behavior different from those of temporal lobe epileptics (66).

The interictal behavior syndrome of temporal lobe epilepsy is also distinguished from behavioral syndromes resulting from other localized neurologic lesions. For example, the deepened emotionality contrasts with the flattened, transient emotions of patients following prefrontal lobe injury, the apathy of patients with Korsakoff's amnesic syndrome, and the indifference following right parietal lobe infarction (71). Perhaps the most cogent argument for the neurologic specificity of the interictal behavior syndrome is its antithesis, the Klüver-Bucy syndrome, which results from structural, nonepileptogenic lesions of limbic structures in the medial temporal lobes (11). In this reproducible, anatomically specific behavioral syndrome, aggression is reduced rather than increased, sexual behavior is increased rather than decreased, social cohesion is diminished rather than heightened, and exploratory behavior rather than viscosity is promoted (1, 4, 11). Thus, it is difficult to attribute the interictal behavior syndrome to "nonspecific" effects of structural damage within the temporal lobe; indeed, beneficial behavioral consequences of temporal lobectomy in the form of reversal of abnormal behavior to the opposite may result from the effects of the destructive lesion upon the epileptic changes (72).

The observations frequently cited to dispute the neurologic specificity of the interictal behavior syndrome are comparisons among patients with differing forms of epilepsy. Most commonly, patients with an EEG-documented temporal lobe focus have been contrasted with "grand mal or generalized" epileptics; both groups may show frequent changes in behavior, and the differences fail to reach statistical significance. The results are summarized as a failure to observe specific behavioral changes in temporal lobe epilepsy (73, 74).

We believe that this type of comparison is a major source of obfuscation. First, the fact that a patient has generalized seizures in no way eliminates the possibility that an epileptic focus is located within the limbic system. Because medially placed foci in the temporal lobe lie far from the usual scalp EEG electrodes, temporal lobe foci may go undetected while secondary cortical dysrhythmias would be observed (1, 29). Second, it has been shown repeatedly that kindling, the creation of new or secondary epileptic foci following repeated electrical stimulation (75), occurs most readily in limbic structures such as the amygdala. There is evidence, both from studies of experimental epilepsy in animals and from clinical observations in humans, that epileptogenic lesions outside the temporal limbic structures may induce daughter foci within the limbic system, following which behavioral deficits associated with limbic foci develop (1, 76, 77).

In our view these anatomic and physiologic realities render behavioral comparisons between temporal lobe and generalized epileptics uninterpretable. The more appropriate, but clinically difficult, comparisons would be with other focal epilepsies or with patients having infrequent generalized seizures of metabolic origin, in which the likelihood of kindling is low. In fact, there is evidence that patients with nontemporal focal epilepsy do not show characteristic behavior changes (1, 38). Patients suffering only generalized withdrawal seizures were differentiated blindly from temporal lobe epileptics because they did not exhibit hypergraphia or other features of interictal behavior in samples of their writing (78).

In summary, we believe that the interictal behavior syndrome is a frequent and specific consequence of limbic epileptic discharge. However, there may be analogous organic syndromes such as those resulting from hallucinogens that chemically affect or even "kindle" similar limbic structures (1, 77). Furthermore, through genetic variation and/or environmental shaping, some fraction of nonepileptic individuals might exhibit a similar behavioral phenotype. As a point of logic, then, the recognition of the specificity of the interictal behavioral syndrome would not imply that whenever the behavioral changes are observed, a temporal lobe focus must be the causative factor.

Psychiatric Specificity of the Interictal Behavior Syndrome

The last controversial issue we shall discuss concerns the behavioral specificity or psychiatric "distinctiveness" of the interictal behavior changes. Are they merely a potpourri of random psychiatric symptoms, indistinguishable from those found in the "typical" psychiatric patient (67)?

Clearly, individual behavioral characteristics such as aggression, sexual dysfunction, and deepened mood occur frequently in psychiatric syndromes. However, the basis of most reports on behavior in temporal lobe epilepsy is, precisely, the unexpected or distinctive quality of the clinical picture; for example, the tendency to write at length, coupled with philosophic or moralistic concerns, preoccupation with details, and aggressivity (9, 10), or the combination of paranoid ideation with warm emotions and a tendency to maintain close social relations (3, 4, 32). The interictal behavior syndrome is a cluster of behavioral features not typically encountered together in other patients. In all likelihood, individual behavioral features like aggression may occur more frequently or extremely in syndromes other than temporal lobe epilepsy. Furthermore, because many of the "traits" sampled by the questionnaire of Bear and Fedio (10) are closely correlated (e.g., temper and overt aggression; circumstantiality, obsessiveness, and viscosity; emotionality and altered mood), patients with other syndromes may endorse multiple associated traits. The critical observation, both clinically and statistically, is the simultaneous occurrence of generally uncorrelated behavioral characteristics among temporal lobe epileptics. The existence of this cluster is not contradicted by the observation that one could obtain an "average" profile that includes many of the interictal behavior features from a mixed group of psychiatric patients. This average profile of "nonspecific psychopathology" would not describe any particular patient. Indeed, it is hard to place any clinical meaning on such a statistical composite of, for example, a depressed patient, a schizophrenic, and a sociopath (67).

In addition to the tendency of these behaviors to cluster in the temporal lobe epileptic, the quality of individual behaviors is often distinctive. For example, the morally justified aggressive acts with subsequent remorse, commonly seen in temporal lobe epilepsy, are quite rare in both idiopathic sociopathy and frontal lobe disease. In a recent study employing structured interviews to examine these and other distinctions among behavioral symptoms, observers blind to diagnosis found highly significant differences among profiles of patients with aggressive character disorder, affective disorder, and idiopathic schizophrenia compared to temporal lobe epileptics (32).

APPROACHES TO MECHANISM AND TREATMENT OF INTERICTAL BEHAVIOR CHANGES

The principal aims of this chapter have been to present a clear picture of the range of interictal behavior changes observed in patients with temporal lobe epilepsy and to clarify misunderstanding that may generate controversy. The elucidation of underlying mechanisms and the development of effective treatments are critical tasks for the future.

We shall only summarize possible approaches to these issues. It has been suggested that an increased tendency to associate drive-related (emotional) responses to many stimuli may underlie the panoply of interictal behavior changes (1, 10, 77). This hypothesis is supported by the finding that autonomic responses to a wide range of visual stimuli appear to be enhanced during the interictal period in patients with temporal lobe epilepsy (68).

Drawing on anatomic and physiologic observations that limbic structures within the temporal lobe, such as the amygdala, link sensory association cortices with drive-controlling centers within the hypothalamus, it has been suggested that an epileptic focus may lower the threshold for the creation of sensory-limbic connections, facilitating fortuitous emotional associations (1, 77). The kindling phenomenon, readily demonstrated within the amygdaloid complex, provides a possible physiologic model for this effect (1, 75, 77).

The formation of such interictal "hyperconnections" (1, 77) may be a process independent of, or even antagonistic to, the ictal synchronization of neuronal firing that results in overt seizures. Thus, the observations that anticonvulsants such as phenytoin do not reverse interictal behavior changes (4) and that seizure frequency may even correlate inversely with the severity of interictal behavior (41, 42) are consistent with this view.

Several approaches to the control of interictal behavior are suggested by this model. Medications reducing the intensity of affects might be expected to reduce the frequency or severity of the fortuitous associations; such agents include lithium carbonate (which may have anticonvulsant effects in a low therapeutic dose range), propranolol, and clonidine (77). Transmitter-active medications shown to inhibit the kindling effect in animals would be worthy of trial, e.g., cholinergic blockers, adrenergic agonists, and dopamine agonists (77). Carbamazepine may be an especially effective psychotropic agent because it combines anticonvulsant, antiimpulsive, and antikindling effects (77).

Clearly, some patients suffer psychotic symptoms, usually within the setting of other interictal behavior changes. These individuals often need antipsychotics. For patients requiring the least increase in limbic excitability, agents such as the dihydroindolone molindone may be preferable (79).

If the mechanisms sketched above are correct, prompt surgical removal of the epileptic focus—preventing both paroxysmal seizures and the development of interictal change in limbic excitability—might be effective therapy (72). Secondary therapeutic lesions within the limbic system, involving the amygdala or the prefrontal cortex, or within the lateral hypothalamus appear to ameliorate particular behaviors, principally aggression (80, 81).

We believe that there is also a role for directive psychotherapy, which might be conceptualized as bringing altered emotional susceptibilities to the attention of intact, higher-order association cortices within the brain. In our experience group therapy meetings with temporal lobe epileptics manifesting interictal behavior changes have been especially efficacious, providing consensual validation of otherwise bizarre experiences and intense emotions, and serving as a forum for the development of innovative coping strategies.

In summary, the existence of distinct changes in ideation, emotion, and behavior has been firmly established. Only further investigations will enable us to refine the typical clinical presentation and its variants, document its incidence and prevalence in the population at large, uncover its pathologic substrate, and ameliorate its disabling consequences.

REFERENCES

1. Bear DM: temporal lobe epilepsy—a syndrome of sensory-limbic hyperconnection. *Cortex* 15:357-384, 1979
2. Davison K, Bagley C: Schizophrenia-like psychoses associated with organic disorders of the central nervous system—review of literature. *Br J Psychiatry* 4:113–184, 1969
3. Slater E, Beard AW: Schizophrenia-like psychoses of epilepsy. *Br J Psychiatry* 109:95–150, 1963
4. Blumer D, Benson DF: Psychiatric manifestation of epilepsy, in *Psychiatric Aspects of Neurologic Disease, Vol 2.* Edited by Benson DF, Blumer D. New York, Grune & Stratton, 1982, pp 25–48
5. Stevens JR, Hermann BP: Temporal lobe epilepsy, psychopathology and violence: the state of the evidence. *Neurology (New York)* 31:1127–1132, 1981
6. Tizard B: The personality of epileptics: a discussion of the evidence. *Psychol Bull* 59:196–210, 1962
7. Lishman AW: Temporal lobe epilepsy, in *Organic Psychiatry*. Oxford, Blackwell Scientific Publications, 1978
8. Bear DM: The temporal lobes: an approach to the study of organic behavioral changes, in *Handbook of Behavioral Neurology, Vol 2.* Edited by Gazzaniga M. London, Plenum Press, 1979
9. Waxman SA, Geschwind N: The interictal behavior syndrome of temporal lobe epilepsy. *Arch Gen Psychiatry* 32:1580–1586, 1975
10. Bear DM, Fedio P: Quantitative analysis of interictal behavior in temporal lobe epilepsy. *Arch Neurol* 34:454–467, 1977
11. Klüver H, Bucy PC: "Psychic blindness" and other symptoms following bilateral temporal lobectomy in Rhesus monkeys. *Am J Physiol* 119:352–353, 1937
12. MacLean PD: Chemical and electrical stimulation of small hippocampus in unrestrained animals, part II: behavioral findings. *Arch Neurol Psychiatry* 78:128–212, 1957
13. Gastaut H, Collomb H: Etude du comportement sexuel chez les épileptiques psychomoteurs. *Ann Med Psychol* 112:657–696, 1954
14. Blumer D, Walker AE: Sexual behavior in temporal lobe epilepsy. *Arch Neurol* 16:37–43, 1967
15. Kolarsky, A, Freund K, Machek J, et al: Male sexual deviation—association with early temporal lobe damage. *Arch Gen Psychiatry* 17:735–743, 1967
16. Jensen I, Larsen JK: Marital aspects of temporal lobe epilepsy. *J Neurol Neurosurg Psychiatry* 42:256–265, 1979
17. Ellison J: Alterations of sexual behavior in temporal lobe epilepsy. *Psychosomatics* 23:499–509, 1982

18. Shukula GD, Srivastava DN, Katiyar BC: Sexual disturbances in temporal lobe epilepsy: a controlled study. *Br J Psychiatry* 134:288–292, 1979

19. Taylor DC: Sexual behavior in temporal lobe epilepsy. *Arch Neurol* 21:510–516, 1969

20. Johnsen J: Sexual impotence and the limbic system. *Br J Psychiatry* 3:300–303, 1965

21. Hierons R, Saunders N: Impotence in patients with temporal lobe lesions. *Lancet* 2:761–764, 1966

22. Blumer D: Hypersexual episodes in temporal lobe epilepsy. *Am J Psychiatry* 126:1099–1106, 1970

23. Epstein AV: Relationship of fetishism and transvestitism to brain and particularly to temporal lobe dysfunction. *J Nerv Ment Dis* 133:247–253, 1961

24. Hoenig J, Kenna JC: EEG abnormalities in transexualism. *Br J Psychiatry* 134:293–300, 1979

25. Currier RD, Little SC, Suess JF, et al: Sexual seizures. *Arch Neurol* 25:260–264, 1971

26. Freeman FR, Nevis AH: Temporal lobe sexual seizures. *Neurology (Minneap)* 19:87–90, 1969

27. Hooshmand H, Brawley BW: Temporal lobe seizures and exhibitionism. *Neurology (Minneap)* 19:1119–1124, 1969

28. Sperber S, Sperber D, Williamson P, et al: Sexual automatism in complex partial seizures. *Neurology (New York)* 33:527–533, 1983

29. Devinsky O, Bear D: Varieties of aggressive behavior in patients with temporal lobe epilepsy. *Am J Psychiatry*, (in press)

30. Pincus JH: Can violence be a manifestation of epilepsy? *Neurology (New York)* 30:304–307, 1980

31. Delgado-Escuetta AV, Mattson RH, King L, et al: The nature of aggression during epileptic seizures. *N Engl J Med* 30:711–716, 1981

32. Bear D, Levin K, Blumer D: Interictal behavior in hospitalized temporal lobe epileptics—relationship to idiopathic psychiatric syndromes. *J Neurol Neurosurg Psychiatry* 45:481–488, 1982

33. Beresford HR: Letters to the editor. *Neurology (New York)* 30:1134–1140, 1980

34. Waxman SA, Geschwind N: Hypergraphia in temporal lobe epilepsy. *Neurology (New York)* 30:314–317, 1980

35. Roberts JK, Robertson MM, Trimble MR: The lateralizing significance of hypergraphia in temporal lobe epilepsy. *J Neurol Neurosurg Psychiatry* 45:131–138, 1982

36. Seidman L: Emotional and cognitive changes in temporal lobe epilepsy. PhD dissertation, Boston University, 1978

37. Bruens JH: Psychosis in epilepsy, in *Handbook of Clinical Neurology*. Edited by Vinken PJ, Bruyn GW. Amsterdam, North Holland Biomedical Press, 1974, pp 593–610

38. Dongier S: Statistical study of clinical and EEG manifestations of 546 psychotic episodes occurring in 516 epileptics between clincial seizures. *Epilepsia* 1:117–142, 1959

39. Glaus A: Ueber Kombinationen von Schizophrenie und Epilepsie. *Z Gesamte Neurol Psychiatr* 135:450–500, 1931

40. Gibbs FA: Ictal and nonictal psychiatric disorder in temporal lobe epilepsy. *J Nerv Ment Dis* 113:522–528, 1951

41. Landolt H: Die Temporallappenepilepsie und ihre Psychopathologie. *Bibl Psychiatr Neurol* 112:1–112, 1969

42. Pond DA: Psychiatric aspects of epilepsy. *J Indian Med Prof* 3:1441–1451, 1957

43. Flor-Henry P: Schizophrenic-like reactions and affective psychoses associated with temporal lobe epilepsy: etiological factors. *Am J Psychiatry* 126:148–152, 1969

44. Taylor DC: Factors influencing the occurrence of schizophrenia-like psychoses in patients with temporal lobe epilepsy. *Psychol Med* 5:249–234, 1975

45. Jensen I, Larsen JK: Psychoses in drug resistant temporal lobe epilepsy. *J Neurol Neurosurg Psychiatry* 42:948–954, 1979

46. Herman B, Dikmen S, Schwartz M, Karnes W: Interictal psychopathology in patients with ictal fear: a quantitative investigation. *Neurology (New York)* 32:7–11, 1982

47. Mesulam MM: Dissociative states with abnormal temporal lobe EEG. *Arch Neurol* 38:176–181, 1981

48. Schenk L, Bear D: Multiple personality and related dissociative phenomena in patients with temporal lobe epilepsy. *Am J Psychiatry* 138:1311–1326, 1981

49. Blumer D, Walker AE: Memory in temporal lobe epileptics, in *The Pathology of Memory*. Edited by Talland G, Waugh N. New York, Academic Press, 1969, p 65–73

50. Glowinski H: Cognitive deficits in temporal lobe epilepsy. *J Nerv Ment Dis* 157:129–137, 1973

51. Quadfasel AF, Pruyser PW: Cognitive deficits in patients with psychomotor epilepsy. *Epilepsia* 4:80–90, 1955

52. Dennerll RD: Cognitive deficits and lateral brain dysfunction in temporal lobe epilepsy. *Epilepsia* 5:177–191, 1964

53. Milner B: Intellectual functions of the temporal lobe. *Psychol Bull* 51:42–62, 1954

54. Lezak MD: *Neuropsychological Assessment*. New York, Oxford University Press, 1976

55. Heilman KM, Valenstein E (eds): *Clinical Neuropsychology*. New York, Oxford University Press, 1979

56. Walsh KW: *Neuropsychology: A Clinical Approach*. London, Churchill, 1977

57. Goodglass H, Kaplan E: Assessment of cognitive deficit in the brain-injured patient, in *Handbook of Behavioral Neurobiology, Vol 2: Neuropsychology*. Edited by Gazzaniga MS. New York, Plenum Press, 1979, pp 3–22

58. Rey A: *L'examen clinique en psychologie*. Paris, Presses Universitaries de France, 1964

59. Osterreith PH: Le test de copie d'une figure complexe. *Arch Psychol* 30:204–356, 1944

60. Milberg W, Greiffenstein M, Lewis R, et al: Differentiation of temporal lobe and generalized seizure patients with the WAIS. *J Consult Clin Psychol* 44:39–42, 1980

61. Coughlan AK, Warrington EK: Word comprehension and word retrieval in patients with localized cerebral lesions. *Brain* 101:163–185, 1978

62. Borod JC, Goodglass H, Kaplan E: Normative data on the Boston Diagnostic Aphasia Examination, Parietal Lobe Battery and the Boston Naming Test. *J Clin Neuropsychol* 2:209–215, 1980

63. Borkowski JG, Benton AL, Spreen O: Word fluency and brain damage. *Neuropsychologia* 5:135–140, 1967

64. Landsdell H: Effects of extent of temporal lobe ablations on two lateralized deficits. *Physiol Behav* 3:271–273, 1968

65. Meyer V: Cognitive changes following temporal lobectomy for relief of temporal lobe epilepsy. *Arch Neurol Psychiatry* 81:299–309, 1959

66. Wilson H, Olson WH, Gascon GG, et al: Personality characteristics in multiple sclerosis. *Psychol Rep* 51:791–806, 1982

67. Mungas D: Interictal behavior abnormality in temporal lobe epilepsy. *Arch Gen Psychiatry* 39:108–111, 1982

68. Bear D, Schenk L: Increased autonomic responses to neutral and emotional stimuli in patients with temporal lobe epilepsy. *Am J Psychiatry* 138:843–845, 1981

69. Kristensen O, Sindrup FH: Psychomotor epilepsy and psychosis. *Acta Neurol Scand* 57:361–369, 1978

70. Mirsky AF, Primac VW, Marsan CA, et al: A comparison of the psychological test performances of patients with focal and nonfocal epilepsy. *Exp Neurol* 2:75–90, 1960

71. Bear DM: Organic alterations in personality, in *Outpatient Psychiatry: Diagnosis and Treatment*. Edited by Lazare H. Baltimore, Williams & Wilkins, 1979, pp 337–352

72. Falconer MA: Reversibility by temporal lobe resection of the behavioral abnormalities of temporal lobe epilepsy. *N Engl J Med* 289:451–455, 1973

73. Mignone RJ, Donnelly EF, Sadowsky D: Psychological and neurological comparisons of psychomotor and nonpsychomotor epileptic patients. *Epilepsia* 11:345–359, 1970

74. Small JG, Milstein V, Stevens JR: Are psychomotor epileptics different? *Arch Neurol* 1:187–194, 1962

75. Goddard G, McIntyre D, Leech C: A permanent change in brain function resulting from daily electrical stimulation. *Exp Neurol* 25:295–330, 1969

76. Stamm JS, Warren A: Learning and retention by monkeys with epileptogenic implants in posterior parietal cortex. *Epilepsia* 2:229–242, 1961

77. Bear D: Interictal behavior in temporal lobe epilepsy: possible anatomic and physiologic basis, in *Epilepsy: Neurotransmitter, Behavior, and Pregnancy*. Edited by Wada J. Vancouver, Joint Publication of Canadian League Against Epilepsy and Western Institute on Epilepsy, 1979

78. Sachdez HS, Waxman SG: Frequency of hypergraphia in temporal lobe epilepsy—an index of interictal behavior syndrome. *J Neurol Neurosurg Psychiatry* 44:358–360, 1981

79. Oliver AP, Luchins VJ, Wyatt RJ: Neuroleptic-induced seizures. *Arch Gen Psychiatry* 39:206–209, 1982

80. Kiloh LG, Gye RS, Rushworth RG, et al: Stereotactic amygdalotomy for aggressive behavior. *J Neurol Neurosurg Psychiatry* 37:437–444, 1974

81. Vaernet K, Madsen A: Stereotaxic amygdalotomy and basofrontal tractotomy in psychotics with aggressive behavior. *J Neurol Neurosurg Psychiatry* 33:858–863, 1970

7

Psychosis in Epilepsy

Shirley M. Ferguson, M.D., F.A.P.A.
Mark Rayport, M.D. C.M., Ph.D., F.A.C.S.

The relationship between psychosis and epilepsy inspires debate concerning such basic issues as the nature of the psychosis, mechanisms of its production, and its correlations with epileptic phenomena. Efforts to provide an explanation of this relationship parsimoniously during the 1950s and 1960s (1–3) have been challenged by the proposition that a multifactorial approach may be more correct (4–6). This chapter will review the problems in the relationship between psychosis and epilepsy and address them in the context of the authors' ongoing clinical experience in a multidisciplinary comprehensive epilepsy program.

PSYCHOSIS IN EPILEPSY: A CRITICAL REVIEW OF THE LITERATURE

Phenomenology of Psychosis in Epilepsy

The association of behavioral disturbances with epilepsy has been recorded since antiquity (7). From the inception of psychiatry

---

We thank W. Stephen Corrie, M.D., for the electroencephalographic and stereo-electroencephalographic data.

until the flowering of neurology in the latter half of the nineteenth century, the behavioral observation and care of epileptic patients remained primarily in the province of psychiatrists. Descriptions of behavioral derangements in patients with epilepsy spanned the gamut of psychiatric symptomatology. The psychiatric diagnoses made by Esquirol (8) among 389 epileptic women hospitalized at the Salpêtrière included hysteria, melancholia, mania, monomania, idiocy, dementia, weakened memory, etc., showing that mental derangements in epileptic patients included disorders of thinking and affect and deficits in higher cerebral functions. Insanity was accepted, with recognition of its organic aspects, as an adjunct of epilepsy.

In the modern era of epileptology, which began with the discovery of the human electroencephalogram (EEG) by Berger (9) in 1929, epilepsy increasingly became a subject for neurologic study despite the evidence of behavioral and neuropsychiatric changes in epileptic patients, particularly in physical attacks (10). Adopting Turner's term "psychomotor" (11), Gibbs and associates (12, 13) advanced the concept of characteristic interictal temporal EEG findings in psychomotor epilepsy. This report seemed to portend a fresh understanding of behavioral symptoms in epilepsy. In 1951 Gibbs (14) wrote that temporal lobe epilepsy and psychosis were "commonly associated": Among 275 epileptic patients with sharply localized spike foci, the focus was in one or both anterior temporal areas in 163 (59 percent); of these patients 95 percent had a history of psychomotor epilepsy, 32 percent had severe personality disorders, and 17 percent had psychosis. He saw the epileptic and psychiatric components of psychomotor epilepsy as "independent . . . physiologically antithetic [yet] anatomically associated."

Contemporaneous studies of the psychosis in patients with temporal lobe epilepsy came from English investigators. Hill (15) in 1953 described a "paranoid hallucinatory psychotic state" that was said to be "a definite clinical entity." Pond (16) in 1957 emphasized the absence of affective impairment as seen in true schizophrenia. Dongier (17) reported on a collaborative study of 536 psychotic episodes in 516 epileptic patients from psychiatric hospitals, outpatient clinics, and private practice. Among centrencephalic epileptics the psychotic episodes were brief (several hours), never chronic or permanently mentally disturbing, and not leading to dementia. The episode often began with a seizure. Confusion was frequent. Psychotic episodes in patients with psychomotor epilepsy were of long duration (days or weeks) and were rarely preceded by a tonic-clonic seizure but often ended in one. Confusion was not always present. Disturbances of affect were prominent.

Although the disciplines of neurology, neurological surgery, neuropsychiatry, and neuropsychology became actively involved in the study and treatment of temporal lobe epilepsy, their intellectual paths joined infrequently. Careful delineation of electrophysiologic events has not often been accompanied by rigorous clinical behavioral descriptions. The dearth of sophisticated collaborative work is reflected in the lack of descriptions of the relationships of psychopathologic and neurophysiologic phenomena. Recently, in the climate of expanding psychobiologic understanding, the pendulum has swung again to an interest, and, in fact, a demand, for precise behavioral description in order to administer correct treatment. The third edition of the *Diagnostic and Statistical Manual of Mental Disorders* (18) represents the culmination of this trend. Similar precision has yet to be extended to the definition of psychosis in epilepsy.

In epileptic patients "psychosis" has been variously applied, sometimes referring to a distinguishable entity, e.g., episodic psychosis (19), at other times to states of impaired consciousness or to chronic psychosis such as schizophrenia and affective conditions. In the recent literature, classifications of psychosis occurring in epilepsy patients have included a broad spectrum of symptomatology (5, 6, 20, 21), while interest has been concentrated on the psychosis resembling schizophrenia.

In 1956 Rodin and associates (22) studied the psychoses of six patients with psychomotor epilepsy and EEG disturbances in the temporal lobes. They concluded that these patients had "schizophrenic reactions associated with 'temporolimbic system' dysfunction." Although Bleuler's fundamental symptoms were not predominant, they designated the psychosis as a "symptomatic schizophrenia." In 1963 Slater et al. (1) introduced the term "schizophrenia-like psychosis" in their highly influential paper. In agreement with the earlier English authors, the schizophrenia-like psychosis in their 69 cases was characterized by the prominence of paranoid ideation that often had a mystical and religious coloring. Although Slater et al. reported that schizophrenia-like psychosis differed from process schizophrenia with its affective impoverishment and clear sensorium by the preservation of affect, the presence of organic findings ("a psychoorganic syndrome"), and the absence of genetic tainting or a premorbid schizoid personality, the term "schizophrenia" entered the literature to characterize psychosis in epilepsy.

In 1974 Bruens (5) reviewed the cases of Slater et al. He noted that primary delusions, a sine qua non for the diagnosis of paranoid schizophrenia, did not occur and, in fact, that the delusions were "empathizable—the patient remains in our world." Bruens concluded that "none of the psychoses fulfill the criteria for the diagnosis of schizophrenia." Subsequently, Scandinavian authors again described psychosis in epilepsy as "paranoid-hallucinatory" (23), "psychosis with paranoid delusions" (24), and "paranoid hallucinatory syndrome of epilepsy" (25).

In 1980 Perez and Trimble (26) sought to remedy the lack of accurate phenomenologic description with a quantitative approach to diagnosis, utilizing the Present State Examination of Wing et al. (27, 28), which is based on the first-rank symptoms of Schneider (29) for nuclear schizophrenia and events in the patient's life during the month preceding the interview. In 24 consecutively referred patients with "unequivocal epilepsy and active psychosis which had continued for more than one month," they found that the psychosis of 11 cases (45.83 percent) fulfilled the criteria of the nuclear schizophrenia syndrome. Seventeen (70.83 percent) of their cases had "complex partial seizures of probable temporal lobe origin." The 11 cases (64.70 percent) of psychosis were all in this subgroup (30). Psychiatrically, the validity of these authors' conclusion is dependent on the acceptance of the Schneiderian criteria as diagnostic for schizophrenia, a position still in question (31–33). Further, as reemphasized by Parnas and Korsgaard (34), Schneider limited the validity of the first-rank symptoms for the diagnosis of schizophrenia to cases without coarse brain damage. Sherwin (35) pointed out that in comparison with process schizophrenia, the psychosis in epilepsy was "more periodic, socially less disruptive, frequently did not require major tranquilizers and did not require chronic hospitalization." He concluded that "it cannot be overstated that the psychosis associated with epilepsy may not be the same disorder as schizophrenia." Betts et al. (21) emphasized the relative frequency of undifferentiated epileptic paranoid psychoses in temporal lobe epilepsy that are organic and develop out of a paranoid personality. The problem is compounded by the phenomenologic difficulty of the definition of schizophrenia in nonepileptic psychiatric patients. Brockington and associates (36) wrote, "The concept of 'schizophrenia' has been particularly controversial, with gross differences in its usage in different parts of the world. . . ."

Among non-schizophrenia-like psychotic manifestations in epilepsy, organic psychotic symptomatology as a possible accompaniment to seizure activity appears to have been largely taken for granted and not often closely studied. In 1969 Ferguson and associates (4) described similarities between seizure content, psychosis, seizures, and responses to electrical brain stimulation. In 1981, nonetheless, Toone (38) wrote that he was "not aware of any attempt to trace the evolution of ictal and postictal experiences into the psychotic state." Affective symptomatology has also been neglected (6, 21, 37). Betts (37) observed that "depressive states have been little described despite the fact that perhaps they are the most important psychiatric complication of epilepsy." Perez and Trimble (26) concluded that the psychoses in patients with temporolimbic epilepsy were heterogeneous and that disorders of affect were prominent in the one-third of their cases who did not have "schizophrenia."

The psychotic mental states above have been presented as chronic. Whether the duration criteria utilized in these studies would exclude episodic psychiatric symptomatology is open to question. Slater et al. (1) accepted a patient into their study population if the psychosis was of weeks' or months' duration. Among their 69 patients, 20 were described as having repeated brief confusional episodes at the onset of psychosis, and 31 were chronic cases. Among Bruens' 19 psychotic patients (5), 9 had an episodic course. Betts et al. (21) took note of such findings in their study population and postulated that there may be two different subpopulations of schizophrenic patients among epileptics: those patients with an organic change in the temporal lobe and those with episodic schizophreniform psychosis that is more clearly related to attack frequency. Kristensen and Sindrup (23) stated that the paranoid hallucinatory epileptic psychosis could be chronic or episodic. Perez and Trimble (26) used for inclusion a duration of psychosis of "more than 4 weeks." The course of the psychosis should help to elucidate the appropriateness of the term "chronic," but outcome has been little studied (38). Slater et al. (1) found that one-third of their 69 cases of schizophrenia-like psychosis had attained a complete remission of their psychosis, whereas another one-third had partially improved. Bruens (5) reported similar outcome findings.

The categorization of the psychosis as interictal also requires examination. Glaser (39) stated that "subictal paroxysms have a role in interictal psychotic episodes." Ferguson et al. (4) emphasized that clinical seizures may be very subtle during psychosis and may erroneously be considered absent. A recent rereading of Gowers (40) has shown that he and J. H. Jackson held a similar view. We agree with Benjaminsen (41) who observed that "epileptic psychosis is frequently not recognized as epileptic in psychiatric units." Ramani and Gumnit (42) stated: "The diagnosis of interictal psychosis and differentiation from interictal confusional states is often difficult to establish in retrospective studies. Crucial information pertinent to the exact type and frequency of seizures and possible anticonvulsant toxicity may not be available because of inadequate documentation."

In short, despite the current emphasis on the "schizophrenia" of temporal lobe epilepsy, the demonstrated phenomenology of psychosis in epilepsy also encompasses affective and organic symptomatology. Few authors have rigorously separated chronic from episodic forms and interictal from periictal occurrence.

Prevalence of Psychosis in Epilepsy

Estimation of the prevalence of psychosis in epilepsy faces substantial problems.

Dongier (17) related 536 psychotic episodes to the clinico-EEG type of epilepsy. She found that 40.2 percent had occurred in cases of centrencephalic epilepsy, 44.0 percent in cases of psychomotor epilepsy, 6.2 percent in cases of focal epilepsy, and 9.6 percent in cases of unclassified epilepsy, whereas in the author's contributed sample of 84 cases, psychosis occurred predominantly in the psychomotor group (63 percent) in contrast to the generalized (30 percent).

Hypotheses have extended from an "affinity" between epilepsy and psychosis to an "antagonism," which culminated in the induction of major seizures for the treatment of psychoses in 1934 (43). As historical perspective on electroconvulsive therapy shows, the antagonism theory was operationally appropriate for schizophrenia of the catatonic type, now thought to be a condition more closely allied to the affective disorders, and for the affective disorders themselves (44). Therapeutic implications are common knowledge and evident in the indications for electroconvulsive therapy today.

Support for the relational hypothesis was implied in findings of increased psychiatric symptomatology in patients with temporal lobe epilepsy (14, 15, 45–47). Subsequently, figures in the literature have ranged widely from a frequent to a coincidental relationship between psychosis and temporal lobe epilepsy: Gibbs and Gibbs (48) reported that among 678 cases with clinical psychomotor seizures, 7.2 percent had unclassified psychosis, 2.1 percent had manic-depressive psychosis, and 0.2 percent had schizophrenia, adding to a prevalence of 9.5 percent. Among 1,806 patients with psychomotor and grand mal seizures, the prevalence of psychosis was, respectively, 9.4, 1.7, and 0.8 percent—total

11.9 percent. Thus, among 2,484 patients with psychomotor seizures, 21.4 percent had psychosis. In contrast, only 0.73 percent of 5,598 cases of grand mal seizures had psychosis. Most of the psychiatric data on these cases apparently became available to the authors secondarily from a broad referral EEG practice. In the general U.S. population, the prevalence of schizophrenia is estimated to be 0.23–0.47 percent; that of well-defined manic-depressive illness 1 percent for men and 2 percent for women (49). Ervin et al. (50), studying patients psychiatrically and neurologically, found that among 42 patients with temporal lobe EEG spiking, 81 percent received a diagnosis of schizophrenia. Stevens (51) found a similar prevalence of psychosis in patients with temporal lobe (31.4 percent) as compared with generalized epilepsy (29 percent), yet each of the two psychotic diagnoses—"schizophrenia" and "paranoid"—was more prevalent in the psychomotor group. Mood disturbances—"dysphoria" and "anxiety"—were three to four times more frequent in the psychomotor group than in generalized epilepsy. Thus, we would conclude that behind the comparable prevalences generated by the authors' quantitative approach, qualitative differences existed in the psychoses of the psychomotor and generalized epilepsy cases. It is necessary further to allow that the smallness of the focal motor-sensory group ($n = 12$) precluded the demonstration of the effect of age on the appearance of psychosis postulated for the psychomotor and generalized groups. Of interest is that similar differences between the results of quantitative and qualitative approaches have appeared in the literature of personality in epilepsy (52).

Despite these discrepancies, a significant consensus has developed in the literature that prolonged psychoses in patients with epilepsy occurred predominantly in patients with temporal lobe epilepsy (1, 2, 20, 39). Some reservations are to be observed. Slater and associates (1) reported that temporal EEG disturbances occurred in 48 (68.5 percent) of their 69 patients with a schizophrenia-like psychosis. Ramani and Gumnit (42), studying both mental state and epileptic phenomena in patients hospitalized on an epilepsy unit, found that among nine patients who developed psychosis, only five had complex partial seizures, whereas four showed evidence of generalized epilepsy.

The difficulty or impossibility of accurate estimation of the prevalence of psychosis is related partly to the phenomenological problems discussed previously. Complicating the issue further is the fact that the prevalence figures largely represent schizophrenia-like psychosis and paranoid states (38), often accepted as the interictal psychosis of temporal lobe epilepsy. Trimble and Perez (30) cautioned against this practice in their description of the psychoses of temporal lobe epilepsy as heterogeneous, schizophrenia-like psychosis accounting for only two-thirds of these cases. Added caution is necessary because of frequent difference in the relative rigorousness of the diagnosis and classification of epileptic and psychotic phenomena.

In view of all these obstacles and uncertainties, Fenton's conclusion (6) appears apposite that "little is known about the prevalence of the psychoses of epilepsy."

Classification of Psychosis in Epilepsy

Reflecting the evolution of the understanding of the psychoses of epilepsy, recent classifications have been based variously upon the state of consciousness, namely, impaired or clear (5, 20), on psychopathology (21), and on the ictal state, that is, ictal-postictal or interictal (38).

Bruens (20) in 1971 divided the psychotic syndromes into four symptomatic categories that he regarded as not sharply defined: paranoid syndrome with delusions; psychoses with mental regression; schizophrenia-like psychoses; and confusional states. In 1974 Bruens (5) presented a classification based on the state of consciousness and duration of the psychosis, as follows:

Psychotic States with Disturbance of Consciousness (twilight states)
- Psychoses in which the disturbance of consciousness is the most prominent feature
  - postparoxysmal twilight states
  - absence status (Lennox), status psychomotoricus
  - twilight states not chronologically related to the seizures
- Delirious states

Psychotic States with Normal Level of Consciousness
- Brief, often periodic psychoses (episodic psychoses)
  - dysphoric states
  - manic states
  - depressive states
  - alternating psychoses with productive symptomatology
- More prolonged or chronic psychoses
  - paranoid syndromes
  - psychoses characterized by marked psychical regression
  - schizophrenia-like syndromes
  - manic-depressive psychoses

In 1976 Betts et al. (21) proposed a classification based on psychopathology. Their three groups were as follows:

> (1) Global disruption of personality. There is disturbance of thinking, behavior, emotional relationships, feeling, and perception. This group includes the schizophrenias and schizophrenia-like states. (2) Primary disturbance of mood. There may be depression or pathologic elation and such secondary symptoms as depressive hallucinations or delusions. (3) Organic psychosyndromes. These include confusional states, changes in behavior, in the context of epilepsy associated with subictal epileptic activity, and delirium.

Only in the organic psychosyndrome is any mention made of epileptic activity. However, as discussed in the sections on phenomenology and mechanisms of psychosis, there is evidence for ictal or minimal ictal involvement in the production of psychotic symptoms resembling schizophrenia or affective disorders. Toone (38) comments on Betts et al.'s omission of brief psychoses. Bruens (5) included brief psychoses under states with normal consciousness, but admitted to the difficulty of differentiating these from twilight states, owing to the problem of deciding whether or not consciousness is impaired.

In 1981 Toone (38) offered a classification in which the psychotic states were differentiated by the presence or absence of seizure activity:

1. Psychoses directly related to the occurrence of seizure activity.
   a. Abnormal mental states that are a direct and immediate consequence of underlying seizure activity and which may have some of the features of a psychotic state:
      i. continuous auras
      ii. petit mal status
      iii. temporal lobe status
   b. Postictal psychoses
2. Interictal psychoses
   a. schizophrenia-like and paranoid psychoses
   b. affective psychoses

Challenge to this classification lies in the uncertainty of the designation "interictal." Glaser (39) stated: "Often it is difficult to separate an ictal or postictal psychotic episode from an interictal behavior disorder. Acute epileptic psychotic reactions have been regarded as actual components of the psychomotor temporal lobe seizure complex since descriptions by French neuropsychiatrists of the 19th century and later by Jackson, Penfield and Jasper,

Gastaut and Lennox." Ferguson et al. (4) observed the role of subtle seizure activity in the production of psychosis.

It can be concluded that a classification recognizing the interrelationship between epileptic and behavioral mechanisms would be desirable.

Etiology and Pathogenesis of Psychosis in Epilepsy

That epileptic seizures can be associated with, or cause, psychosis is widely accepted when the immediate link can be observed. Thus, there is agreement that an epileptic twilight state with impairment of consciousness may follow a recognized seizure or cluster of seizures (postictal psychosis). Another unequivocal relationship is the association of a psychotic state with EEG evidence of generalized spike-wave or focal temporal status epilepticus (ictal psychosis). These psychotic states tend to be of limited duration.

The challenge has rested with the determination of the pathogenesis of the psychotic states that have been described as chronic and interictal. Critical reservations with regard to the latter parameters of the psychotic states have been developed in the previous sections.

Hypotheses in the literature regarding the relationships between psychosis and seizure activity have ranged from age-related coincidence (51) to specific mechanisms, which are summarized below.

Pathophysiologic Hypotheses. Pond's hypothesis (16) related to the impact of limbic seizures on the emotional life of the epileptic patient. He postulated that transient abnormal affect and/or perception become integrated into the psychic life and may become the anlage of psychosis.

Williams (53) implicated the anterior temporal lobe in the production of psychosis, because of its role in the evaluation and interpretation of afferent input, furnishing information necessary to establish the self-concept—the feeling of "I am." He hypothesized that when this process is disrupted by the seizure disorder, erroneous interpretations of ongoing experience may lead to depression or paranoid ideation.

Slater et al. (1) attributed psychosis to the dying cells of an atrophic process (demonstrated by pneumoencephalography in 37 of the 56 cases so studied). They postulated that an "increase in the atrophy as a result of the occurrence of seizures eventuated (over an average period of 14 years) in the changes accounting for psychosis . . . with the tendency of the psychosis in the fullness of time to pass off into an organic deficit." This hypothesis would be consonant with their findings of organic personality changes rather than schizophrenic deterioration and their conclusion that the schizophrenia-like psychosis is a stage in a dementing process. Symonds (54) related the development of psychosis "not [to] loss of neurones in the temporal lobe . . . but [to] the disorderly activity of those that remain, and this disorderly activity is of the kind that is also likely to cause seizures." Fenton (6) called attention to the fact that no systematic psychometric data were available in the work of Slater et al. to substantiate the theory of organic deterioration. However, we noted that among 11 of their patients who had had pneumoencephalograms, 6 showed progressive atrophic changes on repetition of this test. Radiologic studies in 57 patients with psychosis associated with epilepsy (of the temporal lobe type in 30) by Toone et al. (55) have not supported the concept of atrophy.

Taylor (56) examined the association between the location and the nature of the epileptogenic lesion and psychosis in Falconer's patients. He noted that mesial temporal sclerosis was rarely associated with psychosis, whereas an "alien tissue" lesion, such as hamartoma or a cystic tumor, was more frequently found in patients with psychosis. However, the correlation of the lesion with age at onset of seizures (rather than the pathology) seemed the more probable explanation. Thus, mesial temporal sclerosis, which develops very early in life and tends to be associated with onset of seizures in the first decade, was uncommon in cases with psychosis (2 of 41 cases). "Alien tissue" lesions, on the other hand, were correlated with later onset of seizures (past the first decade) and more frequent incidence of psychosis (11 of 47 cases). He concluded that the psychologic consequences of epilepsy beginning in adolescence were the explanation for the psychosis.

Flor-Henry (2) in 1969 stated that he was the first to show that "epileptic activity of the dominant temporal lobe is highly correlated with the emergence of psychosis of a schizophrenic type" in a retrospective study of 100 cases of temporal lobe epilepsy, 50 of whom had had "a documented psychotic episode observed in the hospital setting" and 50 of whom were without psychosis and were matched only for sex, serving as controls. The diagnoses of temporal lobe seizures were based on hospital records and confirmed by extracranial EEG. The psychotic cases had few or no psychomotor seizures and fewer seizures in general than the nonpsychotic controls, a point made earlier by Gibbs (14). Manic-depressive psychosis occurred in patients with foci in the nondominant temporal lobe.

Other investigators reporting on lateralization of the epileptic process before and after Flor-Henry's studies were not in agreement. Slater and associates (1) had not found a laterality effect. Glaser (39) also reported no consistent lateralization in 37 patients with psychomotor seizures and episodes of psychosis. Taylor (56) found, among 15 temporal lobe epileptics with psychosis, 7 with involvement on the left, 5 with involvement on the right, and 3 with bilateral involvement. Kristensen and Sindrup (23) observed 27 patients with left-sided and 29 with right-sided foci among 56 temporal lobe epileptics with psychosis. They emphasized the location of the abnormality in the mediobasal temporal lobe as the crucial factor, rather than lateralization. Trimble and Perez (30) agreed with the increased left-sided involvement in the schizophrenic group, but could not confirm lateralization to the nondominant temporal lobe in patients with affective disorders. The radiologic evaluation of epileptic patients with psychosis by Toone et al. (55) "did not provide firm support for the hypothesis of lateralized structural damage related to the pattern of the psychotic illness."

Sherwin (35, 57) and Sherwin et al. (58) responded to the critical question emerging from the laterality studies, namely, the accuracy of the localization of the epileptogenic focus. They performed retrospective studies for the prevalence of psychosis on two series of patients who had been selected for neurosurgical treatment by temporal lobe excision after rigorous preoperative studies that included stereo-EEG at the University of California, Los Angeles (UCLA), and Sainte-Anne Hospital, Paris. In the UCLA series, laterality of the epileptogenic lesion was established by stereo-EEG recording of ictal episodes. Among 63 cases, indication of psychosis was found in the records of 7. The epileptogenic lesion was on the left in five cases. Six of the cases had a psychosis diagnosed as paranoid or schizophrenic. In the Sainte-Anne Hospital study, more rigorous criteria of laterality required the successful relief of epilepsy by surgical excision. Among 80 qualifying cases, the records of 7 had histories of psychosis. The epileptogenic lesion was on the left in five. In both investigations the relative prevalence of left- and right-sided foci in the psychotic and nonpsychotic groups differed significantly. Sherwin stated that he made no attempt "to validate the psychiatric diagnosis."

It is relevant to note also a study of cerebral hemispheric asymmetries with computed axial tomography (CT) in nonepileptic schizophrenia (59). The comprehensive review of the literature in this article affirmed a left-sided locus of pathology in schizophrenia and relatively little evidence for localization in the temporal lobe. The authors reported that the CT scan methodology provided evidence for abnormalities in the left frontal lobe.

Electrographic and Clinical Seizure Activity. In 1958 Landolt (60) reported on serial scalp EEG recording in 107 cases of epileptic twilight states and psychotic episodes. Clinically, the psychotic episodes were characterized as "epileptic mania." He found an inverse relationship between seizure occurrence and the affective psychotic episodes during which he observed "forced normalization" in the EEG. This finding occurred in 47 of the psychotic cases and was absent in 4. Landolt thought the phenomenon was only loosely connected with temporal lobe epilepsy, although most of these cases had "electroencephalographically focal epilepsy with an epileptogenic focus over one of the temporal lobes." He provided little or no information as to type of seizures in his cases. It is of interest that Landolt's findings approximate the electroconvulsive therapy paradigm. Several authors have pointed out that normalization of the EEG in conjunction with psychosis could be an effect of medication (60–62). Flor-Henry (2), on the basis of extracranial EEG data, stressed the inverse relationship between psychosis and seizure activity. Thus, psychosis was viewed as an interictal event. This view is suspect if one carefully evaluates the interictal period to determine if indeed it is seizurefree as the term implies, or whether subtle clinical seizures "invisible" to untrained observers or electrical seizures in the depth of the brain "invisible" to the scalp EEG are involved in the production of the psychosis. Flor-Henry stated that psychosis tended to occur as seizure frequency diminished and also that abnormal electrical activity in the depth of the temporal lobe could be related to psychosis. This begs the question of the definition of seizure activity. Flor-Henry's statements imply that only seizure activity that is clinically evident is to be so designated. A further explanation for the inverse theory of Flor-Henry may lie in his case selection, which included patients with affective disorders to whom the electroconvulsive therapy paradigm might be applicable.

In contrast, Glaser (39) in his study of psychosis in 37 patients with temporal lobe epilepsy found that EEG correlations occurring with interictal psychotic episodes consisted of more intense focal temporal or bilateral paroxysmal discharge. He suggested that when, on occasion, normalization did occur during the psychotic state, subictal cerebral excitation might be occurring. Evidence of subclinical seizure activity has been reported by Ferguson and associates (4). Chkhenkeli and Geladze (63), whose series of 150 cases included 8 in whom stereo-EEG observations had been obtained, wrote that "in the interictal period prolonged subclinical epileptic discharges can be found in the mediobasal formations of the temporal lobe in patients with temporal epilepsy with marked emotional-affective disturbances, especially in the medio-basal part of the amygdaloid complex."

An opposite or inconsistent relationship between seizure activity and psychosis has been described by other authors. In the series of Slater et al. (1), epileptic seizures persisted up to the onset of the psychosis. "In the great majority, it was not possible to relate the onset of the psychosis to any change in the quality or frequency of the fits." However, in a small number of cases, they found a frequency change—an increase in frequency of seizures in two cases and a decline of frequency in six cases "successfully controlled by medication"—an explanation also advocated by others (30, 61, 64) who stressed the role of antiepileptic drugs in producing an inverse or see-saw relationship. Taylor (3) found no relationship between the frequency of attacks and psychosis. Kristensen and Sindrup (65) found a decrease in complex partial seizures in patients during psychosis. Jensen and Larsen (24) found a higher frequency of grand mal, petit mal, focal seizures, and automatisms in their surgical epileptic populations with psychosis. Shukla et al. (66) noted that both an increase and decrease in seizure frequency were found in association with the onset of psychosis.

Reports of the development of psychosis in patients cured of seizures by surgery (24) have been mentioned (38) as lending support to Landolt's (60) and Flor-Henry's (2) hypotheses with regard to the inverse relationship between seizure activity and psychosis. In explanation of this occurrence, observations of Ferguson and Rayport (67) may be applicable. They emphasized the role of adjustment to living without epilepsy after successful seizure surgery in the production of postoperative psychiatric symptoms. Adjustment problems included loss of identity, exposure to previously hidden hostilities, and premature expectations of the environment for improved performance on the part of the patient. Horowitz and Cohen (68) described patients who developed paranoia and depression after successful seizure surgery. This symptomatology was explained as resulting from a combination of persistent cognitive deficits interrelated with interpersonal difficulties occurring in relation to the changed self-image of the patients.

In the end, it would appear that whether or not seizure activity is prophylactic against psychosis, that is, whether or not it shares an inverse relationship with the psychotic state, may be determined by the type of psychosis, as suggested from electroconvulsive therapy experience. Toone (38) points out the inconsistent occurrence of this "see-saw" relationship as illustrated by the observation that when psychosis precedes epilepsy, the former is not aided by the latter. It should be emphasized that Trimble (62) in his recent survey of psychosis in epilepsy found a significant prevalence of affective disorders.

Post et al. (69) saw a role for kindling in the development of abnormal behavior in patients with temporal lobe epilepsy. They suggested that major motor seizures, such as those artificially induced by electroconvulsive therapy, might be anticonvulsant to seizure activity in the limbic system. It would not then be contradictory that both major seizures and antiepileptic drugs such as carbamazepine may be helpful for the control of affective disorders. If major seizures are controlled, disturbed behavior may occur owing to the persistence of minor limbic seizure activity. This may in part explain the controversy over the antagonism or affinity of psychosis and epilepsy. It may be recalled that Slater and associates (1) noted a decrease in major, not psychomotor, seizures in some epileptic patients who became psychotic.

Neuropharmacologic/Pharmacologic Factors. Specific deficiency of folate has been suggested by Reynolds (64) as a precipitant of psychosis in the epileptic patient. Deficiency of folate as a consequence of high doses of phenytoin may explain the coincidence of seizure control and psychosis. A disturbance of amine metabolism accounting for the inverse relationship between seizures and psychosis was proposed by Trimble (70), who stated that an increase in central monoamine activity may both raise the threshold for seizures and increase the propensity for psychosis.

Psychogenic Factors. Psychosis may have psychogenic components originating in the situational reaction to being an epileptic. In addition, the effect of the intrusion of seizure experiences into conscious life may be the gradual development of psychosis (16). These factors may be compounded by chronic impairments of temporal lobe function, leading to reduced adaptive ability and sometimes to psychosis (4, 5).

Higher Function Impairment. Jackson (10) wrote of the role in behavioral difficulties, including insanity, of impairments of high level cortical functioning as a result of seizures. Glaser (39) described cognitive deficits in patients with temporal lobe epilepsy and psychosis. Horowitz and Cohen (68) observed impairments in language processing and memory as having a role in the development of paranoia in patients with temporal lobe epilepsy. Ferguson et al. (4) called attention to the role of continuous and intermittent higher function impairments in the production of psychosis and "everyday psychopathology." Bruens (5) also mentioned the impairment of integrative processes involved in the production of psychosis.

Multifactorial Hypotheses. A multifactorial basis for behavior disturbance in epilepsy was hypothesized by the present authors (4) who stressed the need for an individual approach. Bruens (5) concurred with both points. He wrote in regard to chronic epileptic psychosis that "a multifactorial genesis has to be considered, the various factors being of differing significance in each individual case." Fenton (6) concluded, after reviewing the possible explanations for the development of psychosis in patients with epilepsy, that "like most psychiatric disorders, it is probable that the psychoses of epilepsy result from a complex interaction of multiple etiologic factors—biologic, physiologic, and social. The relative importance of any one factor varies from individual to individual with an interplay of pathogenic factors."

ORIGINAL OBSERVATIONS

Psychiatric observations regarding the relationship between epilepsy and psychosis were reported by these authors and their colleagues in 1962 and 1969 from studies of patients at the New York Neurological Institute (71) and the Albert Einstein College of Medicine (4). Since 1969 comprehensive studies of patients with epilepsy have been conducted at the Medical College of Ohio by a multidisciplinary epilepsy group, including researchers from the disciplines of neurology and electroencephalography, neuropsychiatry, neurosurgery and clinical neurophysiology, nursing, and social work.

We have proposed, as have others (5, 6, 60), a multifactorial explanation for psychosis in epilepsy. We will attempt to further delineate this concept, by describing our methodology and commenting on phenomenology, mechanisms, the relation of seizure activity to psychosis, and the classification of psychosis.

Methodology

Direct gathering of information, often over a prolonged period of time, is essential. Our behavioral data were obtained directly by members of the team or were communicated to the team by allied personnel; they were not acquired from records of an unrelated observer in another setting and/or at a different time. The contribution of observations by family members was invaluable. Behavioral data were gathered with attention to the precise definition of seizure phenomena and possible relationships between them. These relationships could be missed initially or misunderstood because of their subtleness. Sometimes, hypotheses concerning the mechanisms of observed behavior disturbances evolved slowly. Although patients were followed in a controlled clinical and psychiatric setting, understanding of the behavioral symptomatology remained elusive for a considerable period. In some cases behavior was clarified only as first-hand observations accumulated in the respective domains of information during direct multidisciplinary clinical observation, intensive seizure monitoring with scalp- and stereo-EEG, with split-screen video recording, during electrical brain stimulation, and after cortical resection.

Thus, basic data on each patient consisted of a detailed longitudinal seizure and general behavioral history, a neuropsychiatric examination, a neurologic history and examination, and neuroradiologic studies. Stereotactically implanted cerebral depth electrodes that remain in place from 2 to 3 weeks for stereo-EEG were utilized to solve problems of localization or lateralization of the epileptic seizure mechanism. The sites of stereotactic electrode implantation were chosen on the basis of probable epileptic focus lateralization suggested by the aggregate of the above data, in-hospital seizure observation, scalp EEG studies (including tracings with nasopharyngeal and/or sphenoidal leads during waking and sleep), and bilateral Wada tests. Psychiatric observations of behavior and seizures were made during extended periods: at regular clinic visits with patient and family and/or during prolonged psychiatric hospitalization. During neurosurgical hospitalization, seizure and behavior manifestations were observed on a specialized nursing unit and during recording and electrical brain stimulation sessions in the EEG laboratory. Postoperative follow-ups extended from 15 months to 14 years.

Phenomenology

We define epileptic psychosis as an episodic or chronic alteration of reality contact, which is frequently associated with clearly visible or subtle seizure manifestations and deficits in higher cerebral functions. Psychosis may be manifested by impaired ideation (delusions) and/or perceptions (illusions and hallucinations), mood disturbances, and irrational behavior often of an aggressive type. Elucidation of psychotic phenomenology will be illustrated through presentation of the following case.

Case 1 (KRS)
Complex partial seizures. EEG: left anterior temporal lobe focus. Left temporal lobectomy. Seizurefree on medication.

This case illustrates the misapplication of a schizophrenia diagnosis for a chronic organic behavioral syndrome and for an acute episode that could be shown to be clearly related to subtle ictal discharge. Such a sequence is not uncommon if a patient is treated on a general psychiatry service. In 1969 we reported the case of KRS who had a seizure disorder from childhood. He was viewed by his desperate family as nonfunctional and unable to adequately process everyday situations. He was considered by some as chronically psychotic.

KRS's seizure pattern, indicating a dominant temporal lobe focus involving the posterior speech area as well as affective and integrating processes, was characterized by the sudden inability to understand what was being said or what he read. He would say, "A line keeps coming back; I try to figure it out. I write it down but it doesn't make any sense." After termination of a prolonged behavioral automatism, difficulty in remembering ongoing material would continue for several hours. On two occasions prior to coming under our observation, he had been reported to have suffered a schizophrenic psychosis following a period of epileptic status. We were able to observe the onset of a psychotic episode in the wake of an increase in minor seizures noted only by the more experienced staff members and in retrospect. The first behavioral symptomatology consisted of eating hallucinated food particles after he had refused food offered to him by a nurse. Later this behavior was interpreted as misidentification of the nurse as his mother with whom food had become a major area in the battle for control. When his behavior became unmanageable because of overactive destructive movements, KRS was sent to an isolation room in a general psychiatry ward where a diagnosis of schizophrenia, catatonic type, was made. In the psychiatric records, seizures were said to be absent. However, when the epilepsy group observed the patient extensively on the psychiatric unit, he was clearly having frequent small subtle seizures. His condition was reinterpreted as an acute organic psychosis superimposed on a chronic organic brain syndrome. During gradual recovery over weeks, a resurgence of psychotic thinking was noted whenever small seizures recurred. After he recovered, KRS reported that during the period of isolation necessitated by his hyperactive destructive state, he concluded in concrete fashion that he had misbehaved: "I was separated from my family to keep me out of the way." Items in the environment had been incorporated into his disordered thinking. A travel poster on the wall in the unit made him feel that he was a prisoner in a concentration camp in Europe.

Mechanisms of Psychosis

Endogenous and Exogenous Mechanisms. The case of KRS illustrates that mechanisms accounting for the occurrence of psychosis may be endogenous and/or exogenous. Endogenous mechanisms comprise seizure activity with associated higher cortical function deficits that may result in reduced ability to comprehend, remember, judge, and reason, leading to the appearance of psychosis. Higher cortical function deficits may occur continuously, with exacerbations, or episodically in relation to seizures, resulting in continued or repeated encroachment on the patient's function and adjustment (4, 72).

Another endogenous factor is the anatomical location of the epileptic focus. As previously discussed, controversy has attended claims for a consistent laterality of temporal lobe dysfunction in epileptic patients with psychosis. The present authors (4) believe that intervening variables related to various locations of the seizure focus will determine the precipitation of psychosis: "Our data suggest that the development of psychosis may depend on combined involvement of medial and lateral structures of one or both temporal lobes with disruption of reality contact by interference with the retention, recall, continuity, ordering, and integration of ongoing experience. These functions are essential for the maintenance of ego functioning. Interference with this combination of functions to a mild, chronic degree by a fixed and a discharging lesion may lead to the often heard evaluation of these patients by family and peers as 'different, queer, slow to catch on', showing everyday psychopathology. When further interference with these same functions occurs as a result of increased local brain impairment, psychosis may appear."

The importance of exogenous factors is evident. If a biological explanation alone could suffice to explain the occurrence of psychosis, then similar behavior should be associated more regularly with given pathophysiological events. Exogenous factors include environmental pressures, such as persistent, derogatory, and rejecting attitudes of important others in the patient's environment, and other emotional events affecting the patient. Exogenous events are more apt to adversely affect the individual in whom endogenous mechanisms are operating.

The following two cases illustrate the fact that psychosocial factors may be essential in the precipitation of acute psychosis once disruption by seizure activity has occurred. The similarity between seizure phenomena and psychotic phenomena is evident. The role of religiosity should also be noted in these case histories. Religious experiences were present in the reality situation and in conscious seizure experiences; they were incorporated into the psychosis and later into interictal thinking.

Case 2 (MIR)

Tonic generalized seizures with postictal automatism. EEG: bilateral paroxysmal slow activity, predominant anteriorly.

MIR was a 15-year old boy whose seizure disorder began at the age of 4 years. He was accustomed to frequent seizures, suffering from one to two minor seizures each night, two to three major seizures each week, and episodes of status epilepticus once a month. His seizures were tonic, followed by prolonged automatism during which he could wander outside, up to the altar of the church, etc. He was brought to the Medical College of Ohio Hospital after one of his episodes of status had not responded as usual to treatment in the emergency room of the local hospital. After regaining consciousness, his behavior was bizarre. Although fully oriented and able to recall recent events, he was markedly paranoid with persecutory and grandiose delusions. Psychotic themes were religious and sexual. He thought that the devil was trying to gain control, and he was convinced that he was the transmitter of God's will. He had auditory and visual hallucinations with content related to the themes mentioned. He had illusions, thinking that there were cameras in various corners of the nursing unit taking pornographic pictures.

With the adjustment of antiepileptic medication and the prescription of antipsychotic medication, MIR recovered from the psychosis after several days. Recovery of insight was only partial. He was not sure that the above had not occurred, but felt that God had resumed proper control. Although he continued to have episodes of status about once a month, a full-blown psy-

chosis has not recurred during the last 2 years. Subsequent to the psychotic episode, the patient's mother reported that before this episode of status epilepticus, the family, deeply devoted to a fundamentalist church that accepts the reality of the devil, had relied more than usual on the church for help because of a sexual indiscretion of the patient's younger sister. The patient had been very much involved in the serious feelings of the family.

Case 3 (RUD)

Complex partial seizures. Scalp-EEG: focal, right anterior hemisphere. Stereo-EEG: right temporal ictal focus. Right anterior temporal lobectomy. Seizurefree on medication.

RUD, a 23-year-old man, began to have posttraumatic seizures at the age of 10 years. He described an epigastric sensation with fear associated with a feeling of guilt and a fear of dying. This aura articulated with a traumatic life experience consisting of parental strife that led to divorce despite strong Catholic affiliation. The patient felt guilty, thinking that he was responsible for his seizures and for the marital discord. Early, he sought solace in religion, trusting that the Lord would prevent the disruption at home. As official changes in church ritual appeared, RUD felt abandoned and was in considerable conflict over his religious practice. He finally resolved this by leaving the church. During his psychosis, which followed a period of epileptic status, he became very vocal, declaring that he was threatened by hellfires around him and warned the staff, whom he clearly recognized, to keep their distance for their own safety. He felt that Satan was trying to get control of him. He experienced various illusions that his hands were melting, his feet were like rock, and sounds were "weird." Upon recovery after 5 days, he recognized the abnormality of his thinking, but felt the experience could serve as a reminder that he should return to the church. He said, "I must get my act together." For a time after his psychotic episode, he read the Bible assiduously and attended church services regularly.

Temporal Relationships Between Seizures and Psychosis. Various temporal parameters have been reported in the relationship between seizures and psychosis.

1. A prolonged interval between the onset of the seizure disorder and that of psychosis (e.g., 14 years) (1). In contrast, our data indicate that not infrequently both the seizure disorder and

the psychotic thinking, rather than being separated in time, have an early onset and have altered behavior at times even preceding the officially diagnosed seizures, when subtle seizure manifestations had not been recognized. Common characteristics in the history and experience of chronically psychotic patients in our series included: early onset of seizures in infancy or early childhood; frequent seizures; limbic and/or aphasic auras with vivid, frightening, and/or paranoid feelings; higher cortical function impairment of comprehension, memory, and sequential ordering of thoughts; misinterpretation of and primitive response by the environment to events not identified by them as ictal (see Cases 6, 7, and 8).

2. Onset of seizure disorder during puberty. Accurate designation of the actual age at onset of the seizure disorder would be essential to maintain this hypothesis. Although clear-cut seizures began at puberty in some of our cases, it was not unusual for these patients to have experienced auras, unrecognized as ictal, throughout childhood. In these cases, serious behavioral consequences resulted, especially when the environmental reaction was one of insensitivity to the source of the difficulty and punitive (Case 8).

3. A see-saw mechanism between seizures and psychosis: Landolt (60), Flor-Henry (2), and others have noted that seizures alternated with psychosis; i.e., when seizures were controlled, psychosis might be expected, and vice versa, each being a different expression of a common pathology. Under our working conditions we have more often observed the development of behavior disturbances in relation to ongoing seizure activity.

Case 4 (WAC)

Primary generalized epilepsy with tonic seizures. EEG: generalized polyspikes and waves; slow background.

Only one patient, WAC, a 28-year-old woman, with onset of seizure disorder at 5 years, showed a see-saw relationship between seizure activity and psychosis. Psychosis appeared for the first time at the age of 28 following unusual control of her previously frequent seizures by methsuximide. Illusions were prominent: "The bed is all wrong. There's no top sheet. Every time I try to get it, it's moved." When the drug was discontinued, the seizures recurred, and the psychotic symptoms subsided and did not recur during the subsequent 2 years.

Reduction of seizures did not seem to be the sole precipitant of psychosis. Following earlier (6 years) implantation of a cer-

ebellar stimulator, a 60-fold reduction (20–30 to 2–4/day) in the frequency of seizures had occurred without the appearance of psychotic ideation. In this case it was postulated that a neuropharmacologic mechanism produced the apparent see-saw relationship: As anticonvulsant medication controlled seizures, it also caused behavioral symptoms of a psychotic kind.

The correctness of a lengthy interval between onset of the seizure disorder and that of psychosis (1) and of a see-saw mechanism between seizures and psychosis (2) bears reexamination in view of the recognition problems of subtle ictal activity and the unpredictability with which psychosis follows similar biologic change (e.g., seizure events). In addition, the notion of an unrelated alternating course between seizure activity and psychosis may be supplanted by the observation of an altered mood state and/or paranoid thinking directly preceding or following one or a series of diurnal or nocturnal seizures (Cases 9 and 13). Furthermore, the absence of major seizures is not equivalent to freedom from seizures in view of the behaviorally adverse effects of subtle seizure activity (Case 1).

Phenomenologic Classification of Epileptic Psychosis

To emphasize the interaction between seizure activity and psychosis, we suggest a phenomenologic classification of epileptic psychosis. This classification was derived from an epileptic population of 218 patients among whom 33 had shown psychotic manifestations. No significant cerebral lateralizations were noted. The numbers of patients in each category were as follows: acute psychotic episode(s), 10; chronic psychosis, 4; dysphoric-paranoid syndrome, 8; paranoid-aggressive syndrome, 8; affective states, 3.

Acute Psychotic Episodes. Acute episodes were associated with seizure activity of clear-cut (Cases 2 and 3) or subtle (Case 1) type, occurring prior to or during the psychosis. The seizure activity often resulted in higher function impairments that provided the immediate antecedent of the psychotic reaction. Psychosis lasted for days to weeks. Patients might interpret their location concretely in response to their treatment and/or environmental cues (Cases 1 and 11). On the other hand, the patients might be fully oriented in all spheres but be actively delusional and hallucinatory. The religious theme was prominent (Cases 2 and 3).

Chronic Psychosis. Chronic psychosis was characterized by varying combinations of paranoid and obsessional thinking, hallucinations, somatic preoccupation and illusions, religiosity, magical thinking, and aggressive behavior. Subtle deficits of higher cortical functions were frequent, including impairment of auditory comprehension with easy misinterpretation, compromised memory, concreteness, stickiness, and difficulty getting the point. The intrusion of unusual ictal experiences was also evident in the psychotic state. The following three cases will illustrate these points.

Case 5 (GAD)
Complex partial seizures. EEG: temporal abnormalities.

GAD, a chronically paranoid 35-year-old woman with posttraumatic temporal lobe epilepsy, had grandiose delusions that she had been selected to draw up plans for interplanetary space stations. She interpreted her seizures as instances of care by her guardian spirit. During the amnestic period of her seizure, she would carry out activities she had planned before the ictus. Thus, if hungry, she might continue with preparation of a sandwich during the seizure. On recovery, she would credit the preparation to her guardian spirit. If preparation for a bath coincided with her olfactory aura, she would presume that a fragrant bath had been drawn for her. The magical sense of grandiosity and relationship with an extraterrestrial agency became very real to her.

The possibility of intrusion of seizure experiences into ongoing thinking as a mechanism for psychosis has been described in the literature (16).

Case 6 (WIT)
Complex partial seizures. EEG: bitemporal irregularities.

WIT, a 16-year-old girl, had had a behavioral problem since the age of 3 when she became recurrently aggressive toward other children. For this she would be appropriately punished. At 5 years she had her first recognized psychomotor seizure. During her aura, and also in her dreams, she would feel very afraid, as if being chased. In her general demeanor, she was chronically paranoid. She felt that she was being checked and picked on, and was hypercritical of others. She related poorly to people of any age. Examination of higher nervous functions showed a subtle impairment of comprehension and of sequential ordering. Misinterpretation of normal somatic features (e.g., a freckle) maintained a chronic delusional psychosis.

Early onset of frightening experiences, in both seizure phenomena and environmental response, led to a chronic paranoid state.

Case 7 (WHJ)
Complex partial seizures. EEG: left temporal spike focus progressing to bifrontal paroxysmal slow activity.

WHJ, a 38-year-old man, had a chronic seizure disorder dating from infancy. Seizures would occur as frequently as three to four times a day. During the aura he would have an epigastric sensation, feel afraid and strange, experience receptive aphasia ("I hear you but I don't hear anything you say"), and have auditory hallucinations. After a behavioral automatism, he would find himself in another location, sometimes at a considerable distance from his starting point. The postictal period would last 24–48 h and sometimes up to weeks. At this time he would become increasingly suspicious and aggressive. These feelings became pervasive, developing into a chronic paranoid psychosis. With an increase in seizure frequency, he would have an exacerbation of the psychosis. When the latter was associated with self-neglect or aggressive behavior directed at his "enemies," so called because he thought they had done something morally wrong, a mental hospital admission would be precipitated. Religion became an ongoing component of his thinking. He stated, "God's all through my body," and he pointed to his bilateral Dupuytren's contractures, which he believed to be stigmata. "The seizures help me in doing righteousness. I can live with them. I am one of the afflicted."

The frequency, vividness, and prolongation of the intrusion of unusual experiences into his life formed the basis of the development of the psychosis.

Dysphoric Paranoid Syndrome. A dysphoric-paranoid state was characterized by repeated intrusion of depressive affect in the prodrome of the seizures, sometimes lasting for hours; by auras with fear, suspicion, and even loss of recognition of faces; and by reactive dysphoria and continuous sensitivity, to a paranoid degree, in interpersonal relationships, as the patients mistrusted their environment and/or wondered what people thought of them during their prolonged, dysphoric, withdrawn periods (Cases 12 and 13). Some had experienced a punitive attitude on the part of their environment, which misinterpreted dysfunction associated with seizures as "bad behavior," as in the following case.

Case 8 (BRW)
Complex partial seizures, left temporal, due to astrocytoma. EEG: left anterior temporal interictal and ictal focus. Left anterior temporal lobectomy. Seizurefree on medication for 8 years, then occasional small attacks.

When BRW came under our care as an 11-year-old boy, he had had seizures for 6 years. He was of small stature. His father was a rigid individual who had great expectations of his initially precocious first-born. From the onset of the seizure disorder, the child was punished whenever a seizure occurred, the father interpreting the seizure manifestations as inattentive and resistive behavior. His father continued to be punitive and rejecting throughout the patient's life, being greatly perturbed by the lack of accomplishment.

BRW tried to pursue his education, with great effort and insufficient success. Jobs and on-the-job training had been numerous and unfulfilling as well as providing minimal recognition. Subtle higher function difficulties with stickiness, obsessive thinking, concreteness, and difficulty in "catching on" made interpersonal relationships tenuous and advancement minimal. Dysphoria was evident in that nothing ever seemed right. Gradually paranoid interpretation became pronounced and led to irritability and at times to aggressive behavior.

The seizure phenomena in this case provided negative personal experiences resulting from an aura of existential fear. This recurring experience reinforced distrust and led to increased detachment and misinterpretation. In the postictal period there was prolonged confusion. The repeated seizure experiences nourished the paranoid thinking and dysphoric feeling.

Paranoid Aggressive Syndrome. Patients with paranoid aggressive symptomatology were often referred because of behavioral difficulties manifested by continuous irritability with episodic worsening of aggressive behavior associated with seizures. Other patients showed a course characterized by relatively agreeable periods of days or weeks alternating with periods of comparable length during which they were irritable, critical, paranoid, and sometimes aggressive. When the episodes were examined closely, they were found to be precipitated by an increase in frequency of seizures, sometimes overlooked because of their nocturnal occurrence. Paranoid aggressive syndrome is illustrated by the following two cases.

Case 9 (GRN)

Complex partial seizures. EEG and intensive seizure monitoring: right anterior temporal focus. Right anterior temporal lobectomy. Continuation of seizures on medication.

GRN was a 48-year-old married man whose seizure disorder commenced at the age of 38 following head trauma. Seizures would begin with a smothering feeling and experience of faces "looking different." Subsequently, either a right-sided motor event with falling would occur or he would have a period of automatic behavior characterized by lip smacking, fumbling (with objects at hand or undressing), or wandering (might go several blocks from home). In the postictal period, he was confused: "He sits around, he looks blank. He doesn't seem to understand and doesn't try to talk." Seizure frequency ranged from an average of six per month to five to six per day. The impetus for consideration of neurosurgical treatment related to prolonged periods of behavioral symptomatology consisting of serious paranoid-aggressive behavior, during which he would verbally and/or physically attack family members over a period of days to weeks. At other times he was pleasant and thoughtful.

After considerable study it became evident that a satisfactory period of adjustment (weeks) would be followed by a period of difficult behavior beginning the day after a "restless night." The possibility of a nocturnal seizure mechanism was confirmed by the wife's more careful observation of the patient's sleep and his behavior on the day following the nocturnal seizures, such as sleeping later into the morning and arising in a changed, hypercritical paranoid state.

Case 10 (FER)

Complex partial seizures, left temporolimbic, due to astrocytoma of left fusiform gyrus. EEG: Left temporal spikes. Left anterior temporal lobectomy. Seizurefree on single medication.

FER, a 24-year-old man, had his first seizure at 6 years, a major motor attack. At 9 years a cerebellar tumor was removed. After the operation and despite rejection by his peers, he coped well, engaging in solo activities such as collecting. His chronic temporolimbic seizure disorder began at the age of 11. At the age of 12, his aggressive behavior became prominent, and by the age of 15, psychiatric hospitalization was necessary. Between the ages of 15 and 24, FER attended a school for the emotionally disturbed and a college for the emotionally handicapped, and was studied on the research ward of a state hospital. He was seen by a total of six psychiatrists outside the institutions. Study at a national neurological center led to a conclusion of inoperability. From the ages of 21–24 he lived in a state institution for epileptics, until referred to the authors with the persisting chief complaints of drug-refractory seizures and dyscontrol syndrome.

The pattern of FER's seizures was as follows: After an onset charcterized by receptive aphasia and speech arrest, he stared and became rigid. The family had noted, and in-hospital observations confirmed, that his aggressive behavior would precede a seizure by hours to days. Following periods of demanding, impulsive, aggressive behavior, FER would have one or more seizures and show higher function impairments. For instance, 1 day he wanted coffee. Instead of waiting for the nurse to bring it to him, he went into the hall and grabbed the coffee pot from her, with the result that coffee was spilled on her. When examined after this episode, his speech was not as clear as usual, and later he had several seizures. The following morning, he was confused, restless, and irritable, disoriented for time, did not recognize known personnel, and showed some retrograde amnesia. After recovery, he related that he remembered the examiner's visit the day after the accident. "You were familiar, but I didn't know your name. I was in a fog."

At operation an astrocytoma was found in the left fusiform gyrus. The left temporal lobectomy included also the amygdala and anterior hippocampus. At last follow-up, 12 years later, FER was 36 years old. He had had no behavioral problems, although he had an occasional moment of aphasic arrest. He had been holding a civil service job in the capital of his state and served on the board of directors of the local epilepsy association. He wrote in a letter: "Helping those individuals who are mentally disturbed is like a dream come true. Assisting others who are less fortunate means more to me than money."

The primary aggressivity occurring in the prodromal period of his seizures was eliminated with the removal of the discharging medial limbic structures.

Affective States. Patients with prominent affective symptomatology noted that a negative mood state was relieved by the occurrence of a seizure. They could be described as having a cyclic mood disorder. These patients may in large part account for the see-saw relationship between seizures and psychosis as described in the literature. There is inferential support for this in that authors describing the inverse relationship between seizures and psychosis included in their population patients with episodicity and a strong affective component in their psychosis (1, 2) (Case 16).

Evidence from Electrical Brain Stimulation

Cortical resection of the epileptic focus and electrical brain stimulation through chronically implanted cerebral electrodes provided tools to achieve further clarification of the relation between ictal activity and behavior. Behaviorally significant stimulation responses with regard to psychosis will be described in the context of clinical history and personal longitudinal observations in five patients with temporolimbic epilepsy.

The following case studies will clarify the mechanisms of psychosis in patients undergoing electrical brain stimulation and/or cortical resection. Patients will be described under the various categories of the phenomenological classification of epileptic psychosis: *acute psychosis* (Case 11), *dysphoric-paranoid state* (Cases 12 and 13), *paranoid-aggressive syndrome* (Cases 14 and 15), and *affective states* (Case 16). No patient with chronic psychosis underwent stereo-EEG and eletrical brain stimulation. The reports utilize comparison of clinical seizure manifestations and behavior and their interrelationships with the patient's daily life setting with those observed during brain stimulation in patients with intractable temporolimbic epilepsy.

Case 11 (HAJ): Acute Psychosis
Complex partial seizures, bitemporal, due to calcified hemangioma of left fusiform gyrus. Scalp-EEG: bitemporal spikes. Left temporal lobectomy. Recurrence of seizures. Stereo-EEG and electrical brain stimulation. Radiofrequency amgdalotomy, right. Unimproved.

HAJ, a 41-year-old male farmer, was referred for consideration of further surgical therapy for his seizures. His seizure disorder began at the age of 24 while he was in the military service. At 31 years of age, scalp EEG studies at the Montreal Neurological Institute showed bilateral temporal spike foci. At 32 years of age, left temporal lobectomy at that institute included the amygdala, hippocampus, and a calcified hemangioma of the posterior fusiform gyrus. He was seizure free for 1 year when chronic seizures recurred. The pattern was unchanged from before surgery. He had an aura of jamais vu, which was followed by a prolonged automatic state.

Neuropsychiatric examination revealed chronic impairment of recent memory. During hospitalization on the neurologic-neurosurgical nursing unit, the patient had an increase of seizures, then became disoriented and delusional. He declared himself to be the Lord. He left his bed periodically and strolled around the ward, confidently ministering to "his flock" of fellow patients whom he nonetheless greatly frightened. Attempts at restraint were resisted with blows. HAJ vigorously choked and slapped one of our colleagues and struck and stunned our nurse. He was transferred to a psychiatric facility where he had to be kept in physical restraints for 10 days. The patient was treated with antipsychotic and anticonvulsant medications. He recovered and was discharged after 3 weeks.

Brain stimulation studies were performed 1 year later when persistent seizures led to the decision to proceed with stereo-EEG to localize the intractable seizure mechanism. Prior to a stimulation session, HAJ was oriented and in a positive mood state. Retention abilities were known to be impaired. Following stimulation of the right hippocampus, he was asked about his head dressing. He said, "It's a bandage. I fell. I tried to get away but I ran into a two-by-four." After stimulation of the right lateral temporal cortex, he was asked where he was. He said, "In Hollywood. The police are here to make a film. I'm here to take photos because of blackouts."

In this case brain stimulation produced increased higher function deficits and paranoid thinking, antecedents to his previous psychotic episode. Even though brain stimulation had been kept to a minimum, consistent with diagnostic objectives and avoidance of a possible prolonged psychotic episode, the disorientation and misinterpretation reappeared intermittently over a period of several hours.

This patient was a hard-working, freely moving farmer who had great difficulty in accepting the confinement of hospitalization. He had chronic memory impairment. His seizures were ushered in by an aura of jamais vu, followed by a prolonged automatism during which he carried out his intent or feeling prior to the seizure. In his psychosis, he became "free"—he assumed a powerful stance and wandered masterfully and aggressively around the ward.

Following an increase in electrical activity by electrical brain stimulation, HAJ showed increased memory impairment with disorientation and paranoid thinking.

Case 12 (SHB): Dysphoric-Paranoid State
Complex partial seizures due to unknown cause. Scalp-EEG: right frontotemporal spike bursts. Stereo-EEG: right mesial temporal ictal focus. Electrical brain stimulation. Right anterior temporal lobectomy. Seizurefree on medication.

SHB, a 19-year-old girl, had seizures since childhood. She led a reclusive existence for several years after being expelled from school because of seizures and behavior problems. She became homebound, not involved in meaningful activity, and showed reversal of daytime and nocturnal activities. Her minimal interpersonal contacts were impaired by paranoid feelings.

The patient's seizures began with an aura of epigastric sensation, with a fear for her life as she identified with her mother, a cardiac invalid. During the ictus she pounded her stomach or a nearby object. Seizures occurred from 7 to 20 times a day.

Following electrical stimulation of the left amygdala and afterdischarge, the patient looked and reacted as if afraid. She was disoriented for place and did not recognize familiar people. She struggled to get off the stretcher, saying that she had to "get away." In this patient the great frequency of seizure experiences consisting of fear and misidentification of familiar persons resulted in a paranoid reaction to and withdrawal from her environment. During electrical brain stimulation the sequence was reproduced.

Case 13 (SNJ): Dysphoric-Paranoid State
Complex partial seizures. Scalp-EEG: left temporal spikes. Intensive seizure monitoring: seizure onset not recorded. Stereo-EEG: bilateral hippocampal ictal foci. Electrical brain stimulation.

SNJ, an attractive, bright, 18-year-old girl whose chronic seizure disorder began at 5 years of age, had a seizure frequency of 20/month at the time of the study. Her seizures varied in severity from auras only to seizures lasting up to 20 min.

The seizures began with a prolonged depressive prodrome (sometimes lasting for hours). She described accompanying suicidal impulses—"If someone would tell me to jump out the window, I might do it." During the aura she had a "dizzy and indescribable sensation" in the head and "a sick feeling in the stomach," sometimes followed by auditory illusions and derealization. During her ictus, she stared, turned her head and upper torso to the left, displayed an alimentary pantomime, and spoke in irrelevant, stereotyped fashion. Postictally she had a behavioral automatism.

It was noted that SNJ was not doing as well as before in school: She was slower, comprehended and remembered less well, and had a tendency to be concrete. She became less trusting in interpersonal relationships and eventually paranoid. Her family arranged for psychiatric help because of the admixture of depressive and paranoid manifestations.

During electrical brain stimulation of the mesial temporal structures, the depressive and paranoid feelings were reproduced.

Case 14 (PAB): Paranoid-Aggressive Syndrome
Complex partial seizures, temporolimbic, due to trauma. Scalp-EEG: bitemporal spikes. Stereo-EEG: right hippocampal ictal focus. Electrical brain stimulation. Right temporal lobectomy. Seizurefree on medication.

PAB was a 27-year-old woman at the time of her right temporal lobectomy. Her first seizure occurred at 16 months of age following head trauma. At 2 years she was described as placing a hand on her upper abdomen, presumably indicating an epigastric sensation at the onset of her spells. At 10 years irritability and rage outbursts appeared: "Sometimes, no one knew why she was mad." The seizures and behavior resulted in erratic school attendance. At 18 years old she was assigned to a sheltered workshop where she met a man in his fifties whom she married. He did not understand the illness. Her mother gave her a year's supply of anticonvulsants as a wedding present. At 20, after bearing two children, PAB was admitted to a psychiatric hospital in her home state because of aggressiveness toward herself and others. She remained there for 4 years. At the age of 25, the patient was moved to our psychiatric facility to be within the orbit of our group for possible surgical treatment.

Her seizure pattern was as follows: Aura—Epigastric sensation with fear, paranoid feeling (that she was going to be attacked), visual illusions (walls about to fall), and inability to speak; Ictus—Ran, sometimes encountering dangerous situations. Postictally—Attacked other patients.

After a short period of time in the hospital, the patient met with considerable rejection by patients and staff. She was considered unpredictable in mood, manipulative, not trustworthy, overly complaining, paranoid, and aggressive. Diagnostically,

PAB was regarded by some staff members as a case of character disorder and/or psychosis who also had seizures. Observations on the psychiatric ward helped to identify an organic mechanism for some of these characteristics: (a) One day the patient was found with bruises in an unexpected location on the hospital grounds. She stated that while out walking on the grounds, she had been attacked by a man and had been bruised in the struggle as she attempted to escape. Fortunately, a different, objective version was available. A nurse stated that she saw PAB walking on the grounds at some distance from a male patient. Suddenly the patient began to run at top speed, tripped, picked herself up, and ran into the nearest building. This sequence was consistent with the description of her seizures. (b) PAB would get into frequent fights with other patients. Close observation showed that the individuals attacked were those with whom the patient had had previous negative interactions and that this aggressive behavior occurred following a recognized seizure. (c) The patient was seen during a prolonged period (days) of detachment when she would complain of feeling afraid, point to her epigastrium, and give her location as "a hotel" and the nurses as "maids." An EEG obtained during this time showed increased temporal spike activity.

Marked fluctuations in PAB's mood state were observed on the neurosurgical unit. One day she arrived in the EEG laboratory for electrical brain stimulation morose, sullen, and irritable, exhibiting no spontaneous conversation. The next day she was spontaneous, pleasant, and talking freely. She asked, "How is it you change? Yesterday, you looked sad. Today you are happy. On some days, I feel on top of the world. On other days, I feel terrible, as if the world is against me."

On stimulation of the left hippocampus, PAB had an epigastric sensation with fear. She stated: "People look different." Looking at one of the medical staff she said, "He is double his weight and strength" or "He is small. I could hold him in my hand. I hear people fussing. It is so fast, I can't keep up. The voices are tangled as if someone is trying to overtalk you." On stimulation of the right hippocampus, she said, "Voices are screaming." This was followed almost immediately by her statement that "the tone of voice is soft and pleasant." She then described a feeling of fear and said, "I'm afraid; I don't like to talk. I would like to get away. The words are twisted." On stimulation of the right amygdala, she became dysphoric and irritable: "I feel afraid, someone is after me. I'm going to be captured."

The rapid fluctuations in affect and perception during brain stimulation were similar to those appearing in her spontaneous behavior, which had resulted in a negative reaction from her environment.

Following right temporal lobe excision that included the amygdala and hippocampus, her emotional liability and aggressivity were eliminated. It was possible for gradual rehabilitation to occur. She was helped to separate from the institutional setting and progressed to a sheltered workshop and competitive work. She resided first in a group home, later at the YWCA, and finally in her own apartment. PAB expressed appreciation for her improvement in letters, poems, and during radio interviews, which are part of her active work in support of the cause of patients with epilepsy.

Case 15 (COD): Paranoid-Aggressive Syndrome
Complex partial seizures, temporal lobe. Scalp-EEG: bitemporal independent spikes. Stereo-EEG: bilateral independent hippocampal seizures. Electrical brain stimulation.

COD, a 16-year-old boy, was referred for neurosurgical evaluation because of aggressive behavior and seizures dating from the age of 8 years. The earliest seizures were interpreted as "nightmares." Awakening in the night, he would be found sitting up, staring, screaming, and attacking anyone who approached. Such episodes subsequently appeared during the day. He also manifested extended periods (hours to days) of irritable behavior during which he attacked people and things. Within a year the behavior problem grew to major proportions, and the boy was admitted to a children's general hospital where it was necessary to keep him in a caged bed. A second hospitalization elsewhere was abruptly curtailed when his behavior was so disruptive that the family was asked at 11:00 p.m. to take him home. By the age of 10, COD required admission to a children's psychiatric hospital where he remained for 4 years. When he was 15 years old, a cerebellar stimulator was implanted elsewhere with only minimal benefit. At 16, he was admitted to the Medical College of Ohio Hospital for a second evaluation for possible neurosurgical control of refractory partial epilepsy and behavior.

Close scrutiny of seizure content and behavior difficulty indicated a close association: (a) Prior to a seizure, easy irritability and abusive behavior occurred in response to small stimuli, from hours to as long as 2 days. (b) During his aura he experienced an epigastric sensation with fear associated with visual illusions—the faces of people in sight would look like those of monsters ready to attack—and receptive aphasia. (c) During the ictal-postictal periods, he would stare, scream, run, and attack. (d) After a seizure, he would be tractable and apologetic.

During electrical brain stimulation, rapid shifts from pleasant, reasonable behavior to fearful, paranoid, aggressive behavior were observed during electrically induced afterdischarge and during clinical seizures. In a prestimulation period, COD arrived in the EEG laboratory mentally clear and well oriented, stating that he was "in the hospital, in the recording place. Here for a test." Stimulation of the right amygdaloid nucleus produced a subjective response of disorientation, misidentification, and paranoid, aggressive content. He gave the location as "a garage," identified the doctors present as "police who are after robbers who stole $1,000.00." He made pawing movements if approached. On stimulation of the right hippocampus, the location was again "the garage," but the staff were classified as "family members—cleaning up together." On a different day, he arrived at the EEG laboratory in a pleasant mood, looked around, and commented on the equipment. Stimulation of the left hippocampus produced a clinical seizure that began with a look of great fear. He then sat, drew himself up, and retreated toward the head of the bed and began to thrash against his restraints. He could not speak.

This patient showed two mechanisms of aggressivity: (a) Historically, he had a seizure prodrome with a raised level of irritability and attack behavior in response to minor stimuli. (b) During spontaneous seizures and on brain stimulation, aggressivity occurred in response to the experience of the fear and threatening visual illusions of the aura.

Case 16 (BANS): Affective State
Complex partial seizures, left temporal lobe. Scalp-EEG: bilateral temporal spikes. Stereo-EEG: left hippocampal ictal focus. Electrical brain stimulation. Left temporal lobectomy. Seizurefree on medication.

BANS, a 35-year-old married schoolteacher, had had a chronic seizure disorder since childhood. Her mother had reacted adversely to the problem—resenting and hiding the illness. The patient experienced marked depression with self-deprecation, guilt, and suicidal thoughts when seizures would increase in frequency.

Her seizures began with a feeling in her chest that "something bad is going to happen" and "a wave of strangeness." At times, this wavelike sensation would spread over her body, becoming pleasurable when it reached her genitalia.

After an increase in clinical and electrical seizures during intensive seizure monitoring with depth electrodes, BANS experienced a prolonged (days) period of hypomania characterized by increased psychomotor activity and elevation of mood with unusual giggling. Her speech was characterized by flight of ideas, clanging, paranoid ideation, and impaired social judgment. Electrical stimulation of the left amygdala reproduced the affective content of her spontaneous seizures.

Thus, increase in seizure frequency and electrical brain stimulation produced affective shifts characterized by alternation of depression and pleasurable feelings. The psychosis occurring after an increase in seizure activity was an affective one of the hypomanic type lasting several days.

SUMMARY

Our findings provide explanatory data to support the conclusion that psychosis in the epileptic patient results from a multifactorial mechanism. The majority of the patients had complex partial seizures. Careful clinical observations extended by intensive seizure monitoring, stereo-EEG, electrical brain stimulation studies, and the results of cortical resection of the epileptic focus have indicated the possible links between ictal process and behavior. The significant role of subtle seizure activity in the development of psychosis has been emphasized in contrast to the view found in the literature that seizure activity may be an alternative expression of the brain locus capable also of manifesting psychosis.

Redefinition of terminology is suggested. The terms "schizophrenia-like" and "schizophrenia" are seen as overly inclusive and/or inaccurate. The term "epileptic psychosis," defined by prevailing components of thought disturbance, affective changes, paranoid ideation or aggressive behavior, and higher cortical function impairments, is advocated. A phenomenologic classification has been described, consisting of: acute psychotic episodes; chronic psychoses; dysphoric-paranoid states; paranoid-aggressive states; and affective states.

An intensive interdisciplinary approach can contribute significantly to the understanding of possible links between seizure activity and psychosis and consequently to the treatment of the individual epileptic patient with psychosis.

REFERENCES

1. Slater E, Beard AW, Glitheroe E: The schizophrenia-like psychoses of epilepsy. *Br J Psychiatry* 109:95–150, 1963
2. Flor-Henry P: Psychosis and temporal lobe epilepsy. A controlled investigation. *Epilepsia* 10:363–395, 1969
3. Taylor D: Mental state and temporal lobe epilepsy: correlative account of 100 patients treated surgically. *Epilepsia* 13:727–765, 1972
4. Ferguson SM, Rayport M, Gardner R, et al: Similarities in mental content of psychotic states, spontaneous seizures, dreams, and responses to electrical brain stimulation in patients with temporal lobe epilepsy. *Psychosom Med* 31:479–498, 1969
5. Bruens JH: Psychoses in epilepsy, in *Clinical Handbook of Neurology, Vol 15*. Edited by Vinken PJ, Bruyn GW. New York, American Elsevier, 1974, 593–610
6. Fenton GW: Epilepsy and psychosis. *J Ir Med Assoc* 71:315–324, 1978
7. Temkin O: *The Falling Sickness.* 2nd edition, revised. Baltimore, The Johns Hopkins Press, 1971
8. Esquirol E: *Des Maladies Mentales.* Paris, 1838
9. Berger H: Ueber das Elektroenzephalogramm des Menschen. *Arch Psychiatr Nervenkr* 87:527–570, 1929
10. Jackson JH: *Selected Writings of John Hughlings Jackson, Vol 1: Epilepsy and Epileptiform Convulsions.* Edited by Taylor J. London, Hodder and Stoughton, 1931. Reprinted: New York, Basic Books, 1958
11. Turner WA: *Epilepsy, A Study of the Idiopathic Disease.* London, Macmillan, 1907, p 130
12. Gibbs FA, Gibbs EL, Lennox WG: Cerebral dysrhythmias of epilepsy; measures for their control. *Arch Neurol Psychiatry* 39:298–314, 1938
13. Gibbs EL, Gibbs FA, Fuster B: Psychomotor epilepsy. *Arch Neurol Psychiatry* 60:331–339, 1948
14. Gibbs FA: Ictal and non-ictal psychiatric disorders in temporal lobe epilepsy. *J Nerv Ment Dis* 113:522–528, 1951
15. Hill D: Psychiatric disorders of epilepsy. *Med Press* 229:473–475, 1953
16. Pond DA: Psychiatric aspects of epilepsy. *J Indian Med Prof* 3:1421–1451, 1957
17. Dongier S: Statistical study of clinical and electroencephalographic manifestations of 536 psychotic episodes occurring in 516 epileptics between clinical seizures. *Epilepsia* 1:117–142, 1959
18. American Psychiatric Association: *Diagnostic and Statistical Manual of Mental Disorders.* 3rd edition. Washington, DC, APA, 1980

19. Strauss H: Epileptic disorders, in *American Handbook of Psychiatry, Vol 2.* Edited by Arieti S. New York, Basic Books, 1959, pp 1109–1144

20. Bruens JH: Psychoses in epilepsy. *Psychiatr Neurol Neurochir* 74:175–192, 1971

21. Betts TA, Merskey H, Pond DA: Psychiatry, in *A Textbook of Epilepsy.* Edited by Laidlaw J, Dickens A. Edinburgh, Churchill Livingstone, 1976, pp 145–184

22. Rodin EA, DeJong RN, Waggoner RW, et al: Relationship between certain forms of psychomotor epilepsy and "Schizophrenia." I. Diagnostic considerations. *Arch Neurol Psychiatry* 77:449–463, 1956

23. Kristensen O, Sindrup EH: Psychomotor epilepsy and psychosis: III. Social and psychological correlates. *Acta Neurol Scand* 59:1–9, 1979

24. Jensen I, Larsen JK: Psychosis in drug-resistant temporal lobe epilepsy. *J Neurol Neurosurg Psychiatry* 42:948–954, 1979

25. Parnas J, Korsgaard S, Krautwald D, et al: Chronic psychosis in epilepsy. A clinical investigation of 29 patients. *Acta Psychiatr Scand* 66:282–293, 1982

26. Perez MM, Trimble MR: Epileptic psychosis—diagnostic comparison with process schizophrenia. *Br J Psychiatry* 137:245–249, 1980

27. Wing JK, Cooper JE, Sartorius N: *The Description and Classification of Psychiatric Symptoms.* London, Cambridge University Press, 1974

28. Wing JK, Sturt E: *The PSE-ID-CATEGO System. A Supplementary Manual.* London, Institute of Psychiatry, 1978

29. Schneider K: *Clinical Psychopathology.* Transl. by Hamilton MW. London, Grune & Stratton, 1959

30. Trimble MR, Perez MM: The phenomenology of chronic psychoses of epilepsy. *Adv Biol Psychiatry* 8:98–105, 1982

31. Carpenter WT Jr, Strauss JS, Muleh S: Pathognomonic symptoms in schizophrenia? An empiric investigation of Schneider's first-rank symptoms. *Arch Gen Psychiatry* 28:847–852, 1973

32. Abrams R, Taylor MA, Gaztanaka P: Manic-depressive illness and paranoid schizophrenia. A phenomenologic, family history, and treatment-response study. *Arch Gen Psychiatry* 31:640–642, 1974

33. Pope HG Jr, Lipinski JF Jr: Diagnosis of schizophrenia and manic-depressive illness: a reassessment of the specificity of "Schizophrenic" symptoms in the light of current research. *Arch Gen Psychiatry* 35:811–828, 1978

34. Parnas J, Korsgaard S: Epilepsy and psychosis. *Acta Psychiatr Scand* 66:89–99, 1982

35. Sherwin I: Psychosis associated with epilepsy: significance of the laterality of the epileptic lesion. *J Neurol Neurosurg Psychiatry* 44:83–85, 1981

36. Brockington IF, Kendell RE, Leff JP: Definitions of schizophrenia: concordance and prediction of outcome. *Psychol Med* 8:387–398, 1978

37. Betts TA: A follow-up study of a cohort of patients with epilepsy admitted to psychiatric care in an English city, in *Epilepsy: Proceedings of the Hans Berger Centenary Symposium*. Edited by Harris P, Maudsley C. Edinburgh, Churchill Livingstone, 1974, pp 326–336

38. Toone B: Psychoses of epilepsy, in *Epilepsy and Psychiatry*. Edited by Reynolds EH, Trimble MR. Edinburgh, Churchill Livingstone, 1981, pp 113–137

39. Glaser GH: The problem of psychosis in psychomotor temporal lobe epileptics. *Epilepsia* 5:271–278, 1964

40. Gowers WR: *Epilepsy and Other Chronic Convulsive Diseases: Their Causes, Symptoms and Treatment*. New York, Williams Wood, 1885, p 100

41. Benjaminsen S: Temporal lobe epilepsy and schizophreniform psychosis. *Ugeskr Laeger* 142:168–169, 1980

42. Ramani V, Gumnit RJ: Intensive monitoring of interictal psychosis in epilepsy. *Ann Neurol* 11:613:622, 1982

43. Meduna L von: *Die Konvulsiontherapie der Schizophrenie*. Halle Marburg, 1937

44. Fink M: Behavioral effects of induced seizures (ECT). Presented at the workshop "Epilepsy and Psychosis: Affinity and/or Antagonism," Fifteenth Epilepsy International Symposium, Washington, DC October 1, 1983

45. Green JR, Duisberg REH, McGrath W: Focal epilepsy of psychomotor type. A preliminary report of observations on effects of surgical therapy. *J Neurosurg* 8:157–172, 1951

46. Mulder DW, Daly D: Psychiatric symptoms associated with lesions of the temporal lobe. *JAMA* 150:173–176, 1952

47. Hill D, Pond DA, Mitchell W, et al: Personality changes following temporal lobectomy for epilepsy. *J Ment Sci* 103:18–27, 1957

48. Gibbs FA, Gibbs EL: *Atlas of Electroencephalography, Vol 2: Epilepsy*. Reading, Addison-Wesley, 1952, pp 114, 169

49. Nicholi AM Jr: *The Harvard Guide to Modern Psychiatry*. Cambridge, Harvard University Press, 1978

50. Ervin F, Epstein AW, King HE: Behavior of epileptic and nonepileptic patients with "temporal spikes." *Arch Neurol Psychiatry* 74:488–497, 1955

51. Stevens JR: Psychiatric implications of psychomotor epilepsy. *Arch Gen Psychiatry* 14:461–471, 1966

52. Guerrant J, Anderson WW, Fischer A, et al: *Personality in Epilepsy*. Springfield, Charles C Thomas, 1962

53. Williams D: Man's temporal lobe. *Proc R Soc Med* 61:335–336, 1966

54. Symonds C: The schizophrenic-like psychoses of epilepsy [Discussion]. *Proc R Soc Med* 55:314, 1962

55. Toone B, Dawson J, Driver MV: Psychoses of epilepsy: a radiologic evaluation. *Br J Psychiatry* 140:244–248, 1982

56. Taylor DC: Factors influencing the occurrence of schizophrenia-like psychoses in patients with temporal lobe epilepsy. *Psychol Med* 5:249–254, 1975

57. Sherwin I: The effect of location of an epileptogenic lesion on the occurrence of psychosis in epilepsy. *Ad Biol Psychiatry* 8:81–97, 1982

58. Sherwin I, Person-Magnan P, Bancaud J, et al: Prevalence of psychosis in epilepsy as a function of the laterality of the epileptogenic lesion. *Arch Neurol* 39:621–625, 1982

59. Newlin DB, Carpenter B, Golden CJ: Hemispheric asymmetries in schizophrenia. *Biol Psychiatry* 16:561–582, 1981

60. Landolt H: Serial electroencephalographic investigations during psychotic episodes in epileptic patients and during schizophrenic attacks, in *Lectures on Epilepsy*. Edited by Lorentz de Haas AM. Amsterdam, Elsevier, 1958, pp 91–133

61. Blumer D, Benson DF: Psychiatric manifestations of epilepsy, in *Psychiatric Aspects of Neurologic Disease, Vol 2*. Edited by Benson DF, Blumer D. New York, Grune & Stratton, 1982, pp 25–48

62. Trimble MR: The interictal psychoses of epilepsy, in *Psychiatric Aspects of Neurologic Disease, Vol 2*. Edited by Benson DF, Blumer D. New York, Grune & Stratton, 1982, pp 75–91

63. Chkhenkeli SA, Geladze TS: Forced normalization of the EEG and some mechanisms of psychopathological manifestations in epileptics. *Neurosci Behav Physiol* 2:113–117, 1982

64. Reynolds EH: Epilepsy and schizophrenia: relationship and biochemistry. *Lancet* 1:398–401, 1968

65. Kristensen O, Sindrup EH: Psychomotor epilepsy and psychosis: I. Physical aspects. *Acta Neurol Scand* 57:361–369, 1978

66. Shukla GD, Srivastava BC, Katiyar BC, et al: Psychiatric manifestations in temporal lobe epilepsy. *Br J Psychiatry* 135:411–417, 1979

67. Ferguson SM, Rayport M: The adjustment to living without epilepsy. *J Nerv Ment Dis* 140:26–37, 1965

68. Horowitz M, Cohen FM: Temporal lobe epilepsy. Effect of lobectomy on psychosocial functioning. *Epilepsia* 9:23–41, 1968

69. Post RM, Uhde, TW, Ballenger JC, et al: Carbamazepine, temporal lobe epilepsy, and manic-depressive illness. *Adv Biol Psychiatry* 8:117–156, 1982

70. Trimble MR: The relationship bgetween epilepsy and schizophrenia: a biochemical hypothesis. *Biol Psychiatry* 12:299–304, 1977

71. Ferguson SM: Psychiatric and behavioral aspects of temporal lobe epilepsy. *Bull NY Acad Med* 38:668–677, 1962

72. Hermann BP: Deficits in neuropsychological functioning and psychopathology in persons with epilepsy: a rejected hypothesis revised. *Epilepsia* 22:161–167, 1981

8

Major Mood Disorders Related to Epileptic Changes

Jonathan M. Himmelhoch, M.D.

> *do you get me?) according to such supposedly indigenous throstles Art is o World o Life a formula*
>
> —e.e. cummings

The diagnosis of the affective disorders is in danger of becoming a formula. Descriptors of depression or mania are selected from one diagnostic system or another as if from a Chinese menu [Research Diagnostic Criteria (RDC), *Diagnostic and Statistical Manual of Mental Disorders*, 3rd edition (*DSM-III*), International Classification of Diseases-9, Diagnostic Interview Schedule]. Diagnosis turns into simple description, and diagnostic categories into neoplatonic Procrustean beds into which heterogeneous affective syndromes are forced to fit regardless of their obvious differences from one another regarding premorbid development, course, and outcome. Diagnosis as description, therefore, displaces the notion of diagnosis as hypothesis. As a result, what Kety (1) has called the "process of the medical model" is destroyed—i.e., that process by which a diagnostic hypothesis, no matter how absurd, is ever more refined by the cruel realities of clinical experience, until by dint of accident or accumulated knowledge, speculations become syndromes that in turn become etiologically defined illnesses.

Formulaic invocation of diagnostic systems has probably obscured detection of those affective illnesses that are closely related to the epilepsies, particularly those occurring in patients with epileptiform changes on electroencephalograms (EEG) and/or in behavioral patterns who do not manifest seizures of any kind. The initial hypothesis of a relationship between epilepsy and mood appeared in the Hippocratic corpus, where the unknown author of *Epidemics* stated (2):

> Most melancholics usually also become epileptics, and epileptics melancholics. One or the other [condition] prevails according to where the disease leans: if towards the body, they become epileptics, if towards reason, melancholics.

Nineteenth century German psychiatrists expanded considerably on these vague behavioral correlations by describing specific psychopathological manifestations occurring during the course of epilepsy. [Kety (1) has noted that "the process of the medical model" usually takes centuries and, as in this case, can take millenia.] Their observations came from extremely ill epileptic populations, housed in institutions because of frequent, clinically obvious grand mal seizures that seemed to be producing profound aberrations in interictal behavior. Their descriptions preceded, for the most part, the discovery of temporal lobe abnormalities and limbic system neurophysiology. But even without this knowledge and even though they have been criticized for their failure to recognize the importance of institutionalization in producing characterologic and mental changes in their patients, middle-European clinicians such as Samt, Kraepelin, and Gruhle produced descriptions (3) that foreshadowed the discovery, during the second half of the twentieth century, of the interictal behavioral syndromes of psychomotor epilepsy. They noted the difference between "postepileptic (interictal) insanity" and "psychic epileptic equivalents" (ictal mental changes). In reference to the affective disorders, they described interictal dysphoric lability, religious euphoria, and depressed, anergic, semistuporous periods—mental changes that link epilepsy to both the bipolar and unipolar major affective disorders. Finally, they described the inverse relationship of these interictal affective changes to seizure frequency.

> Yes, physician and attendants do hope for a seizure in these often very difficult patients, which comes like salvation for everybody: the patient is much more bearable for weeks thereafter (4).

Increasing knowledge of the phenomenology of psychomotor epilepsy and the resultant understanding of the role of the temporal lobes and the limbic system in the emotional life of the individual have, during the twentieth century, considerably honed present conceptualizations of the specific interictal, psychopathological syndromes associated with epilepsy. It is now generally accepted [Stevens et al. being one group of hold-outs (5)] that patients with temporal lobe epilepsy suffer more frequent and specific interictal behavioral sequelae than do other epileptics (6). The following four major traits or syndromes have been well described: global hyposexuality (7); deepened emotionality ranging from episodic intense anger to hyperreligiosity (8, 9); viscosity-circumstantiality (8, 9); and a schizophrenia-like cognitive disorder (10). These characteristic changes are thoroughly analyzed in other chapters of this volume. It is the purpose of this chapter to describe and explain the importance of the mood disorders associated with epileptic changes (11, 12).

Whereas the above-listed changes produced by epileptiform activity have been described frequently and in much detail, the affective sequelae are clearly the most overlooked. Some of these disorders were well described by Samt and Kraepelin 100 years ago, and consist of affective lability, periodic dysphoria, and/or euphoria. Many clinicians would write off such patients as "dysthymic," "hysteroid," or "atypical," if, as is often the case, they were unaware of associated epileptic changes. However, the occurrence of episodes that meet criteria for major bipolar or unipolar affective disorders is also not uncommon. Betts (13) found that almost one-third of 72 epileptic patients admitted to psychiatric hospitals were suffering from major mood disorders. Although some of these patients showed no evidence of mania or hypomania, the incidence of driven or euphoric symptomatology during the course of an affective episode was quite frequent. Hence, manic-depressive illness represents the most important differential diagnosis for patients with epilepsy-related affective syndromes that meet criteria for major affective disorders, just as dysthymia, or atypical depressive disorder, is the major differential diagnosis in such patients with minor affective illnesses.

Flor-Henry (14) has found that temporal lobe epileptic patients with associated labile and/or bipolar affective syndromes show a preponderance of foci in the nondominant temporal lobe when compared with temporal lobe epileptics with schizophrenia-like, interictal behavioral syndromes who have a greater dominant temporal lobe involvement. This is a most important and fascinating observation from a theoretical point of view. But his finding that patients with affective syndromes have far fewer seizures is even more significant from a clinical point of view. It leads directly to the hypothesis that there is a group of patients with epileptic changes, but without clinical epilepsy, whose clinical presentation consists solely of a minor or major affective episode.

This hypothesis, which serves as the fulcrum for this chapter, extends the ancient Hippocratic speculation and, at the same time, refines the relationship between epilepsy and the affective disorders even further. If it is true, it is unlikely that the cavalier and reflexive use of modern psychiatric diagnostic systems will uncover such subtle mood disorders because the clinician cannot rely on manifest epilepsy as a diagnostic clue. Such failure to discern epileptiform affective syndromes would not only confound research in affective diagnosis, it would destroy the design of effective treatment for this hypothesized subgroup.

IN SEARCH OF THE SUBICTAL MOOD DISORDER

> *It is often necessary to forget one's doubts and to follow the consequences of one's assumptions wherever they may lead—the great thing is not to be free of theoretical prejudices, but to have the right theoretical prejudices.*
>
> —Steven Weinberg, *The First Three Minutes* (15)

Gruhle's observation (4) that the behavioral syndromes of epilepsy occur in inverse proportion to seizure frequency forms the basis for most theories of subictal and/or interictal psychiatric disease. Blumer (16) and Walker (17) both defend the notion that the anterior temporal lobe produces inhibitory effects on hypothalamic activity, which, in turn, strongly suggests that chronic subictal firing of an epileptic focus must depress diencephalic nuclei important to the determination of vegetative behavior and cognition. The affective, cognitive, and sexual syndromes described above ensue pari passu. This concept has also been invoked to explain the worsening behavior of epileptics whose pharmacological treatment has been so successful that they experience no manifest ictus. Indeed, it is Landolt's observation (18) that interictal psychopathological syndromes form because of a mechanism called "forced normalization"—the brain's adaptive attempt to normalize synchronous electrical activity. A full-blown seizure cuts through this physiologic adaptation and thereby produces temporary relief of interictal or subictal behavioral changes. It is only a small step from Landolt's hypothesis to the central thesis of this chapter, which is the end result of the work of many other investigators. The following paraphrases the hypothesis of Stevens et al. (5, 19): The association of altered psychic states with subcortical spike discharges permits the conjecture that sustained nonictal depolarization, hyperpolarization, increased unit activity, or enhanced synchrony manifest as rhythmic theta spikes and high voltage spindles may be the electrical signals associated with autochthonous subjective distortions and behavioral and cognitive aberration. Suppression of frank seizures with anticonvulsants may lead to a relative increase in catecholamines over cholinergic substances at receptor sites, which in turn increases seizure threshold allowing subcortical spiking to continue at even a higher level as well or possibly producing those affective and cognitive changes frequently noted in catecholamine excess states.

According to this theory, both labile dysthymic and major bipolar affective syndromes could readily occur in patients who never experience ictus. The variations in their moods (rapid and evanescent in the former; longer lasting and more stable in the latter) are explained by alternating diencephalic inhibition and release, according to changes in subictal electrical activity. During periods of greater activity, dysphoria, anergia, and depression prevail, but in periods of lesser inhibition, euphoria develops, often with that beatific religious coloration described by nineteenth century clinicians.

Ballenger, Post, and Kopanda (20–22) expanded this theory by introducing the concept of neuronal sensitization, which they labeled "kindling." According to this model, repeated subictal firing and repeated neuronal exposure to agonists (both naturally occurring neurotransmitters and synthetic substances such as amphetamine or cocaine) may abnormally facilitate pathways that can disrupt or radically alter behavior. Complete facilitation would, in the end, lead to a seizure, but Post and Kopanda (20) are careful to explain, "Although we are using a seizure model of kindling to explicate possible limbic and cortical mechanisms mediating some progressive behavioral effects (in this case from cocaine), seizures per se are not a prerequisite of the kindling model." It is no coincidence that these investigators used their theory to accurately predict the effectiveness of carbamazepine, a limbic anticonvulsant and antikindling agent, in the treatment of refractory and/or rapid-cycling manic-depressive illness. They conclude from their experiments that this effect of carbamazepine reflects the importance of limbic kindling in the etiology of manic-depressive and schizoaffective illness. But the converse explanation is also possible; namely, that among severe or refractory bipolar patients, there is a subgroup of patients sensitive to carbamazepine who have subictal affective syndromes. Both interpretations are probably valid, as Silberman et al. (23; part of the same investigating team) so report, after comparing 44 patients with RDC major affective disorder with 37 patients with complex partial epilepsy with 30 hypertensive but neurologically normal controls:

> Considerable attention has been given to the possible occurrence of behavioral disorders secondary to epilepsy. In this study we report evidence for a converse relationship. . . . There may be a spectrum of symptoms spanning epilepsy, affective illness, and possibly other psychiatric syndromes which arise from neuronal disregulation in the limbic system. . . .

CLINICAL CONSIDERATIONS

Two and one-half millenia have distilled the hypothesis to the straightforward idea that limbic neuronal disregulation produces a distinct affective coloration of behavior whether it occurs in a patient with: obvious temporal lobe epilepsy; subictal limbic foci, who either experiences no ictus whatsoever or ictal activity so subtle as to meld with his or her personality and be clinically unrecognizable; or a limbic syndrome that is not epileptic as suggested by Post and his coworkers (20–22). Even in patients with the other interictal behavior syndromes, affective disregulation follows, by necessity, since the combination of a cognitive disorder, heightened emotionality, and global hyposexuality looks clinically identical to an atypical affective syndrome. This similarity is highlighted when psychiatric patients with abnormal EEGs are compared with those with normal ones (24). The cognitive distortions, peculiar affect, religiosity, somatic delusions, and labile irritability of the former group (24) looks like a review of the behavioral observations of Samt, Kraepelin, and indeed, of every clinician from the last 100 years who has investigated the relationship between epilepsy and psychiatric illness.

Thus, the theoretical prejudice that there is a set of mood disorders etiologically associated with epileptic changes, either ictal or subictal, bids fair, in Weinberg's words (15), to be the "right theoretical prejudice." Seven case reports follow of patients who either had affective syndromes accompanied by hard EEG evidence of subictal limbic epilepsy or had clinical symptom profiles identical to those described by a century of clinicians as typical of interictal affective illness. All seven patients failed to respond to traditional treatments for mood disorders, but responded to anticonvulsants or, as would be predicted by the nature of their illness, to anticonvulsants plus antidepressants (often the very antidepressant that failed before introduction of an anticonvulsant).

The patients are divided into two groups, those who come closest to the *DSM-III* description of dysthymic disorders, and those who come closest to *DSM-III* descriptions of bipolar and/or schizoaffective syndromes. Although one must, perforce, use this diagnostic system, there is little doubt that careful history taking and attention to detail could readily identify almost all of these patients' mood disorders as either subictal or interictal. Routine examination, carried out by inexperienced personnel using "standard instruments," would not only mislabel this unique subgroup, but push it into a long series of ineffective treatment trials.

"DYSTHYMIC" SUBICTAL MOOD DISORDERS

The long-standing clinical descriptions of this group of patients by Samt, Kraepelin, and Gruhle have been reviewed above. Clinical data derived from experience with >3,000 affectively ill patients in affective disorders clinics at Yale University and the University of Pittsburgh have allowed us to distill an even more complete clinical description of this dysthymic syndrome (Table 1).

The description still resonates with the words of Kraepelin and Samt. Lability of mood is the key clinical feature for the detection of the "dysthymic" subictal syndromes. As transient mood changes are stretched out into longer and longer cycle length, "rapid cy-

TABLE 1. *"Dysthymic" subictal mood disorders*

1.	Chronic depressive baseline
2.	Brief "euphorias," often with beatific religious coloration
3.	Brief severe depressive dips with impulsive suicide attempts (frequently wrist cutting)
4.	Unusual amount of irritability and hostile outbursts
5.	Marked premenstrual exacerbation in women
6.	Paradoxical reactions to standard mood-active drugs
7.	Severe cases often diagnosed as severe and/or rapid-cycling bipolar affective disorder, schizoaffective disorder, or, rarely, delusional depression; milder cases often diagnosed as dysthymic disorder, atypical or hysteroid depression, or cyclothymia
8.	Range from frank temporal lobe epilepsy to behavioral disorders with paroxysmal EEG, or EEG may be normal, but patients fit above clinical descriptors

cling" replaces "lability" as the proper descriptive term marking dysrhythmic affective syndromes, and "dysthymia" becomes "bipolarity." But even in patients with bipolar presentations, mood swings tend to last for <6 weeks, and switches occur frequently. Among the dysthymics, however, mood changes can last for only minutes or even seconds, a phenomenon that should create an index of suspicion for the dysthymic subictal diagnosis.

Case 1

SC was a 21-year-old white female college student who came to the Affective Disorders Clinic after treatment for depression and irritability with tricyclics, chlordiazepoxide, and psychotherapy had failed. Indeed, she complained that her high-strung irritability and her labile mood became worse, testified to by a 22-lb weight loss during treatment. Relationships with family and friends had deteriorated under the assault of her impulsive irritability. Particular difficulty arose around her family's disapproval of her boyfriend, and stressful telephone calls from her family were followed by self-destructive behavior on two occasions: the first time by superficial wrist cutting; the second by slamming her fist ferociously into a wall, resulting in a Colles' fracture. Her moodiness became worse during each premenstrual period.

Her developmental history revealed she had been delivered 1 month prematurely after a very difficult pregnancy, that she was left-handed, and that she had great trouble separating from her mother to go to school. All this settled down by the age of 13, at which time she became a driven overachiever. During her senior year, her dysphoria, impulsivity, and irritability became chronic, interrupted only briefly by 3- to 4-day periods of outgoing, overachieving cheerfulness. One of her sisters had experienced Devic's multiple sclerosis and thyroid cancer but had seemingly recovered from both. A second sister had been successfully operated on for a chondrosarcoma.

Her mood lability, developmental history of soft neurologic signs, family history of neurologic illness, and paradoxic response to antidepressants all suggested the presence of a subictal dysthymia. EEG confirmed this impression, showing a bilateral grade II temporal dysrhythmia. Treatment with phenytoin stabilized her mood, but left her chronically mildly depressed. Changing her treatment to carbamazepine 600 mg daily produced a complete remission. A year after graduation, she left for Houston, Texas, where she has developed a successful career as an advertising executive.

Case 2

TF, a 29-year-old married woman, presented with a chief complaint of uncontrollable depression for which she could see no precipitating event. Her symptoms included difficulty falling asleep, sleep continuity disturbance, nightmares, early morning awakening, loss of weight, extreme tenseness, anxiety, and occasional panic attacks. She experienced an alternation of libido between global hyposexuality and driven promiscuous hypersexuality. Despite her symptoms she was competent, organized, and effective. She showed marked affective lability. She would joke and laugh through her tears as she related sad events, and cry sentimentally as she related pleasant ones. TF was a chic and seductive woman with an energy level that belied her low self-esteem.

The patient had once been hyperthyroid, but had been successfully treated. She had no family history of any major affective syndromes. TF was originally treated for major depression with cognitive behavioral therapy and adequate doses of imipramine. She experienced a moderate reduction of anxious and depressive symptoms, but became more labile, with bursts of manialike hyperactivity and hypersexuality. When imipramine was increased beyond 200 mg at bedtime to attain fuller symptomatic control, fleeting hypnagogic phenomena with mild disorientation and hyperarousal were induced. Imipramine was decreased and she was rediagnosed as having a manic-depressive mixed state. Lithium was added to her regimen. She improved somewhat. After a few months, however, her symptoms began to recur. She became more agitated, depressed, hyperactive, and hypersexual.

Consultation was obtained from the Affective Disorders Clinic. The patient's lithium and imipramine were stopped and an EEG was performed. TF was given an interim diagnosis of hysteroid dysphoria, and phenelzine was begun. As a result, some of her symptoms diminished, but her lability increased, accompanied once again by panic attacks. When her EEG showed slowing and rare paroxysmal spike-wave discharges, carbamazepine was added to her regimen. Within 14 days virtually all symptoms, including her lability and hyperactivity, disappeared. She remains asymptomatic 5 years later on the combination of a monoamine oxidase inhibitor and an anticonvulsant.

Case 3

PM, a 24-year-old white female nursing student, became depressed in the wake of discovering she had multiple sclerosis. Actually, she became affectively ill when all of her multiple sclerosis symptoms had lysed (except for some residual cerebellar signs), after she had been successfully treated with prednisone. Her affective syndrome consisted of mixed symptoms of dysphoria and irritability against a constant background of hypomanic denial. Indeed, on one occasion she experienced what she called a "beatitude"—a religious sensation warmly suffusing her body, signifying Christ's intent to cure her multiple sclerosis. Her developmental and family histories were noncontributory.

PM was referred to the Affective Disorders Clinic by her local hospital because physicians there felt she could benefit from lithium salts. When her EEG returned "normal," she was placed on 600–900 mg lithium carbonate daily. She markedly improved, but after 7 weeks began to develop staring spells, absences, and more "beatitudes." PM's dysphoria also worsened. Repeat EEG showed diffuse, nonspecific slowing and was interpreted as a borderline record. Lithium was stopped and replaced with carbamazepine 400–600 mg daily. Except for occasional nausea and ongoing cerebellar signs, all of her symptoms disappeared.

Without carefully harvested medical and neurologic histories and without good EEGs, all three of these cases might have been diagnosed as pure affective syndromes, either dysthymia, cyclothymia (minor affective illness), or one of the major atypical depressive syndromes. Yet, even without such additional information, the clinical presentation of each patient so closely approaches those classic descriptions of interictal affective illness that the klaxon should have sounded under any circumstances. The clinical presentation of mood lability, dysphoria, and irritability should always raise the index of suspicion for a subictal affective disorder. When such symptoms are accompanied by a family or personal history of neurologic illness, a medical history of any disease that involves the CNS, or a developmental history of prematurity or soft neurologic signs, the clinician should assume the diagnosis to be a subictal or interictal mood disorder until proven wrong.

The nature of mood lability in these patients is particularly important to note. Anergic, chronic depression, punctuated by irritable and/or self-destructive agitated outbursts, is the most common form. But careful attention must be given to tease out the history of those typical but very brief euphoric experiences. These euphoric periods can be as short as 2 or 3 s, and rarely last longer than a few hours. They often are euphorias of thought, not action, typically taking on religious and beatific coloration. Sudden religious conversions are not uncommon in the life history of interictal and subictal affectively ill subjects (25). Sexual arousal, though less frequent than religious sensations, can also be part of the euphoric experience of these patients (as exemplified by Case 2). Neither sexual nor religious euphoric experiences will be volunteered to the clinician, both because the patients' experiences are so brief and because they are so personal yet simultaneously so embarrassingly peculiar.

The final clinical feature shown by each of these patients, which is of great importance in the recognition of dysrhythmic affective disorder, was their paradoxical response to mood active drugs. Many investigators have previously noted that "atypical," "hysteroid," and/or "unstable" mood disorders respond poorly or paradoxically to tritetracyclic antidepressants (26–28). Surely part of the reason for this phenomenon is that a significant number of such patients have subclinical epileptiform disorders that are made worse by pharmacological treatment because, by one means or the other, each of these substances lowers the seizure threshold. Davies et al. (29) and Neil et al. (30) have shown the differences in clinical presentation between schizophrenics with and without phenothiazine-induced dysrhythmic changes on their EEGs. Even though these patients are schizophrenic, their phenothiazine-evoked spike-wave discharges seem to augur the identical, labile, dysphoric, affective coloration seen in more "purely affectively ill" patients. Recent problems with the tetracyclic maprotiline (31) and a recent paper by Preskorn et al. (32) have refocused attention on the ability of tritetracyclics to produce subictal EEG and behavioral changes. Lithium salts also are known to make abnormal EEGs worse (33), and sedatives, alcohol, and minor tranquilizers all lower the seizure threshold when they produce tolerance. Alcohol and/or sedative habituation is almost "an occupational hazard" among patients with affective illness. Therefore, any paradoxical or unexpected reaction to traditional antidepressants, particularly in a patient with a labile mood disorder, should raise suspicion of either a subictal mood disorder or a sedative/alcohol tolerance or both. Ballenger and Post (34) were quite correct to invoke kindling as a model for alcohol/sedative withdrawal syndromes. The irritability and labile moodiness that are the affective markers of alcohol, sedative, and minor tranquilizer withdrawal are readily understood in terms of this model.

MANIC-DEPRESSIVE-LIKE SUBICTAL MOOD DISORDERS

It is probable that these bipolar dysrhythmic syndromes differ from the previously described dysthymic, labile, and atypical ones merely according to the intensity and length of reciprocating temporohypothalamic inhibition and disinhibition, or, in other terms, according to the "kinetics of 'kindling'." On occasion these disorders can be clinically inseparable from typical bipolar illness, but there are usually clinical differences from primary major bipolar affective disorder. In the first place, the subictal syndromes tend to be more rapidly cycling and to display more often mixed symptomatology (simultaneous presentation of manic and depressive symptoms). What was mood lability and instability in the dysthymic presentations has intensified and lengthened to the point that each mood swing meets criteria for major affective disease, but the cycles are still short and the switch phase may dominate the clinical picture, producing mixed episodes. As a result the manic phase in these patients is often much more dysphoric and uncomfortable than it is for many primary bipolar patients. In the second place, the manic and/or hypomanic phase is much more likely to be linked to compulsive or to peculiar driven symptomatology. Inserted thoughts or classic compulsions are frequently observed. Indeed, the combination of hypomania and compulsivity should push the clinician to think about a subictal major mood disorder. Compulsive eating is also a strong clue. Bulimia, nighttime gorging, and food fetishes are linked to this syndrome. Finally, any pronounced tendency for a patient to develop confusional or organic symptomatology during either the manic or depressive phase of his or her illness should at least raise suspicions.

Not all subictal affective syndromes are labile or bipolar in their presentation. However, they usually have enough atypical or organiform symptoms to vitiate a simple diagnosis of "major depressive illness." The vast majority of seriously ill subictal patients referred to our clinic came with the diagnosis of manic-depressive illness or schizoaffective disease.

Case 4

JK was a 28-year-old married woman who came to the Affective Disorders Clinic because of unstable mood. She reported that for 2 years she had alternating 2- to 3-week periods of anergia and depression with 1- to 2-week periods of accelerated energy that she described as a "natural" high. However, even during the high periods she felt anxious and uncomfortable. This period of unstable mood had been ushered in by what seemed to be a classic mixed psychotic manic-depressive episode that had begun 1 week after the birth of her first child. She felt herself to be "Earth Baby," possessed by supernatural powers. She had been chosen by God as one of three "Earth Babies" in the United States. She felt she could transcend all common concerns and could make things right for people and nature. During all this time, she still felt depressed and believed she was dying. She would experience sudden losses of energy, which made her feel that there were evil forces trying to kill her and her baby. She had a confusional edge, and she slept very little. After 2 weeks her mixed state began to resolve into a pure psychotic depression with multiple somatic complaints and delusional pain. She asserted she was dead. Butyrophenones had little effect, but the episode gradually abated on its own. Two months later the alternating mood states that prompted her to come for treatment recurred.

Because she was adopted, there was no family history helpful to diagnosis. But she had experienced two discrete depressive episodes at ages 16 and 20 and one clear-cut hypomanic episode at age 19. Her depressive episodes became worse on tricyclic antidepressants, and her manic episode was untreated. After age 20 she became affectively labile. Along with her affective history, she reported that she experienced frequent blackout spells in late childhood and early adolescence. Moreover she described underlying intermittent feelings of mild depersonalization and derealization, which occurred whether she was high, low, or euthymic.

An EEG was performed and showed occasional bilateral temporal paroxysmal spike-wave discharges. JK was started on a trial of lithium salts, but carbamazepine was substituted when she developed a chronic depressive baseline on lithium. A complete remission was obtained on carbamazepine.

JK's case is the first example of quasi-bipolar illness chosen because it represents a "transitional" case in the sense that JK originally experienced typical manic-depressive episodes, which in turn may have been influenced by the simultaneous presence of a temporal dysrhythmia. In other words, she may have been afflicted by two separate affective illnesses—typical bipolar disease and a subictal mood disorder. This author (35) has noted that neurologically soft "second factors," such as sedative habituation or paroxysmal limbic epileptiform activity, tend to push bipolar mood swings into more rapid-cycling and mixed symptomatic clinical presentations. The mechanism of this phenomenon forms the central hypothesis of this chapter: namely, that lowered seizure thresholds and subictal limbic activity suffuse behavior with a labile affective coloration—an effect that is readily deducible from the affective changes associated with epilepsy, particularly psychomotor epilepsy. The putative powers of the tricyclics to produce rapid cycling (36) may well be derived from the same mechanism. Indeed, it may be possible to construct a spectrum of bipolar mood disorders beginning with typical bipolar illness and ending with pure subictal or interictal syndromes where cycle length and frequency are the best clinical determinants of each subtype subsumed within the spectrum. Limbic neuronal instability becomes increasingly involved as one moves from patients with interrupted, well-demarcated major bipolar mood swings to rapid cyclers (to 24- to 48-h cycles) to the typical labile dysphorias and euphorias of the interictal epileptic affective syndromes. Dunner and Fieve (37) have shown that rapid-cycling manic-depressive illness responds poorly to lithium, and Himmelhoch et al. (38) have demonstrated a similar poor response to lithium in patients who present with mixed states. It is precisely in this segment of the above-hypothesized bipolar spectrum that carbamazepine has been shown to be the effective pharmacologic treatment.

The next case describes a bipolar adolescent with severe rapid-cycling illness who responded neither to lithium nor to carbamazepine when each was used separately, but achieved remission when the two were used in combination. Interestingly, this patient showed no EEG evidence of subictal limbic activity.

Case 5

CF was a 16-year-old white male high school student who had been perfectly well until the early spring of 1982. At that time he developed a severe anergic depression for which he was hospitalized and treated with imipramine. Shortly thereafter, he exploded into psychotic mania. Over the next year he cycled without surcease between anergic withdrawal and delusionally grandiose euphoria. Episodes lasted between 2 and 6 weeks. He was admitted to the Adolescent Psychiatric Unit during a manic swing. His mother reported that for the previous week he felt he could do anything and everything. His thought content had become increasingly bizarre and violent. He was obsessed with the violence and bloodshed in two movies, "The Deer Hunter" and "Deliverance." He refused blood drawing for lithium levels because "his Kool-Aid looked like blood." When the staff insisted that his blood be drawn, he requested a knife so that he could supply the staff all the blood it would ever need. Over the previous year he had failed to respond to 2,700 mg daily of lithium salts—even when this was combined with 300 mg thioridazine or 30 mg butyrophenone.

Despite the severity of his mental illness, CF had shown no developmental difficulties nor any previous behavioral problems. His family history showed major depressive illness in his older brothers and alcoholism in his maternal grandmother. EEGs done as an outpatient and during his subsequent stay on the unit were all normal. Further attempts to manage him with large doses of lithium salts and neuroleptics only produced lithium toxicity, nephrogenic diabetes insipidus, and rigid pseudo-parkinsonism.

It was decided to place the patient on carbamazepine 200 mg t.i.d. while his large dosage of lithium was being tapered. When his lithium dosage reached 1,500 mg daily, he stabilized in a normal mood. One week later his lithium was stopped on the assumption that carbamazepine was the effective agent. He gradually became severely anergically depressed. When lithium salts 1,500 mg daily were reinstituted, his depression again lifted and he attained full remission after 2 weeks. CF has remained stable on daily doses of 600 mg carbamazepine and 1,500 mg lithium carbonate.

The only clinical features that distinguish CF's symptoms from those of typical primary manic-depressive illness are age at onset, rapid cycling, and severity of the illness. This rapid-cycling and psychotic profile, however, forms the most typical presentation of adolescent-onset bipolar disease. The ferocity of the syndrome often leads to its misdiagnosis as schizophrenia, a misperception that is further propagated by its poor response to lithium salts. In this case it is possible to hypothesize, along with Ballenger and Post (22), that limbic "kindling" unrelated to epilepsy is the soil in which this primary bipolar syndrome grows. This hypothesis is much harder to defend in typical lithium-responsive primary bipolar illness, where rapid cycling is not present and each mood swing is a discrete entity, separated from both preceding and succeeding episodes by measurable periods of euthymia. CF's need for both carbamazepine and lithium salts is, perhaps, a pharmacologic marker indicating that his illness is midway in the above-described spectrum leading from pure primary affective illness to pure subictal and interictal syndromes. Patients of CF's type usually require both lithium and carbamazepine (22, 39). There is, however, some overlap between the pharmacologic action of lithium salts and the various anticonvulsants. Indeed, Squire (40) observed in 1908 that lithium bromide was the best anticonvulsant available during that era. Modern investigations, however, suggest that lithium is a poor anticonvulsant. Although on occasion it has been used successfully to treat psychomotor seizures (41), it usually makes them worse (33). The following case describes a phenytoin-responsive subictal quasi-bipolar illness, in which phenytoin had similar, but superior, effects to those of lithium on erythrocytic sodium-lithium exchange mechanisms.

Case 6

PD, a 32-year-old single woman, was referred to the Affective Disorders Clinic with a diagnosis of possible manic-depressive illness. She had been experiencing episodic changes in mood for 8 years. She received insight-oriented psychotherapy for most of this time, and although her therapy proved a life-saving support when she felt suicidal, it had not stabilized her mood swings. She had also received trials of several psychopharmacologic agents. Tricyclics invariably made her more dysphoric and irritable. Neuroleptics produced unbearable akathisia. Lithium, in one low-dose trial, had produced relief from her depression, but this effect dissipated within 3 weeks. Electroconvulsive therapy had also provided dramatic, but very short-lived, relief.

PD's clinical picture was not altogether typical of bipolar illness. She had a chronic depressive baseline, manifested by anergia, motor retardation, mild hypersomnia, and social withdrawal. From this baseline she suffered severe and precipitous dips in mood lasting 12–72 h. During these periods she was profoundly hyposomnic, severely dysphoric, and suicidal. She would go on eating binges, particularly at night, which resulted in an 80-lb weight gain over the 8-year period, and she consequently consulted numerous nutritionists, endocrinologists, and diet doctors. She would also experience occasional brief 12- to 72-h euphoric episodes marked by increased social and sexual activity, hyposomnia, and spending sprees. On one occasion this euphoric period lasted 3 weeks.

The patient's developmental history was unremarkable until age 15, when she began to experience occasional fainting spells that were attributed to "hypoglycemia." EEGs were marginally abnormal because of mild generalized slowing and some sharp transient spikes. No frank seizure discharges were observed. All-night polysomnography revealed an absence of delta sleep and some shortening of rapid eye movement latency, suggestive of a mild or remitting primary depressive episode.

Because the sleep laboratory evidence suggested a primary affective diagnosis and the patient had previously responded (albeit transiently) to lithium carbonate, treatment with this drug was initiated (600 mg/day). After 10 days the patient experienced a remission, but over the next 2 weeks her symptoms recurred. At this point she experienced a severe dysphoric hyperphagic episode and had to be hospitalized for 3 days because of suicidal ideation. Tranylcypromine (30 mg/day) was added to her regimen, but symptomatic postural hypotension and severe headaches ended this trial. The patient was made drugfree, and after 2 weeks phenytoin was started. Within 1 month she was in remission, and has remained so for 7 years. During this period PD has lost 80 lbs, excelled in her profession, and married.

This patient was initially considered to have a subictal affective syndrome, but because her sleep studies suggested a primary depressive episode, she was started on lithium and placed in a research protocol where intraerythrocytic sodium and lithium concentrations were measured in correlation with psychiatric rating scales of depression. Figure 1 shows that her depressed mood (measured in terms of motor retardation) correlated very closely with her intraerythrocytic sodium. Lithium's transient positive effects were paralleled by transient decreases in sodium concentration. When her treatment was changed to 400 mg phenytoin daily, her depression remitted and her intraerythrocytic sodium concentration fell again, this time permanently. Erythrocytic sodium and lithium concentrations are known to reflect the activity of a recently discovered lithium countertransport system (42). Alterations of this transport system have been diagnostically correlated with bipolar illness (43). Phenytoin is known to affect the movement of ions across cell membranes in ways that would also tend to reduce intracellular sodium content. Whereas lithium affects the lithium-sodium countertransport system, phenytoin stimulates outward sodium transport from the cell by the sodium pump (Na^+,K^+-adenosine triphosphatase) (44). Any relationship of such effects to the clinical action of lithium or phenytoin is strictly speculative. Nevertheless, the clinical and theoretical overlap between subictal and primary affective syndromes probably extends to their pharmacology.

PD displayed a number of markers for a subictal bipolar diagnosis—compulsive eating patterns, sexual arousal states, chronic depressive baseline with hyposexuality, transient euphorias—but her suicidality also deserves special notice. Prior to her response to phenytoin, PD had to be protected against violent suidical plans

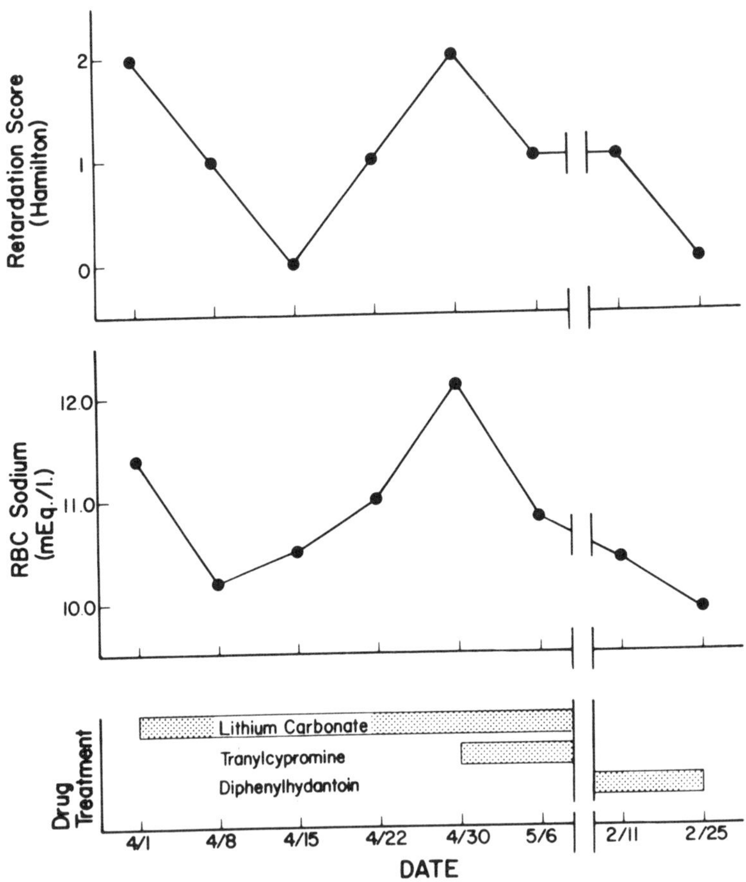

FIGURE 1. *Correlation of depressed mood (motor retardation) and intraerythrocytic sodium level. (A. G. Mallinger, J. M. Himmelhoch, and J. F. Neil, unpublished observations)*

by hospitalization. The chronic depression, rapid and unpredictable changes in mood, transient disturbances in consciousness, affect flooding, and impulsivity that are inherent in limbic system disorders form a rich soil in which violent self-destructive intent grows luxuriantly. It has been our experience that these patients represent the greatest suicide threat among the affectively ill. The final case demonstrates this lethality.

Case 7

SL, a 24-year-old white married woman, presented to the Affective Disorders Clinic with a 6-month history of anergia, hypersomnia, global hyposexuality, and depression. Although her apathy and disinterest had been almost constant, they were punctuated with outbursts of irritability and suicidal rage. She had determined to kill herself with her husband's .357 magnum pistol and actually walked with the weapon to an isolated place 3 miles from any habitation, but suddenly relented and "turned herself in to her husband."

Prior to the onset of her depression, the patient led a very active life, filled with hobbies and activities. She had a particular interest in sports and was an excellent tennis player, golfer, and horseback rider. She also raced sports cars and won many trophies. When her local internist treated her with imipramine, she became so explosively temperamental that her husband called his in-laws to sit with her. Two years before she had had an EEG compatible with minor head injury, which demonstrated right temporal epileptic firing. She had been placed on phenytoin, but quit after 2 days because of oversedation. The diagnosis of interictal secondary bipolar illness was therefore made, and SL was placed on 600 mg daily carbamazepine. She entered remission for 2.5 years, resuming the hectic, physically active, hypomanic schedule she had always enjoyed.

Unfortunately, between races at the local speedway, SL fell from a 6-ft grandstand and was knocked unconscious. After she recovered consciousness, she first became chronically depressed, and then began experiencing bursts of absences, automatisms, spontaneous orgasms, and other phenomena associated with psychomotor seizures. After she attempted suicide three times in 1 week, her husband brought her back to be admitted to the inpatient unit. EEGs on the unit showed continuous right temporal lobe discharges. All attempts to treat her epilepsy and her associated behavioral abnormalities failed. She was referred to a Massachusetts hospital to be evaluated for temporal lobectomy. Implanted electrodes showed a mirror focus. She returned home to the Pittsburgh area, probably still in status partialis. Two weeks after returning home, SL killed herself with a shotgun blast into her right temple.

CONCLUSION

> *A science which orders its thought too early is stifled. Modern science cannot develop a system of ordering its observations . . . until . . . [it] has passed through a long observation and trial.*
>
> —Jacob Bronowski

The existence of the subictal mood disorders is still somewhat theoretical. But as knowledge of the limbic system and psychomotor epilepsy has grown, so has the evidence that there exists a considerable subset of affective syndromes that are either interictal or subictal in nature. Moreover, there seem to be important pathophysiologic relationships between these syndromes and certain primary affective illnesses—particularly rapid-cycling, lithium-refractory bipolar disorders. These concepts are the end result of a hypothesis that began in the Hippocratic corpus. A review of this long-developing literature and experience with >3,000 affectively ill patients has led inexorably to the following conclusions:

1. The presence of subictal epileptiform activity augments behavior with an intense, unstable, affective bias.

2. There is a considerable number of affectively ill patients who have epilepsy-related mood disorders and who have not experienced manifest convulsions. In an epidemiologic survey of our clinic, 75 (10 percent) of 748 patients had a final diagnosis of subictal and interictal affective illness. Only 3.8 percent of this group arrived with this diagnosis. Around 60 percent had been diagnosed as bipolar, about 30 percent as atypical or dysthymic, and about 10 percent as unipolar affective disorder.

3. The bipolar affective syndromes are part of a spectrum that starts with typical bipolar illness, passes through rapid-cycling, lithium-refractory states, and ends in labile, rapidly changing mood disorders that are either subictal or interictal in nature.

4. The vast majority of such patients are clinically recognizable in that they have had a history of epilepsy, an abnormal EEG, or the interictal symptom profiles that have been described in the literature by a century of clinical investigators. In this sense the simple descriptive categories of the RDC and *DSM-III* have "stifled" the recognition of this affective subgroup.

5. The antiepileptic medications, particularly the limbic anticonvulsant carbamazepine, are effective for many of these patients. These drugs often have to be combined with monoamine oxidase inhibitors, tritetracyclics, or lithium salts to achieve optimum results. The need for combined treatment may be partially explained by the sometimes inverse relationship of interictal behavioral symptoms to seizure control. Proper treatment of subictal affective states and rapid-cycling primary bipolar illness is critical because these syndromes are accompanied by high suicidal risk.

REFERENCES

1. Kety S: From rationalization to reason. *Am J Psychiatry* 131:957, 1974
2. *Oeuvres complètes d'Hippocrate, Epidemics, VI, 8, 31, Vol 5*. Edited by Littré É. Paris, 1839–1861, pp 354–356
3. Blumer D: Psychiatric aspects of epilepsy, in *Interdisciplinary Seminar Program—1965: Temporal Lobe Function in Man*. Edited by Mishelevich DJ, Chase RA. Baltimore, The Johns Hopkins University School of Medicine, Department of Psychiatry, 1965
4. Gruhle HW: Epileptische Reaktionen und epileptische Krankheiten, in *Handbuch der Geisteskrankheiten, Bd. 8/IV*. Edited by Bumke O. Berlin, Julius Springer, 1930, pp 669–728
5. Stevens JR, Milstein V, Goldstein S: Psychometric test performance in relation to psychopathology of epilepsy. *Arch Gen Psychiatry* 26:532–538, 1972
6. Pincus JH, Tucker G: *Behavioral Neurology*. New York, Oxford University Press, 1974
7. Gastaut H, Collomb H: Sexual behavior of epileptics of the psychomotor type. *Ann Med Psychol (Paris)* 112:657–696, 1954
8. Bear DM, Fedio P: Quantitative analysis of interictal behavior in temporal lobe epilepsy. *Arch Neurol* 34:454–467, 1977
9. Blumer D: Temporal lobe epilepsy and its psychiatric significance, in *Psychiatric Aspects of Neurologic Disease*. Edited by Benson DF, Blumer D. New York, Grune & Stratton, 1975, pp 171–198
10. Slater E, Beard AW: The schizophrenia-like psychoses of epilepsy. *Br J Psychiatry* 109:95–105, 1963
11. Lishman WA: *Organic Psychiatry*. Oxford, Blackwell Scientific Publications, 1978, pp 360–361
12. Lorentz de Haas AM, Magnus O: Clinical and electroencephalographic findings in epileptic patients with episodic mental disorders, in *Lectures on Epilepsy*. Edited by Lorentz de Haas AM. Amsterdam, Elsevier, 1958, pp 134–167
13. Betts TA: A follow-up study of a cohort of patients with epilepsy admitted to psychiatric care in an English city, in *Epilepsy: Proceedings of the Hans Berger Centenary Symposium*. Edited by Harris P, Mawdsley C. Edinburgh, Churchill Livingstone, 1974, pp 326–336
14. Flor-Henry P: Psychosis and temporal lobe epilepsy: a controlled investigation. *Epilepsia* 10:363–395, 1969
15. Weinberg S: *The First Three Minutes: A Modern View of the Origin of the Universe*. New York, Basic Books, 1977, p 119
16. Blumer D: The sexual behavior of patients with temporal lobe epilepsy before and after surgical treatment. Observations on the part played

by the limbic system in the regulation of sexual activity. *J Neuro Visc Rel (Suppl)* 10:469–476, 1971

17. Walker AE: The libidinous temporal lobe. *Arch Suiss Neurol Neurochir Psychiatr* 111:473–484, 1972
18. Landolt H: Die Temporallappenepilepsie und ihre Psychopathologie. *Bibl Psychiatr Neurol* Fasc 112, 1960
19. Stevens JR, Mark VH, Erwin F, et al: Deep temporal stimuation in man. Long latency, long-lasting psychological changes. *Arch Neurol* 21:157–169, 1969
20. Post RM, Kopanda RT: Cocaine, kindling, and psychosis. *Am J Psychiatry* 133:627–634, 1976
21. Ballenger JC, Post RM: Therapeutic effects of carbamazepine in affective illness: a preliminary report. *Commun Psychopharmacol* 2:159–175, 1978
22. Ballenger JC, Post RM: Carbamazepine in manic-depressive illness: a new treatment. *Am J Psychiatry* 137:782–790, 1980
23. Silberman EK, Post RM, Nurnberger J, et al: Epileptic-like symptoms in affective illness. American Psychiatric Association Annual Meeting, poster paper, 1983
24. Tucker GJ, Detre T, Harrow M, et al: Behavior and symptoms of psychiatric patients and the electroencephalogram. *Arch Gen Psychiatry* 12:278, 1965
25. Dewhurst K, Beard AW: Sudden religious conversions in temporal lobe epilepsy. *Br J Psychiatry* 117:497–507, 1970
26. Klein DF, Davis JM: *Diagnosis and Drug Treatment of Psychiatric Disorders*. Baltimore, Williams & Wilkins, 1969, pp 308–309
27. Paykel ES, Parker RR, Penrose RS, et al: Depressive classification and prediction of response to phenelzine. *Br J Psychiatry* 134:572–581, 1979
28. Robinson D, Nies A, Ravaris CL, et al: The monoamine oxidase inhibitor, phenelzine, in the treatment of depressive-anxiety states. *Arch Gen Psychiatry* 29:407–413, 1973
29. Davies RK, Neil JF, Himmelhoch JM: Cerebral dysrhythmias in schizophrenics receiving phenothiazines: clinical correlates. *Clin Electroencephalogr* 6:103–115, 1975
30. Neil JF, Merikangas JR, Davies RK, et al: Validity and clinical utility of neuroleptic-facilitated electroencephalography in psychotic patients. *Clin Electroencephalogr* 9:36–48, 1978
31. Hoffman BF, Wachsmuth R: Maprotiline and seizures. *J Clin Psychiatry* 43:117–118, 1982
32. Preskorn SH, Othmer SC, Lai CW, et al: EEG abnormalities due to high antidepressant level. American Psychiatric Association Annual Meeting, paper session, 1983

33. Himmelhoch JM, Neil JF: Lithium therapy in combination with other forms of treatment, in *Handbook of Lithium Therapy*. Edited by Johnson FN. Lancaster, MTP Press Limited, 1980, pp 51–67

34. Ballenger JC, Post RM: Kindling as a model for alcohol withdrawal syndromes. *Br J Psychiatry* 133:1–14, 1978

35. Himmelhoch JM: Mixed states, manic-depressive illness, and the nature of mood. *Psychiatr Clin North Am* 2:449–459, 1979

36. Wehr TA, Goodwin FK: Rapid cycling in manic-depressives induced by tricyclic antidepressants. *Arch Gen Psychiatry* 36:555–559, 1979

37. Dunner DL, Fieve RR: Clinical factors in lithium carbonate prophylaxis failure. *Arch Gen Psychiatry* 30:229–233, 1974

38. Himmelhoch JM, Mulla D, Neil JF, et al: The incidence and significance of mixed affective states in a bipolar population. *Arch Gen Psychiatry* 33:1062–1066, 1976

39. Okuma T, Kishimoto A: Anti-manic and prophylactic effects of Tegretol, in *Abstracts of the Sixth World Congress of Psychiatry, Honolulu, Hawaii, 1977*. Summit, Ciba-Geigy, 1977, p 134

40. Squire P: *Squire's Companion to the Latest Edition of the British Pharmacopoeia*. 18th edition. London, J & H Churchill, 1908

41. Shopsin B, Gershon S: Pharmacology—toxicology of the lithium ion, in *Lithium: Its Role in Psychiatric Research and Treatment*. Edited by Gershon S, Shopsin B. New York, Plenum Press, 1976, pp 107–146

42. Duhm J, Eisenried F, Becker B, et al: Studies on the lithium transport across the red cell membrane. I. Li^+ uphill transport by the Na^+-dependent Li^+ countertransport system of human erythrocytes. *Pflugers Arch* 364:147, 1976

43. Mallinger AG, Mallinger J, Himmelhoch JM, et al: Transmembrane distribution of lithium and sodium in erythrocytes of depressed patients. *Psychopharmacologia* 68:249, 1980

44. Woodbury, DM, Fingl E: Drugs effective in the therapy of the epilepsies, in *The Pharmacological Basis of Therapeutics*. 5th edition. Edited by Goodman LS, Gilman A. New York, Macmillan, 1975, pp 201–226

9

Behavioral Effects of Temporal Lobectomy for Temporal Lobe Epilepsy

A. Earl Walker, M.D.
Dietrich Blumer, M.D.

The wealth of psychopathology that tends to be associated with epilepsy and epileptiform abnormalities involving the temporal lobes has been shown to range from more or less subtle personality and behavioral changes, disorders of sexuality, mood changes, anxiety, hysteriform comportment, and schizophrenia-like psychoses to a heightened risk of suicide. One may be tempted to conclude that chronic and excessive neuronal discharges in the temporolimbic system produce all the manifestations of the known mental disorders. However, more careful scrutiny indicates a more specific constellation of psychic manifestations consisting of: an excessive and labile emotionality with heightening of both an angry, irritable disposition and the ethical and religious sense; decreased sexual interest and arousal; and a viscous and circumstantial mental reaction. With proper inquiry such basic characteristics can be identified almost invariably in patients with temporal lobe epilepsy of some severity and duration.

The much less common psychoses, termed "schizophrenia-like," occur not in schizoids, but in individuals with the above-listed basic "epileptoid" characteristics and thus are clearly different from schizophrenic disorders (Chapter 7). A similar statement can be made about those with mood changes, whose sudden, relatively brief, and highly labile moods are distinct from those observed in manic-depressives (Chapter 8).

Changes in personality and conduct that developed on the basis of chronic epileptogenic lesions in the temporal lobe may be reversed with successful resection. The results of the therapeutic procedure thus may clarify the role of such lesions in the genesis of a temporal lobe personality. However, it must be kept in mind that individuals who have undergone temporal lobectomy for partial seizures have had intractable epileptic manifestations, probably pathologic changes throughout the temporal lobe, and have been taking pharmacologic agents, often in toxic amounts, for years—all of which may have contributed to the development of certain personality traits to varying degrees.

In spite of acknowledged limitations, interesting observations can be made on the emotionality and behavior of patients who have had the temporal lobe resected for epilepsy. This report is based upon a series of 50 patients who have been followed from 12 to 30 years (average 17 years) since the resection of a temporal lobe for intractable seizures.

The primary manifestation of temporal lobe epilepsy is the spike focus in the temporolimbic system. Experimental lesions producing such effects have been studied in a number of species. A review of these studies will provide a basis for the discussion of the human material.

THE EXPERIMENTAL MODEL OF TEMPORAL LOBE EPILEPSY

Although experimental epilepsy has been studied for more than a century, the seizures induced by the application of physical and chemical agents to the temporal lobe have been analyzed only recently. Previously the electric stimulation of and the analeptic drugs applied to the temporal cortex have given sparse results. It was only after Gibbs et al. (1) demonstrated that many of the epilepsies had a temporal lobe origin that researchers explored the epileptogenic characteristics of the temporal lobe in animals.

The early studies of Naquet (2) demonstrated that alumina cream injected into the amygdala could induce a variety of clinical manifestations including immobility, pupillary dilatation, facial spasms, and automatisms. Gastaut et al. (3) confirmed these findings. Andy and Akert (4) used the electric current to induce amygdaloid and hippocampal afterdischarge, the clinical effects of which were being observed. The injection of epileptogenic substances into temporal lobe structures was the most popular technique used to study the induced epilepsies. Mayanagi and Walker (5) have reported on the clinical, electroencephalographic (EEG), and steady potential shifts as seizures evolved from the injection of alumina cream in the cortex, amygdala, and hippocampus of the macaque monkey:

> The attacks, either spontaneous or induced by the intravenous injection of Metrazol, were characterized by arrest of movement, staring, unresponsivity to most stimuli, wandering conjugate eye movements, automatisms, twitching of the ear contralateral to the side of alum injection, and, less commonly, vocalization, chewing, hiccoughing, vomiting, adversive head movements and twitching of the face. The associated spiking propagated from the anterior temporal cortex to the hippocampus and amygdala; from the amygdala and hippocampus, which usually fired together, to the temporal cortex and multiple subcortical structures including the hypothalamus, anterior perforated space, anteromedial thalamus, cingulate gyrus, putamen, globus pallidus, and subthalamus. Generalization of the attack, when it occurred, was accomplished by progressively greater involvement of the cerebral cortex and subcortical structures. (p 445)

Chronic behavioral correlates of experimental temporal lobe seizures, unfortunately, have been documented poorly, if at all.

PATHOPHYSIOLOGY OF TEMPORAL LOBE EPILEPSY

Since the recognition of distinct types of epilepsy, many explanations have been expounded to describe the physiologic mechanisms at work. With the demonstration of the origin of psychomotor seizures, usually in the temporal lobe, several investigators have proposed theories to account for the physiologic basis of the various components of these attacks. Unquestionably the best known is the thesis of Penfield based upon the teachings of Hughlings Jackson. According to Penfield, the highest level of functional integration is the centrencephalic system "which has a functional relationship with the cortex of the two cerebral hemispheres" (6, p 473). The greater part of the temporal cortex represents the middle level of differentiation, although functionally distinct from the other components of this level—the sensory and motor areas. This theory has been discussed in detail by a number of Penfield's associates who have attempted to bring these concepts into conformity with modern physiologic thinking (7).

Other hypotheses to explain certain aspects of epilepsy have also been carefully developed. The concept of an epileptic neuron as the basis of most convulsive states has been propounded by Ward (8) and his associates. This thesis has stimulated a great deal of careful investigation that has given a better understanding of epileptic mechanisms.

To account for some psychologic effects of seizure activity, Bear (9) suggests that sensory-limbic hyperconnections may be responsible. "The psychologic changes occurring interictally in temporal lobe epilepsy emphasized extensive and progressive investment of stimulus complexes with intense affective significance. It was suggested that this phenomenon is produced by the formation of new, extensive and excessive sensory (or polysensory) limbic bonds . . ." but, he admits, "it is not possible to establish the existence of such connections directly at the present time."

Based upon these new concepts of the pathogenesis of temporal lobe seizures, a number of investigators have instigated therapeutic procedures to sever lines of discharge propagation, to activate inhibitory mechanisms, and to depress the general excitability of the cortex.

Thus, new theories of the mechanisms of temporal lobe epilepsy are opening avenues for exciting exploration.

EXPERIMENTAL TEMPORAL LOBE RESECTION

Much of the knowledge of the effects of temporal lobe resection in humans has been the result of unilateral operations for the relief of epilepsy. Until recently, the experimental work on temporal lobe extirpation has been carried out on normal animals. For that reason, the results of the excision of human temporal cortices, obviously abnormal, will differ from the findings of experimental animal temporal lobectomy.

The earliest report of abnormalities resulting from temporal lobe excisions came from Schäfer and Brown (10) in 1888. After deep bilateral excision of a monkey's superior temporal gyri (Figure 1), they reported:

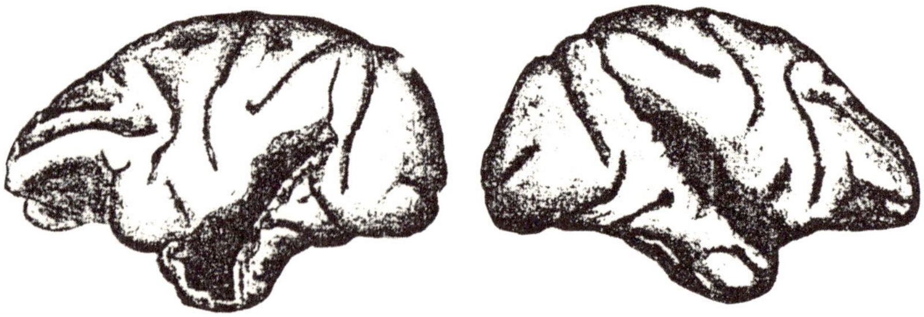

FIGURE 1. Illustrations showing the extent of the lesions of the superior temporal gyri of the monkey. Left: left aspect of the brain; right: right aspect of the brain. (From Schäfer and Brown, [10]).

> This monkey made a rapid recovery; indeed the double operation produced no perceptible effect upon its general health. . . . She appears to have lost, in great measure, intelligence and memory. She investigates all objects, even the most familiar, as if they were entirely unknown, tasting, smelling and feeling all over everything she comes across. She is tame and exhibits no fear of mankind, but shows uncontrollable passion on the approach of other monkeys. . . . She now invariably devours her food by putting her head down to the platter, instead of employing the hands to convey it to her mouth. Moreover, her appetite is insatiable, and she crams until her cheek-pouches can hold no more. She evidently still sees, hears, tastes and smells perfectly well, but her understanding of the impressions which she derives from her senses is unquestionably small. Cutaneous sensibility shows no appreciable diminution. . . .
>
> Recovery proceeded but gradually; . . . there was never, during the whole time that the animal was kept . . . complete return of intelligence. . . . Her appearance remains stupid, and her movements lethargic; she is still savage towards her fellow monkeys; her attention is not easily attracted, either by sights or sounds although an abrupt movement or a sudden and unusual noise will produce signs of perception. She usually takes her food up with her hands; but is still markedly greedy.

Although the authors commented that this preparation was a close approximation of a psychotic individual, the observations were forgotten for 50 years. Then, in a very carefully studied and anatomically well-controlled preparation, Klüver and Bucy (11) reported that bilateral temporal lobectomy in the monkey produced a typical picture: psychic blindness; oral tendencies; tendency to attend to every object in sight ("hypermetamorphosis"); loss of anger and fear; increased sexual function; change from a herbivorous to a carnivorous diet. This report stimulated considerable interest, and a number of investigators attempted to fractionate the syndrome, with marginal success. In cats, Bard and Mountcastle (12) found that the removal of comparable temporal structures produced a savage reaction amounting to rage. The explanation of this apparent paradox is not obvious, for subsequent researchers reported different results. However, the manifestations of the syndrome have been reproduced in cats, monkeys, and humans. Attempts to analyze the neural substance of the individual components of the syndrome have not been entirely successful, although Pribram and Bagshaw (13) believe they were able to do so.

The locations of the lesions responsible for rage are variously placed in the basal nuclei just rostral to the optic chiasm, the olfactory tubercles, the amygdala, and the hippocampal-fornix system. Probably a number of factors, such as species, age, environmental background, etc., play important roles in the varying genesis of emotional discharges in experimental animals.

CLINICAL OBSERVATIONS OF THE FUNCTION OF THE TEMPORAL LOBE

The voluminous literature on the effects of stimulation and ablation of all or parts of the temporal lobe for tumors, inflammatory lesions, or epilepsy has failed to elucidate complex functions of this structure. Nevertheless, some aspects of temporal lobe integration have been clarified; it is apparent that the lateral cortices of the lobe play a different role in the higher mental functions than the medial periamygdaloid and hippocampal structures. However, the precise mechanism involved in the several activities has not been defined. In Table 1 some of the differences in response to electric stimulation are enumerated, and in Table 2 the effects of surgical ablation of the medial and lateral parts of the temporal lobe are presented.

Occasional observations of fragments of the Klüver-Bucy syndrome in humans after bilateral lesions to the temporal lobes have been documented in the literature (14).

TABLE 1. *Effects of electric stimulation of medial (periamygdaloid and hippocampal) and lateral (cortical) aspects of the temporal lobe in patients with psychomotor epilepsy*

	Site of stimulation	
Type of response	**Lateral temporal cortex**	**Medial temporal structures**
Motor	Arrest of speech or dysphasia	Automatisms
Sensory	Nil	Olfactory, visceral (may be complex)
Autonomic	Nil	Varied but abdominal common
Emotional	Simple or complex	Fear, anger with psychic elements
Perceptual	Hallucination, illusions	Hallucinations associated with behavioral acts
Memory	Rarely complex events	Blocked (amnesia)
Consciousness	Unresponsive, confused, or drowsy	Rarely blocked

BEHAVIORAL PROFILE OF PATIENTS WITH TEMPORAL LOBE EPILEPSY

The patients were observed during periods of hospitalization both before and after temporal lobectomy. A history of their behavior was obtained both from the patient and from at least one family member. The patients were interviewed on many occasions and under various circumstances.

Based on our studies, the characteristic traits of the patients can be grouped into several behavioral categories.

Emotionality

If met with a considerate and kind attitude, patients with temporal lobe epilepsy tend to be exceptionally good natured and cooperative. Physicians with a good bedside manner will never incur the wrath of their patients. However, the families will often relate that patients experience recurrent episodes of moodiness, during which they tend to be highly sensitive and increasingly irritable, with explosive anger at times generated by minor slights, whether real or imagined. The angry moods and outbursts tend to be followed by remorse, which may be verbalized or evident by an extraordinarily good-natured attitude. This characteristic emotional

TABLE 2. *Effects of unilateral ablation or destruction of medial and lateral aspects of temporal lobe in patients with psychomotor epilepsy*

	Site of ablation	
Effect	**Lateral temporal cortex**	**Medial temporal structures**
Motor	Nil	Nil
Sensory	Nil	Quadrantanopsia
Autonomic	Nil	Nil
Emotional	Nil (few placid)	Placidity
Perceptual	Nil	Nil
Memory	Rarely impaired	Rarely impaired[a]
Consciousness	Nil	Nil
Sexuality	?	Increased sexuality in the previously hyposexual

[a]Except for subtle verbal memory deficits upon ablation of the dominant temporal lobe and subtle visual memory deficits upon ablation of the nondominant temporal lobe. The deficits can be assessed with special neuropsychologic tests.

lability may be described by the family as a "Jekyll-and-Hyde personality." However, many patients remain persistently good natured. Over many years of repeated and sometimes prolonged contact with patients with temporal lobe epilepsy, only one patient became physically aggressive, and this occurred only on some provocation.

Case 1

A 24-year-old single male patient, who had been brooding over the thoughtless remark of an admitting clerk (that he was "a charity case") and had acted defiantly toward the nursing staff on the research ward, exploded in fury when he was very brusquely approached by a resident physician whose background in boxing made him confident he could handle a tough case, and who attempted to lift the patient off a cart, thus triggering a combat.

The heightened trend to pent up anger and discharge explosively must then be ascertained by taking the history. Often the patient may not report this trait at all and a family member must be questioned. The trait was clearly present in a majority of our patients (29 of 50).

The patients' outbursts are never driven by cold-blooded aggressivity. The terms "irritability" and "heightened anger" describe this trait far better than the term "aggressivity." Only with extreme anger and usually upon some provocation will a patient get carried away sufficiently to attack an opponent, and rarely is anyone injured. More often, rage tends to be vented on inanimate objects. Because of their paroxysmal nature, the outbursts of anger may be referred to as "seizures" by the family. However, they occur in the setting of an angry mood, are triggered by a series of events, are recalled, and are regretted. They are not usually related to any clinical seizure events, except that in a few patients this angry mood may be enhanced in the prodromal phase of a seizure. Occasional acts of postictal violence, usually reflex responses to restraint in a confused patient, may result in injury to a bystander. They are clearly different in nature from the common interictal angry episodes.

Characteristically, an angry outburst may be provoked over an ethical or religious issue. In spite of the emotional lability evident in a majority of patients, their good-natured, helpful, cooperative, and religious attitude prevails by far. The intensification or deepening of their emotionality is occasionally evidenced by intense anger, but most of the time by their deepened feeling toward their family, preoccupation with right and wrong, and their hyperethical and frequently hyperreligious attitudes. Upon sympathetic inquiry the patients willingly relate their intense feelings toward family and others and preoccupations with right and wrong and with religious matters.

Half of our patients, irrespective of the laterality of the temporal lobe focus, had an intense religiosity. Their interest in religion would be manifest in a number of ways: a passion for prayers, reading the Bible, a devotion to church affairs, a marked sense of closeness to God, an urge to follow biblical teachings (such as to care for the sick, handicapped, or poor), and a trend to intersperse their conversations with "God bless you" or similar interjections.

Viscosity

Intertwined with the deepened emotionality is a tendency for patients with temporal lobe epilepsy to exhibit a slow circumstantial mentation and adhesive behavior. This viscosity compels them to carefully consider every minute detail. In contrast to patients with other forms of epilepsy, who may be impulsive in their judgments, the psychomotor patient slowly deliberates each triviality. This trait results in certain characteristic aspects of personality.

In the first place, the patients tend to be entirely sober and have no sense of humor, which relies upon quick associations. Their necessity for detail leads to verbosity and often to hypergraphia, manifested by circuitous letters and documents that temporal lobe patients prepare for their doctor. Another manifestation is the long list of written questions that these patients want to discuss during their interviews. Finally, in their interpersonal relationships this viscosity may be manifested in the permanence of their marital emotional bonds.

The patients in our series showed different degrees of this viscosity. The adherence to each detail, compounded by the deepened emotionality, makes it difficult to expedite a conversation—and, in some, to terminate any conversation—not only representing a peculiar characteristic of many temporal lobe epileptics, but prompting others to avoid them and leading to their isolation. It leads to their being judged "different" or "odd."

Case 2

One of our patients complained bitterly that the boss of his print shop would avoid him whenever he came by to shake hands and exchange a pleasantry with his employees. It turned out that our patient would seize this occasion to elaborate at great length upon issues that appeared very important to him, all the while keeping hold of the boss' hand.

The viscosity, however, is not immutable. The same patient who would hold forth on a single topic in prolonged circumlocution, if left to do so, will often be able to respond more expediently if pressed for answers in a firm and rapid manner. It also appears that such patients may be more straightforward when they are in great anger. Furthermore, we have observed an occasional patient conversing with unusual fluidity following a seizure.

Sexuality

A considerable volume of literature has accumulated regarding the sexuality of patients with temporal lobe epilepsy. In this series 26 patients were considered to be hyposexual before lobectomy. This is a global depression of all sexual experience, not just the impairment of genital arousal. It includes the lack of appreciation of erotic art and literature, the inability to appreciate sexually tinged jokes, and the general lack of appreciation of gender. This hyposexuality is uniquely associated with temporal lobe epilepsy. An individual who develops epilepsy before puberty may never be aware of psychosexual experiences.

The naive sexuality of a 40-year-old male who did not suffer from the common global hyposexuality is illustrated by the following excerpt from one of his numerous letters. He began to have seizures in childhood, masturbated frequently since puberty, yet had remained immature in his relationship to women.

> Another emotional phase is sexual life. Never having relationship with the female sex, being removed from school at thirteen years of age due to numerous auras and mild seizures, I missed the opportunity of socializing with females. Lacking the sexual facts of life, which most boys gain from a father, the subject never entered my thoughts. Following neurosurgery (15 years ago), gradually gaining self-confidence, I spoke with my married friends intimately, learning numerous facts of sex life. Though craving sexual relationship with the female sex, I will not submit to paying a "stranger" for same, which in my opinion, is a pleasurable, passionate experience, not an "over the counter" business. Respecting the opposite sex, having pride and being naive, I could never approach a female (sexually) "on my own" and am hopefully awaiting seduction by the opposite sex.

Psychotic Disturbances

It has been known for some time that chronic epileptic patients tend to develop psychoses. Temporal lobe epileptic patients having seizures for more than a decade may develop peculiar schizophrenia-like disorders. Paranoid traits, often with religious delusions, are common. Yet these patients do not lose their affect and ability to relate nor do they deteriorate mentally. Thus, they present a type of disorder clearly distinguishable from schizophrenic disorders. In this series five patients showed persistent psychotic behavior prior to the operation.

The reasons for psychiatric hospitalization in 14 of our patients are listed in Table 6, in the section on the behavioral profile of the patients after temporal lobectomy (below). Schizophrenia-like psychosis and angry-aggressive behavior are listed as the main reasons for hospitalization, with equal frequency.

PROBLEMS IN UNDERSTANDING THE BEHAVIORAL EFFECTS OF LOBECTOMY FOR TEMPORAL LOBE EPILEPSY

It is apparent that the chief characteristics of the temporal lobe epileptic patient are essentially a reversal of some of the elements in the Klüver-Bucy syndrome, and as such might be considered to represent the results of continuous hyperstimulation of temporal lobe structures by the epileptic discharges.

Obviously not all patients with temporal lobe epilepsy exhibit the full range of these deviant behavioral patterns. Furthermore, the premorbid personality of the individual must to some extent bias the unusual and deviant personality that develops. The changes may be appreciated only with the perspective afforded when the subject is surveyed over a long period of time.

The investigation of the effects of temporal lobectomy is much more difficult to control, anatomically and physiologically, in the clinic than in the laboratory. This is due to the fact that the candidates form a highly select but heterogeneous group who must meet certain criteria for neurosurgery.

First, the various anticonvulsant drugs available must have failed to control the seizures. The majority of the simple cases of temporal lobe epilepsy are controlled medically. Patients with complicating factors, such as personality difficulties, family incompatibilities, and work problems, constitute most of the surgical cases.

The second criterion is that the attacks must originate from a single or localized temporal lobe focus. Only a minority of patients with temporal lobe epilepsy will show predominantly unilateral temporal epileptic activity. Even if there was not early bilateral temporal seizure activity, a mirror focus has often been established before a patient is referred for surgical therapy.

Patients whose temporal lobe seizures have remained refractory to drug treatment are considered candidates for temporal lobectomy only if their epileptogenic zone, in a series of EEGs, appears entirely or predominantly unilateral and is confined to the anterior aspects of one temporal lobe. To document that contralateral EEG changes are insignificant or secondary to the primary focus, special studies with depth EEG may be essential.

Finally, the attacks must be the candidate's major problem. Some patients with temporal lobe epilepsy have serious physical and mental disabilities that make them unsuitable for a serious brain operation designed to relieve what is only a minor phase of their handicap. Such complicated epilepsies must be treated medically.

Gastaut et al. (15, 16) have documented that anticonvulsant medication, by suppressing temporal lobe seizures, may calm an irate disposition or relieve hyposexuality. However, if a drug merely suppresses the overt seizures, some patients, especially children, may become much more temperamental, as if an avenue for the discharge of pent-up energies had been obstructed.

If the surgeon is successful in eliminating the epileptogenic zone, the seizures may be abolished, the EEG normalized, and conduct and personality improved. In clinical terms, one would then expect a mitigation of the hyperemotional-angry behavior, an increase of sexual activity, and a decrease of the viscous-circumstantial behavior.

However, in any given series of patients treated by unilateral anterior temporal lobectomy for epilepsy, the theoretic expectations are bound to be limited. While neurosurgeons may list many who no longer suffer episodes of unconsciousness among their surgical successes, all epileptic activity (aura and EEG spiking) will be abolished in only a minority of surgically treated patients. Thus, fewer patients will show a reversal of a preoperative temporal lobe syndrome.

As was first pointed out by Gastaut (17), the temporal lobe syndrome in epileptic patients represents a reversal of some aspects of the Klüver-Bucy syndrome (Table 3): The excessive tendency to attend immediately to each new stimulus perceived ("hypermetamorphosis") contrasts with the tendency to adhere to one and the same stimulus ("hypometamorphosis" or viscosity); tameness and lack of fear with irritability and deepened emotionality;

and finally, excessive sexual arousal with decreased erotic and genitopelvic response. Psychic blindness and oral tendencies are characteristic of the Klüver-Bucy syndrome, but opposite phenomena are not present in temporal lobe epilepsy. Nor do the changes in dietary habits, listed by Klüver as a specific result of bilateral temporal lobectomy, have a reverse correlation with changes found among temporal lobe epileptics. Anorexia, however, has been reported rarely in temporal lobe epileptic patients.

The Klüver-Bucy syndrome is based on the analysis of behavior changes after ablation of both temporal lobes in primates. Behavioral changes in humans with chronic temporal lobe epilepsy obviously must be of a much more complex nature. Nevertheless, a remarkable congruity is suggested between these opposite versions of the temporal lobe syndrome.

BEHAVIORAL PROFILE OF PATIENTS AFTER TEMPORAL LOBECTOMY

This chapter, which deals primarily with behavior, will not emphasize the principal goal of the unilateral lobectomy, the amelioration of seizures. The effects of the surgical procedure on the seizures in our 50 patients are given in Table 4.

On only two occasions have patients been obstreperous and disturbing to other convalescents after the removal of a discharging temporal lobe. These two postoperative psychic complications were confusional episodes that cleared in a few days without sequelae in one case and after a few weeks in the other. The usual postresection patient was able to leave the hospital within 1 week or 10 days after operation. At that time the patient was well oriented, calm, and cooperative.

An enhanced sense of well-being and optimism is naturally expected in the patient whose seizures have abated after surgical

TABLE 3. *Disorders of the temporal lobe*

Klüver-Bucy syndrome: Hypoactivity	Temporal lobe epilepsy syndrome: Hyperactivity
Psychic blindness	—
Hypermetamorphosis	Hypometamorphosis (Viscosity)
Loss of anger and fear	Increased anger and emotionality
Hypersexuality	Hyposexuality
Oral tendencies	—
Changes in dietary habits	(Anorexia)

TABLE 4. *Effects of temporal lobectomy on seizures*

	Side of lobectomy		
Postoperative seizures	**Right**	**Left**	**Total**
None[a]	9	9	18
Isolated	6	8	14
Fewer	5	9	14
Same	2	2	4
Total	22	28	50

[a]Patients free of any attacks associated with loss of consciousness but who may still have sensory or psychic auras (18).

intervention. A few patients, on the other hand, may experience difficulties in adjusting to a life without the chronic ailment to which they had adapted (19). These circumstances tend to differ from patient to patient. We will review here the effects of temporal lobectomy on the specific behavioral changes that could be related to the presence or absence of the chronic epileptogenic focus. Illustrative case histories will be appended to this discussion.

Effect on Emotionality

An anterior temporal lobectomy may improve irritable behavior dramatically immediately after surgery or gradually over a period of time. Relatives and friends may refer to this change as a mellowing of the individual, who becomes easier to live with and more affectionate. The religiosity tends to persist unless the horizons of the individual are so widened that other interests replace religion.

Irritability is most marked in the very young temporal lobe epileptic, where it has been referred to as "catastrophic rage" (20). The effect of a successful temporal lobectomy on the irritability is therefore most dramatic in this age group (see Case 2).

In this series 22 of 29 preoperatively irritable patients showed less temper, anger, and rage after operation. On the other hand, six of the entire series, some of whom had not been considered aggressive before operation, had more irritability, temper outbursts, and brusque behavior after the operation than before. However, these emotional episodes did not become so severe as to be socially unacceptable. Although generally associated with relief of seizures, the taming effect sometimes occurred when attacks persisted.

Effect on Viscosity

It is difficult to quantify the speed and manner of mentation of patients with temporal lobe epilepsy. Perhaps for this reason a demonstrable effect of lobectomy on viscosity was not apparent. Even patients free of seizures maintained their peculiar slow and circumstantial mental processing.

Effect on Sexuality

Previously hyposexual individuals developed an interest in sexuality after a period of weeks or months following surgical elimination of an epileptogenic focus (see Table 5). In a few cases, a hypersexual swing occurred, sometimes requiring treatment. Four patients in this series developed excessive eroticism, requiring psychiatric hospitalization in one case (see Case 1). This global change persisted for 2 years in one case, and regressed to the original hyposexual state in the others when temporal lobe seizures recurred.

Individuals with normal sexuality before operation rarely experienced change in their sexual appetite even if their attacks were eliminated. Two patients thought they had a decreased libido.

Effect on Psychotic Disorders

Psychiatric hospitalization, so dependent on environmental and economic factors, nevertheless gives a general estimate for the presence of severe psychiatric disorders. Fourteen patients had psychiatric admissions. Six were hospitalized both before and after the operation, four only before surgery, and four only after the lobectomy. It ought to be noted that a few other patients were never hospitalized, despite psychiatric disorders that were no less

TABLE 5. *Sexuality in patients with temporal lobe epilepsy before and after lobectomy*

	Preoperative	Postoperative
Normal	21	29
Hyposexual	26	17
Hypersexual	—	1[a]
Unknown	3	3

[a]Three additional patients had transient postoperative episodes of hypersexuality terminating with recurrence of seizures.

severe than those in patients who were hospitalized. Table 6 lists the reasons for the psychiatric hospitalization.

Apart from three patients with recurrent angry-aggressive episodes, two with postoperative confusional states, and one with a late alcohol-related psychosis, the high incidence of psychiatric hospitalization after surgery was related to the persistence or development of a chronic schizophrenia-like psychosis (four cases). Two further cases suffered from a similar psychosis, without hospitalization after surgery. The temporal lobectomy, regardless of its outcome, did not seem to have a significant effect on the psychosis. In three patients, however, the psychosis became fully manifest only some time after the operation.

One patient, and possibly a second, committed suicide years after the lobectomy. Depression tends to be a significant problem in chronic temporal lobe epileptics.

We conclude as have other writers (21, 22), that schizophrenialike psychoses are not improved, and may be worsened, by temporal lobectomy, even though all epileptic manifestations may be eliminated by the operation. A brief case history will illustrate this conclusion.

Case 3

A 33-year-old married male mechanic underwent a right temporal lobectomy after suffering from psychomotor and occasional generalized seizures since age 14. He also had been admitted to a psychiatric hospital on several occasions over the past years because of delusional, hallucinatory, and at times angry-ag-

TABLE 6. *Reasons for psychiatric hospitalization (14 patients)*

Reasons	No. of patients
Exacerbation of a chronic schizophrenia-like psychosis	5
Transient psychosis (postoperative, confusional)	3
Angry-aggressive behavior	5
Seizures with disturbing behavior	1
Suicide attempt	1
Alcohol-related psychosis	1
Total	16[a]

[a]Two patients were hospitalized for two different reasons, on separate occasions.

gressive behavior. He was intelligent, capable, and usually of a friendly disposition, but would maintain jobs for only a limited time because of his temper. The patient was preoccupied with delusions of personal messages transmitted to him by certain radio stations. His wife remained very devoted to him, despite frequent despair over his erratic behavior.

The operation eliminated all attacks, and all his postoperative EEGs were free of seizure activity. He was perhaps somewhat less irritable, and temporarily showed more sexual interest in his wife. His psychotic preoccupations, however, continued unabated. He worked only sporadically. Three years after the lobectomy he died from a rapidly growing bone cancer. Cerebral metastases had caused renewed seizures that were, however, strictly of the cortical focal-motor variety.

CASES DEMONSTRATING LONG-TERM BEHAVIORAL EFFECTS OF TEMPORAL LOBECTOMY

We earlier reported more quantitative analyses of the long-term behavioral effects from our series of 50 patients with temporal lobe epilepsy treated by unilateral temporal lobectomy (23, 24). These patients have now been followed for 12 to 30 years, with a mean follow-up period of 17 years. The neurologic and psychiatric course of the disorder before and after surgical treatment has emphasized the striking changes that may occur in some patients. The case histories that follow are representative of these changes and serve to highlight aspects of this complex subject.

Case 4

RB was the second youngest child in a large family. He was a healthy, happy, good-natured, and conscientious youngster. He was not adventuresome; in fact, his main interest was singing with the church choir his father directed.

At age 14 RB had an episode of loss of awareness, which might have been a seizure. It could not be determined if similar attacks recurred in the following years. RB graduated from high school and later entered military service at the age of 20. While in a jeep on military maneuvers, he was struck by the limb of a tree and was rendered unconscious for an unknown period of time. Shortly after his accident, he had a generalized seizure, and began to have periods of impaired consciousness as often as once a week. During these episodes he would stare, look upward, and extend his head for about 1 min, after which he would become confused for 10–15 min. This was followed by a sleepy feeling. These episodes occurred two to three times per week, and three or four times a year would be followed by trembling and falling. Once a year he had a generalized seizure.

Following his head injury, RB's seizures were recognized and he was discharged from the military service. After a short period in college, he went to work as a clerk to provide extra income for his family. Later, he obtained similar employment with the government. RB was well liked, devoted, but not fanatically religious. At one time he considered joining a prominent evangelist group. RB sang in the church choir, never drank or swore, and was a model boy around the house. At age 27 he had to be hospitalized for status epilepticus. Two years later, during a seizure, he drove off the road. RB then voluntarily surrendered his driver's license.

He was considered more emotional than his siblings. His sister recalled that he was the only one who cried at her wedding. Apart from this emotionality, his devotion to his family, unusual friendliness, lack of irritability, and exceptional virtue and religiosity, one other trait was outstanding: He showed little interest in sexual matters. RB experienced his first sexual response at the age of 14 or 15, while looking at a pornographic magazine at his brother's home. He masturbated only rarely, as, for instance, after seeing girls in bikinis on the beach. He did little dating and petted on only two occasions. He abhorred "low talk," and moved away from his coworkers whenever they started to exchange improper stories. He had no sexual relations until the time of his marriage at age 37. In the church choir he met a woman, 4 years his senior, who had been left with her six children by an unfaithful first husband. She took a liking to this considerate, gentle, and friendly bachelor and they soon married.

His wife tried to coax him into having sexual relations, but she finally gave up because he didn't seem to enjoy it at all. During their rare attempts at sexual relations, perhaps once a year, he was not active in spite of his wife's seductive maneuvers.

After about 2 years of marriage and following his father's death, RB's seizures became more frequent. Concomitantly he began to suffer marked mood changes, from depression to elation, usually as a prodrome to his attacks. Other prodromal phenomena were irritability, overfriendliness, and hyperreligiosity. Following a seizure he would be his usual self for several days. He became less accurate at work. He talked in loud tones, was overbearing, and lost his sense of humor.

In the ensuing year RB became exceedingly religious, reading or quoting the Bible continually, much to the annoyance of his friends. He was loud, verbose, and rambled in a circumstantial manner. However, he still had periods of cheerful and constructive behavior.

At this time an episode of marked irritability occurred. After a weekend in their cabin, during which RB continuously listened to a radio station that transmitted sermons, the family was driving home. He turned to his wife and told her that she was not saved, but that he was. When his 13-year-old stepson questioned him, he slapped him, and when his wife objected, he slapped her and shouted: "For two cents, I'd kill you both." His wife panicked, obtained a police escort, and had him hospitalized.

At this time the increasing frequency of psychomotor seizures (two or three a week) and the occurrence of two generalized convulsions led to a neurosurgical evaluation (including depth electrode studies) for a temporal lobectomy. The presence of a right temporal lobe focus was established, and he was advised that he might benefit from surgical removal of his temporal lobe.

While waiting for readmission to the hospital, RB had no seizures. He read the Bible continuously and claimed that the voice of the Lord spoke to him "in common language," telling him, among other things, that he should not have the operation. He became so confused and combative that he was committed to a psychiatric hospital where he soon improved but remained contrary, arguing about rules and regulations, for several days.

Upon recovery from this acute psychotic state, at the age of 42, a standard right anterior temporal lobectomy was performed, with resection of about 6 cm from the tip to the anastomotic vein of Labbé, including the amygdala and hippocampus. The temporal lobe appeared tough, suggesting gliosis, but the pathologic report was normal brain tissue with occasional subarachnoid varices. RB had no postoperative complications and was discharged 3 weeks after surgery.

When he returned home, RB slept a lot and had to be coaxed some to take care of his basic hygiene. He was even tempered, quiet, and friendly, and regained his sense of humor.

During the fifth and sixth weeks after the operation, for the first time in 18 months, RB became sexually aroused when his wife seduced him. When he returned to work, his colleagues were surprised to see him whistle at girls. He told his wife that two girls at work were "driving him crazy" and that he felt like *pawing them. The following morning he informed his wife that all he had in mind was sex. He spent the entire day in bed, having erections for as long as 2 h and demanding that his wife relieve him. The next day he remained in bed, having intercourse on two occasions. By this time he was having almost a continuous erection, and his wife felt that his venery was excessive. The following day, in the presence of his mother, he made lewd puns and allusions to men his wife knew, as if they were having improper relations.*

On the first day of the eighth postoperative week, RB worked all day; in the evening, however, his sexual excitement heightened so much that he had an erection whenever he saw a girl, and he incessantly used obscene language, regardless of who was present. The patient ranted about his wife in reference to other men, and "raping all the girls." But he had more rational periods in which he wondered why he was making up such lewd stories. He spent the second and third day of that week at home, claiming the girls at work were bothering him. He remained in bed and wanted his wife. On the evening of the third day, RB seemed confused. He was unable to sleep, was up at 1:30 a.m., dressed and ready to go to work. When his wife got him back to bed, he demanded to be relieved sexually. As always, it was very difficult for him to obtain an ejaculation, and he finally told his wife to "get one of the children to help." The following morning he made references to homosexual practices and made sexual advances to his 15-year-old stepson. After a brief stay at work, he had to be brought home because of his uninhibited foul talk. At home he admonished his stepson: "Come on, hit me for talking to your mother like that, come hit me." RB said he wanted to beat the son, "to get a hold of those big muscles and beat them." His face turned all colors. As his wife and their minister drove him to the hospital emergency room, he would shout "Hi, doll" to women passing in the street and talked about raping them. After 2 days in the hospital, although heavily tranquilized with chlorpromazine, he still used obscene language and expressed the opinion that all his problems would be solved if the interviewer would comply with his (homosexual) desires. Three days later, in the ninth postoperative week, while he was apologizing to his wife over the phone, he became confused and was found dazed outside the booth. His seizures had recurred.

When he was seen 5 days after this event, the patient was reading a book about St. Paul. His sexual excitement as well as the "smart talk" had stopped. He still derived a certain pleasure from describing the obscene vocabulary used by other patients on his ward, but was otherwise very composed. Six weeks later, 3.5 months postoperatively, he had three minor seizures in 1 day and then continued to have about one seizure per month.

Four months after the operation, an EEG showed midtemporal spike discharges on the right side, which were more abundant in sleep. Five days later another EEG showed right temporal sharp potentials, chiefly over the right midtemporal and anterior temporal areas.

With the recurrence of seizures, RB returned to his preoperative self. The frequency of his seizures increased to two to four times per month, although he would not fall and the attacks never became generalized again. He was maintained on Dilantin 100 mg q.i.d., phenobarbital 32 mg q.i.d., and chlorpromazine 25 mg b.i.d. He returned to his work 6 months after surgery.

RB was again uninterested in sexual matters, although he had two separate periods of sexual arousal. During the first period, sexual arousal on 2 consecutive days was followed by a seizure in each instance. His wife asked him not to seek sexual gratification during the second episode, and although "his organ and vocabulary came alive," he showed no desire for intercourse. Thereafter, sexual arousal occurred less than once per year.

RB's religious fervor, on the other hand, was again intense after the recurrence of his seizures. He was never as loud and obtrusive as he had been during the year prior to the operation, but he would still elaborate extensively on his religious experiences whenever he was seen. However, he would usually stop after having described his communion with God or his state of "spine-tingling" religious ecstacy. He would leave religious pamphlets in the office. RB was usually verbose, emphasizing many details, ardently praising his wife, mother, and physician, and thanking the Lord that he had these wonderful people.

Every 1 or 2 months, he would become angry and argumentative at home, lash out at others verbally, declare his independence from his wife, or remain mute and glare at her with hostility. Then after a few days he would resume his good-natured, considerate, and subservient attitude. About 9 years after surgery, his wife had him committed to a psychiatric institution when she could no longer cope with his episodes of moodiness. Six months later he was discharged, but she refused to live with him and moved out of the state.

RB was reevaluated 10 years after surgery, 1 year after his

psychiatric hospitalization. He had rented a room for himself near his church and had returned to work. As usual, he offered no complaints. Apart from work, his life was devoted to religion and music, but particularly to religion. He said, "Music has been with me all my life. Religion I try to use all 24 hours. . . . The whole world is in a tailspin, Christ only can straighten out this mess!" He sang in the church choir, went to Sunday School, and prayed often.

He visited his aged mother frequently, and met his wife for dinner every 2 weeks, whenever she was in town (they had kept the separation unofficial). However, his social activities were limited. He had no interest in sports and rarely went to the movies. Occasionally he looked at television.

RB was pleasantly calm and composed when seen. He was, as usual, unaware of any seizures. When we called his supervisor at work, we were given the following report: "He had no attacks since returning to work 1 year ago. His work is being done more quickly; he can get from one thing to another faster. He was always accurate, but is now very accurate. His work has been excellent. He doesn't seem to bother other people like he used to, and has not gotten involved in arguments at all. I have worked with RB for 20 years, and he is now as good as he has ever been. He is now interested in his work, and seems to be able to put personal problems behind him. He has been far better than we expected when he came back. He shows more control, is less nervous, has good timing, is very intelligent and very thoughtful. . . . He doesn't look depressed. He must have conquered his personal problems."

RB was on Dilantin 100 mg q.i.d., phenobarbital 32 mg q.i.d., and Mellaril 50 mg q.i.d. Dilantin and phenobarbital levels were within therapeutic limits. The EEG was abnormal with excessively diffuse slow activity and recurrent delta runs over the right temporocentral area; sporadic right posterior sharp waves were also seen (awake tracing only).

He stated that he had some interest in women but had not had intercourse nor erections for some years.

Case 5

PM was 3 years old when her mother made the father leave the home. Her father was an alcoholic and had become physically abusive toward the family.

At the age of about 2, PM had two brief episodes of "spasms." At age 6 she suffered a series of about eight convulsions. At 10 years old, she had two convulsions followed by weekly "episodes of staring." At times, the staring episodes initiated erratic and combative behavior of 15- to 30-min duration of which she was amnesic. Almost daily, from that time on, she would become angry with little or no provocation. Thus, she once picked up a board and hit three smaller children riding their tricycles. At other times she hit her playmates with a lead pipe and a baseball bat. She attacked her twin sister with scissors during an argument. She hit or threw things at her mother. "She didn't seem to care if she killed someone. . . . She didn't want anybody close, just wanted to fight. . . . Something in her was driving her, made her mean," said her mother. She did not obey, was uncontrollable, and used foul language. Between her mean spells she would be apologetic and very sweet and would let others have the "shirt off her back," but she would get mad again at the drop of a pin. She even set fires. When her behavior worsened, there was often no apology. She was so very hyperactive that she ran into furniture and was unable to pour a drink without spilling it.

When hospitalized, PM's EEG showed right temporal spiking, and a pneumoencephalogram revealed a dilated right temporal horn. Since her behavior had been the main problem and her seizures relatively infrequent, there was some hesitation before a decision to operate was made.

At the age of 11, a right temporal craniotomy was performed, and a cyst extending from the temporal pole back to the vein of Labbé was identified. There was no communication between the temporal horn of the lateral ventricle and the cyst. Some identifiable temporal cortex formed the wall of the cyst and calcium agglomerations were identified. The cyst wall was resected together with the anterior part of the atrophic hippocampus, but the thin and transparent medial wall adherent to the insula and overlying the middle cerebral artery was left. The pathologic diagnosis on the specimen was cyst with calcified lesion resulting either from a venous angiomatous malformation or an old trauma.

The patient never had another seizure. Her hyperactivity and outbursts of temper ceased promptly with the operation.

In school she was an average student but was rated a "good citizen." She graduated from high school and for 2 years stayed at home, occasionally babysitting. She wanted to become a nurse, and from ages 20–23 worked as a nurse's aid in a neighborhood Youth Corps. She then got a job as a laundry worker, and later as a kitchen helper in a restaurant. When seen 15 years after her lobectomy, she was still working in the restaurant. She had discontinued all medications 5 years earlier. PM felt some tension at work, and she attributed her occasional irritability at home to this. She had smacked her mother a couple of times, then kissed and apologized. PM felt quite independent and had her own car.

As a teenager she liked Sunday School but found church boring. At home she kept a picture of Jesus in her room and often talked about religion. However, as she became more engrossed in her restaurant work, she lost interest in church.

When PM was in the third or fourth grade, a boy had dragged her into some bushes and torn off her clothes. From that time she had been afraid of boys. This had carried over to her teen years, during which she chose only female friends. Perhaps her apprehensions were enhanced by her subsequent experiences with men. On two occasions she had become "engaged" only to find that the men were married. She broke off the relations because, still a virgin, she did not care to become sexually involved.

Case 6

MJ began having seizures at the age of 13 years. When first seen by a physician for the problem, he was having minor seizures one to four times per day and was advised to use phenobarbital at this time. By 14 years of age, MJ's seizures were occurring once a day to once every 2 weeks. When seen again at the age of 16, MJ reported no seizures during the preceding 2 years; however, the following year the attacks recurred. He experienced the seizures for 18 months, and then had a 6-month seizurefree period. The seizurefree period occurred after he began using potassium bromide. When it was discontinued, the attacks recurred. At the age of 24, MJ was having seizures several times per week. At 25 years old he had only occasional attacks. The frequency of the attacks again increased to several times per week and remained unchanged to age 30. The wavering frequency of MJ's seizures was always associated with an alteration in medication, but the positive effects were always temporary.

When he was 30 years old, MJ had a major attack while driving and drove off the road. An attack witnessed by his physician was described: "The patient suddenly shouted, head turned slightly to the left, and some chewing movements were noted."

MJ had two types of seizures that were nearly identical except *that the more severe attack had no aura associated with it. The mild attack was characterized by a "butterfly feeling" in the epigastrium, followed by an involuntary cry after a few seconds. In the mild attack he would reach for his handkerchief and cover his mouth to suppress the cry. He was successful and the seizures were generally not noticed by observers. The more severe attack was characterized by walking several steps in any direction before regaining awareness of his environment. It was during a similar episode that MJ drove his car off the road. The character of the seizures remained unchanged over the years.*

During the 16 years that MJ had seizures prior to surgery, he used phenobarbital, potassium bromide, Dilantin, Luminal, Tridione, Mesantoin, and Mebaral, all of which offered only poor control over the seizures.

MJ was the youngest child in a solid Catholic family. From 13 to 19 years of age, he served as an altar boy in their church. He was also a boy scout from 13 to 22 years of age, and then worked as a Red Cross volunteer for a time. MJ completed high school when he was 19 years old. He was employed in a land office for 4 years, then acquired employment with the state government working in a garage. He had some aspiration to become a firefighter, but realized that his seizures would prevent such an endeavor.

MJ and his parents both reported no significant changes in behavior and temperament after the onset of his seizures. His school performance was average, and MJ said he enjoyed school. He had no close relationships with girls. He reported "having sexual feelings on occasion" but never had an erection or ejaculation, neither while awake nor while asleep. In fact, MJ did not enter full puberty until after the operation, at 30 years of age.

It was not until the patient was 30 years old that a right temporal tip focus was identified. He was then hospitalized for surgical treatment of his persistent attacks. The temporal lobe was excised for a distance of 6 cm from the temporal tip. Two spike foci were located in the lateral aspect of the lobe. A small discharging area below the Sylvian fissure was then resected. The total resection extended from the lower margin of the Sylvian fissure back to the anastomotic vein of Labbé and included the amygdala and rostral hippocampus. The postoperative course was uneventful, and MJ was advised to use phenobarbital and Dilantin.

The patient was not seen again for about 12 years. He had

been using medications (Dilantin and phenobarbital) since the operation but had recently discontinued them. He reported no seizures or auras since the operation. An EEG taken about 2 years postoperatively showed no discrete discharges, but there was a generalized, moderate dysrhythmia. The EEG taken during the follow-up showed abnormality caused by diffuse disorganization in the right temporal region, but no seizure discharges were recorded. His neurologic and physical exams were normal.

Shortly after the operation MJ secured employment as a stock clerk. He was promoted, but after 3 years with the firm, left and took employment as a mail carrier.

MJ felt more confident after the operation, dressed neatly, and attended more social affairs. Six months postoperatively, while on the dance floor, he was greatly embarrassed when he experienced his first erection ever. His first ejaculation occurred about a year later when he had escorted a girl home and gave her a goodnight kiss at the door.

At 42 years of age MJ married. He described his first experience of a climax with sexual intercourse, on the honeymoon, as something akin a volcanic eruption. For many years MJ continued to have sexual relations at least once a night.

When we saw MJ again 22 years after the operation, he reported that he had frontal headaches on rare occasions. About 14 years after the operation, MJ's wife had been awakened by a shaking of the bed. MJ did not have any nervous feelings in his stomach nor any loss of consciousness but resumed use of Dilantin. MJ's memory, hearing, and eyesight were all good. His conversation was somewhat slow and viscous, as he willingly relayed all details of a situation, but he had no trouble with speech.

MJ reported that people frequently asked him what he was so happy about. He was very pleased with his operation, saying that he felt "reborn." MJ attended church services regularly and prayed every morning. He enjoyed fishing, watching television, and reading newspapers. MJ had several close friends, and he and his wife were close to both of their families.

SUMMARY

It is apparent that the psychic effects of a temporal lobectomy for psychomotor epilepsy depend upon a number of factors: the preoperative integrity of neurologic and psychologic functions; the degree of relief from seizures; and the presence or absence of somatic disorders. Some patients, although still having a few mild attacks, have, by reason of a less rasping personality, made excellent adjustments at work and home and are enjoying a life that they could not appreciate before the operation. Other individuals consider their psychosexual renaissance to be the most beneficial effect of their operation. Some patients in this series have been relieved of seizures but have continued to suffer from preexisting psychiatric or neurologic disorders. A few who have not achieved complete freedom from seizures still harbor an irritating personality, and perhaps obtain an inward satisfaction from a preoccupation with religion.

The beneficial effects of a temporal lobectomy on personality and behavior correlate closely with the success in eliminating the seizure manifestations:

1. With the elimination of seizures, angry-irritable moods and aggressive outbursts tend to be mitigated, at times dramatically, immediately after the operation. Even if seizures continue, a diminution of these negative traits may be observed. The hyperethical and religious attitudes tend to remain.
2. The viscosity seems to be unchanged, although a few patients relieved of their seizures seem to have a somewhat more fluid personality. There is need for quantitative measures for this trait.
3. With elimination of the seizure activity, the preoperative hyposexuality tends to be replaced by normal sexual arousal and response or, at times, by hypersexuality. The sexual awakening usually occurs in the second postoperative month. Hypersexual periods may last for as long as 2 years or until the recurrence of seizures.
4. Schizophrenia-like psychoses are not improved by temporal lobectomy, even though all epileptic manifestations may have been eliminated.

REFERENCES

1. Gibbs E, Gibbs FA, Fuster B: Psychomotor epilepsy. *Arch Neurol Psychiatry* 60:331–339, 1948
2. Naquet R: Sur les fonctions du rhinencéphale d'après les resultats de sa stimulation chez le chat. Thesis, Marseille, 1953
3. Gastaut H, Naquet R, Meyer A, et al: Experimental psychomotor epilepsy in the cat: electroclinical and anatomopathological correlations. *J Neuropathol Exp Neurol* 18:270–293, 1959
4. Andy OJ, Akert K: Seizure patterns induced by electrical stimulation of hippocampal formation in the cat. *J Neuropathol Exp Neurol* 14:198–213, 1955
5. Mayanagi Y, Walker AE: Experimental temporal lobe epilepsy. *Brain* 97:423–446, 1974
6. Penfield W, Jasper H: *Epilepsy and the Functional Anatomy of the Human Brain.* Boston, Little, Brown, 1954
7. Gloor P: Electrophysiological studies of the amygdala (stimulation and recording): their possible contribution to the understanding of neural mechanisms of aggression, in *Neural Bases of Violence and Aggression.* Edited by Fields WS, Sweet WH. St. Louis, Green Inc, 1975, pp 5–40
8. Ward AA Jr: Perspectives for surgical therapy of epilepsy, in *Epilepsy.* Edited by Ward AA Jr, Penry JK, Purpura D. New York, Raven Press, 1983, pp 371–390
9. Bear DM: Temporal lobe epilepsy—a syndrome of sensory-limbic hyperconnection. *Cortex* 15:357–384, 1979
10. Schäfer EAS, Brown SM: An investigation into the functions of the occipital and temporal lobes of the monkey's brain. *Philos Trans R Soc Lond (Biol)* 179:303–327, 1888
11. Klüver H, Bucy PC: Preliminary analysis of functions of the temporal lobe in monkeys. *Arch Neurol Psychiatry* 42:979–1000, 1939
12. Bard P, Mountcastle VB: Some forebrain mechanisms involved in expression of rage with special reference to suppression of angry behavior. *Res Publ Assoc Nerv Ment Dis* 27:362–404, 1947
13. Pribram KNH, Bagshaw M: Further analysis of the temporal lobe syndrome utilizing fronto-temporal ablations. *J Comp Neurol* 99:347–375, 1953
14. Marlowe WB, Mancall EL, Thomas JJ: Complete Klüver-Bucy syndrome in man. *Cortex* 18:53–59, 1975
15. Gastaut H, Morin G, Lesèvre N: Etude du comportement des épileptiques psychomoteurs dans l'intervalle de leurs crises. *Ann Med Psychol (Paris)* 113:1–27, 1955

16. Gastaut H, Collomb H: Etude du comportement sexuel chez les épileptiques psychomoteurs. *Ann Med Psychol (Paris)* 112:657–696, 1954

17. Gastaut H: Interprétation des symptômes de l'épilepsy psychomotrice en fonction des données de la physiologie rhinencéphalique. *Presse Med* 62:1535–1537, 1954

18. Walter AE: Critique and perspectives, in *Advances in Neurology, Vol 8: Neurosurgical Management of the Epilepsies.* Edited by Purpura DP, Penry JK, Walter RD. New York, Raven Press, 1975, p 344

19. Ferguson SM, Rayport M: The adjustment to living without epilepsy. *J Nerv Ment Dis* 140:26–37, 1965

20. Ounsted C, Lindsay J, Norman R: Biological factors in temporal lobe epilepsy, in *Clinics in Developmental Medicine 22.* London, Spastics International Medical Publication with William Heinemann Medical Books, 1966

21. Falconer MA: Effects of temporal lobectomy on personality in epilepsy, in *Personality and Science.* Edited by Ramsey IT, Porter R. Ciba Foundation Symposium. New York, Longman, 1971, pp 41–44

22. Jensen I, Larsen JK: Psychoses in drug-resistant temporal lobe epilepsy. *J Neurol Neurosurg Psychiatry* 42:948–954, 1979

23. Blumer D, Walker AE: Sexual behavior in temporal lobe epilepsy. *Arch Neurol* 16:37–43, 1967

24. Walker AE, Blumer D: Long term effects of temporal lobe lesions on sexual behavior and aggressivity, in *Neural Bases of Violence and Aggression.* Edited by Fields WS, Sweet WH. St. Louis, Green Inc, 1975, pp 392–400

10

Dostoievsky's Epilepsy

Norman Geschwind, M.D.

Although many famous people throughout history have been identified with more or less assurance as sufferers from epilepsy, there is possibly no example in which the personal documentation is so complete as it is for the great Russian author Dostoievsky. Although epilepsy appears again and again in literature, there is perhaps no well-known author in whose fictional work this disorder played so important a part as in the case of this Russian master novelist. As a result his works have special interest for the neurologist and psychiatrist.

It would probably be an error to speculate too freely on the basis of an analysis of his personal epilepsy and the descriptions in his writings. It would be an error of greater magnitude not to consider tentatively just what role epilepsy might have played in forming his personality and the character of his literary productions. This topic has aroused interest over many years. Sixty-five years ago,

The work reported here was supported in part by a grant from the Essel Foundation and by a grant from NINCDS (06209) to the Boston University Aphasia Research Center.

This article is based on lectures delivered at the Boston Society of Psychiatry and Neurology on March 16, 1961, and at the Johns Hopkins Medical School on February 16, 1972.

in *Le Progrès Médical*, a brief article appeared under the initials P.M., indicating, one might speculate, the distinguished French neurologist Pierre Marie. More recently, Théodor Alajouanine (1), one of Marie's most important students, wrote an article on the same topic. Perhaps the best-known discussion is that which appears in Freud's famous essay "Dostoevsky and Parricide" (2).

DOSTOIEVSKY'S LIFE

Fyodor Mikhailovitch Dostoievsky was born in 1821 and died in 1881. His life was miserable during almost the whole interval from birth to death, "a long Calvary" as one author put it. His father, a physician and small landowner, described by his famous son as a brutal and difficult man, was murdered by his serfs when Dostoievsky was 18 and a student at a military engineering school. Dostoievsky decided not to join the army but began to write and to be involved in socialist politics. At the age of 28 he was arrested and condemned to death by firing squad, but was reprieved by a decree of clemency from the czar announced only after he had been placed before his intended executioners with his eyes bandaged. His sentence was commuted to 4 years of imprisonment in Siberia to be followed by military service. While in exile he married, but the relationship was not a happy one. Permission was given to him, after 10 years of exile, at the age of 38, to return to St. Petersburg. Five years after his return, in 1864, both his wife and his brother Mikhail, also a writer and to whom he was very attached, died, leaving him with the obligation of supporting two sets of children.

The year 1866, when he was 45 years old, saw the publication of the first of his great novels, *Crime and Punishment*. Over the next 10 years there appeared a succession of other masterpieces. In 1867 Dostoievsky married again, much more successfully than the first time. For 4 years the couple lived mostly in Germany, trying to get ahead of their debts. Unfortunately, a compulsive addiction to gambling again and again wrecked his attempts at financial restitution.

During the last 10 years of his life, following the return to Russia in 1871, Dostoievsky was famous, relatively happy, and prosperous. However, even this period was darkened by the death of his young son, Alyosha, on May 16, 1878, we are told, after epileptic seizures recurring over 3 hours and 10 minutes.

Dostoievsky died in 1881, at the age of 60, following an episode of coughing up blood. A great public funeral was held at St. Petersburg, the site of his eventual success.

Within the opening pages of his essay, Freud provides a brilliant summary of Dostoievsky as a writer and human being. Freud's admiration for his literary talent is unbounded since he rates him as not far behind Shakespeare and calls *The Brothers Karamazov* the most magnificent novel ever written. On the other hand, he is extremely critical of Dostoievsky's personal moral standing. He writes:

> A man who alternately sins and then in his remorse erects high moral standards lays himself open to the reproach that he has made things too easy for himself. After the most violent struggles to reconcile the instinctual demands of the individual with the claims of the community, he landed in the retrograde position of submission both to temporal and spiritual authority, of veneration both for the Tsar and for God, and of a narrow Russian nationalism—a position which lesser minds have reached with smaller effort.

EPILEPSY IN DOSTOIEVSKY'S OWN LIFE

It is not exactly clear when Dostoievsky's seizures began, since the available data are conflicting. It is sometimes said that they began after his father's murder. Yet in his request to the czar for a pardon he stated that they had begun in Siberia. Still other accounts, however, claim that his disease dated back to early childhood. It appears that epilepsy was present before his exile, and that Dostoievsky probably altered the facts to make his appeal for clemency stronger.

By any standard Dostoievsky's epilepsy was severe, with attacks occurring at intervals ranging from a few days to several months. Although there was no episode of prolonged status epilepticus, there were several episodes of repeated seizures. In my own readings, I have found no mention of the use of any medication. Nor was any evidence found of his having consulted any distinguished specialists. Yet one must recall that at the time of Dostoievsky's death in 1881, neurology was a very young field even in Western Europe. The accounts of his trips to Germany do not mention his seeking out of any of the German professors so admired among the educated in Russia at that period. On the other hand, he did go to many doctors and frequently read medical books.

The seizures stopped completely in 1877, 4 years before his death. His illness had thus lasted for at least 40 years.

Dostoievsky described his attacks frequently, and accounts also appear in the writings of acquaintances and family members. Characteristically he could predict the imminent occurrence of a seizure by an indescribable sense of well-being that might be present for a few moments. He is quoted as saying that others have no idea of the bliss that epileptics experience in the moments preceding their attacks. Observers commented on his appearance at this moment; e.g., he is described as glowing with the most transcendent inspiration, after which there were a cry, a fall, and a major convulsion with frothing at the mouth and frequent injuries. Following his awakening he would have a sense of intense depression and guilt, which might last for several days.

Dostoievsky contrasted his feelings preceding and following attacks. Before, there were an extraordinary inner light that flooded the soul and a few seconds of felicity, for which he could give 10 years of his life. On the other hand, after the attack it seemed to him that he had committed a monstrous crime.

EPILEPSY IN DOSTOIEVSKY'S WRITINGS

At least four major characters in Dostoievsky's writings are epileptic. Of these, one of the most interesting is Kirillov, an important figure in *The Possessed*. Speaking to Shatov, another of the major figures, he says, "There are seconds—they come five or six at a time—when you suddenly feel the presence of the eternal harmony perfectly attained." When Shatov asks how often this happens, Kirillov replies perhaps once in 3 days or once a week. His response is negative to the question of whether he suffers from epileptic seizures. Shatov goes on to say, "I've heard that's just how fits begin. An epileptic described exactly that sensation before a fit, word for word as you've done." Kirillov, who at this time is planning his eventual suicide, lets Shatov know that there will not be time for him to develop epilepsy.

The novel in which epilepsy plays the greatest role is, of course, *The Idiot*: the title character, Prince Myshkin, is an epileptic. The description of Myshkin's seizures corresponds very closely to Dostoievsky's personal accounts. Myshkin has a sudden flash of light in his brain and feels as if all of his senses are working at the very highest level. In this moment he is possessed by the same sense of serenity and harmony that Dostoievsky described in his own seizures. Myshkin reflects on the fact that it is disease that leads to these moments of supreme serenity, but decides in the end that this is a fact of no importance in the face of the attainment of insight into a supreme sense of personal completeness.

Dostoievsky was, on the other hand, acutely sensitive to the fact that every attack is not epileptic. The distinction between the epileptic and the nonepileptic attack is a classic problem in differential diagnosis, which must have been far more difficult in Dostoievsky's time than it is now. Indeed, today some attacks remain a problem for even the most sophisticated clinician. In *The Friend of the Family*, the character Foma Fomitch would suddenly stop and stare blankly for as long as an hour, following which he would wake up and state that he had no awareness of what had gone on during all of that time. As lay readers come to this point, they are, of course, expecting that the author will be sympathetic with this unfortunate character. There is, however, a sudden change of tone in the text as Dostoievsky asserts that Foma must have been so anxious to impress others and attract their attention that he voluntarily put on this elaborate act. This is another example of astute clinical judgment, since there are few neurologists today who would regard these attacks as typically epileptic.

Dostoievsky's clinical acumen shows up again clearly in *The Brothers Karamazov*. In this novel, considered by many to be Dostoievsky's greatest work, a brutal murder is committed. It eventually becomes clear that the father of the Karamazov brothers has been killed by his illegitimate son, the epileptic Smerdyakov, a twist to the plot that must recall the murder of Dostoievsky's own father by his serfs. One day before the murder, Smerdyakov tells Ivan Karamazov, the eldest son, that he is certain that he will have a long seizure on the next day. Ivan challenges him with the fact that it is impossible to tell when a seizure can be expected, and Smerdyakov agrees, pointing out that he might therefore have a seizure the very next day. In response to Ivan's question of whether he is going to pretend to have a seizure, Smerdyakov replies that if he wanted to do so it would not be difficult.

Smerdyakov does apparently have a seizure the next day just at the time, it appears, that the father of the Karamazovs is being murdered. The police surgeon, much more interested in the epileptic who is apparently in status than in the murdered old man, comments on the rarity and great interest of such repeated seizures. It is, of course, worth recalling that at that time the lack of any effective treatment for status must have led often to its persistence over many hours or days.

Smerdyakov is removed to the hospital because of these repeated severe seizures. In a later interview, he admits to Ivan that he and not Demitri Karamazov had murdered the old man, that he had then shammed a series of seizures, but that just before being taken to the hospital the next morning, he had had a real seizure.

THE NATURE OF DOSTOIEVSKY'S EPILEPSY

Let us now turn to the question of the type of epilepsy from which Dostoievsky was suffering. Freud used the term "hystero-epilepsy" for the novelist's attacks. There are many reasons for rejecting the possibility of hysterical epilepsy in the usual sense of the term. The individual attacks were brief, stereotyped, and associated with frothing at the mouth. In particular, Dostoievsky was frequently injured in these attacks, a feature that would be most unusual for hysterical seizures. It would furthermore be very unusual in a person of high sophistication and particularly in someone who was so clinically astute about epilepsy. A careful reading of Freud makes it likely that he was not, in fact, suggesting that Dostoievsky was suffering from hysterical pseudoseizures, but was instead using the term "hystero-epilepsy" in the sense of psychosomatic epilepsy, i.e., organic epilepsy resulting from unresolved inner conflicts. Although one cannot totally reject this possibility, the concept of psychosomatic epilepsy has not been well documented.

It seems that one must diagnose Dostoievsky as a sufferer from temporal lobe epilepsy. The argument has been raised that Dostoievsky's aura, i.e., a sense of intense elation, is very unusual. It is indeed the case that when an emotion makes up part of a temporal lobe seizure, it is most frequently unpleasant, e.g., fear, anger, or a sense of vague dread. On the other hand, the very occurrence of an intense emotion itself points strongly to a focal involvement of limbic structures. Furthermore, whereas pleasant sensations are rare either in spontaneous seizures or in stimulation of the structures of the mediotemporal lobe, both have been documented to occur. Any alternative to epilepsy arising in the limbic system thus would appear difficult to accept.

There is also considerable evidence to suggest that Dostoievsky possessed several of the personality features that are now known to be common among those with epilepsy arising in the temporal lobe. Although extremely frequent, they are by no means universal nor are the manifestations of these personality changes always as severe as they were in Dostoievsky's case. Yet the occurrence of the typical pattern is extremely difficult to dismiss. A very common feature is an intense concern with philosophical or religious issues, which are dealt with at great length. No reader of Dostoievsky could be unaware of his preoccupation with problems of this type. He manifested another feature often found among temporal lobe epileptics, i.e., a great emphasis on morality and proper behavior that is often in striking contrast to the actual pattern of daily relationships with others. Freud commented on this specifically, pointing out the increasing depth of religious belief with the passage of the years that did not manifest itself in increased saintliness of personal behavior. Instead Dostoievsky adopted the very worst aspects of nineteenth century Russian narrow panslavism and intense devotion to the czar. One repeatedly finds descriptions, by both himself and others, of his tendency to get embroiled in petty arguments. Although his fellow Russian author Turgenev had befriended him many times, Dostoievsky, on a visit in Germany, appears to have gone out of his way to be insulting. Similarly, he became embroiled in a heated dispute with a guard at the Sistine Chapel, who told him that he could not stand on a chair in order better to view the Michelangelo paintings on the ceiling.

Another striking feature of Dostoievsky's writings is the lack of humor. Neither the biographies that I have read, nor the portions of his published diaries that I have seen, nor his published writings contain any evidence of a sense of gaiety. By contrast, one is constantly made aware that all events are of great importance and that there are no minor incidents. Even the occasional approach to humor is bizarre, e.g., the character in *The Idiot* who, having offered to whisper something to the local governor, bites his ear.

Another intriguing characteristic is the lack of concern with sex or with female beauty. It is easy to contrast Dostoievsky with Tolstoy in whose writings beautiful women are described in detail and passionate sexual attachments are of major importance, as in *Anna Karenina* and *War and Peace*. Physical beauty and sexual passion appear to play very little role in Dostoievsky's books; the bonds between men and women are predominantly at the level of spiritual attachments. This atypical attitude toward sex may well reflect some of Dostoievsky's own features. His daughter pointed out in her biography that she found it astonishing that in his youth there was no woman in his life—no betrothed, no mistress, not even a flirtation. Hyposexuality is well known as a common personality trait in temporal lobe epilepsy. Dostoievsky did marry and father children, so that it cannot be asserted that he remained hyposexual throughout his life. The evidence from his fiction, his diaries, and his daughter's comments all point, however, in this direction.

Another of Dostoievsky's traits, one that appears repeatedly in characters in his novels, was a readiness to become angry on slight provocation. We have already noted this tendency in his own life and in his writings; it is clear from the accounts of others that this was a cardinal feature of his behavior.

The use of these personality traits in Dostoievsky's fiction is of particular interest. In the author himself we have the evidence for a typical mixture of these personality characteristics, i.e., a profound concern with philosophical, religious, and moral issues, combined with intolerance for others and extreme irritability that readily erupted into anger. It is intriguing that in his writings Dostoievsky separated these traits from each other and assigned them to different characters. Although Prince Myshkin describes his seizures in words essentially identical to those used by Dostoievsky in reference to his own, one cannot regard Myshkin as otherwise similar to Dostoievsky. He shares a deep concern for religion and morality, but Myshkin is above all a saintly figure with infinite tolerance and sympathy for the faults of others. However, other characters in the same novel reflect those aspects of Dostoievsky's own character on which Freud commented so unfavorably, i.e., his intolerant moralizing and his ready precipitation into anger even over trivialities. Again and again his tendency is found in Dostoievsky's writings. He assigned his own wish for saintliness to some characters and placed his own unfavorable characteristics in others. A personal sense of disunity appears to have been exorcised by the creation of some characters in which unity is achieved.

It is curious that, in the many years since Dostoievsky's death, the books written about him often do not mention the epilepsy at all, or simply deal with it in passing. This is understandable in light of the caution of literary and art critics in accepting explanations of the greatness of an artist on the basis of disease. Yet one must conclude that students of Dostoievsky have overlooked one of the most important influences on his work. There is as yet no adequate theory of genius, and discussions of the source of greatness, whether based on medical facts or on other aspects of an artist's life, have been inconclusive. Those who frequently see patients with temporal lobe epilepsy are familiar with the tendency of many of them toward hypergraphia, i.e., the production of extensive writings often of a philosophical or religious nature. Although these writings often reveal many of the same concerns and characteristics as found in Dostoievsky's creations, the great majority of them are of little or no literary worth. Epilepsy may help to account for the content, but it cannot explain genius.

On the other hand, the absolute or relative neglect of epilepsy in the hands of Dostoievsky's critics and biographers reflects a failing at a simple scholarly level. Whereas the sources of an author's compositions do not explain his or her genius, they are frequently of passionate interest to literary historians. One need only recall that an entire book was devoted to tracing the sources of Coleridge's poem "Kubla Khan." Since epilepsy is a central source of the themes, personalities, and events in the corpus of Dostoievsky's creations, it deserves far more consideration than it has been afforded in the past.

The importance of epilepsy transcends that of the other sources of Dostoievsky's production. In the hands of the untalented, the translation of the epileptic experience to the printed page fails to achieve literary greatness. However, epilepsy arising in the temporal lobe is of unique interest since the abnormal neural activity affects many of the structures in the nervous system that mediate human emotions. When this tragic disease is visited upon a man of genius, he is able to extract from it a depth of understanding that could be obtained from few other sources. The epilepsy of Dostoievsky and the asthma of Proust are not comparable. Each of these great writers suffered, and the suffering of each increased his understanding of human behavior. Dostoievsky's illness, however, enabled him to see some of the most primitive and powerful sources of human behavior. When Prince Myshkin realizes that the experience of epilepsy cannot be dismissed simply as manifestations of disease, he is speaking to the reader on behalf of his creator.

POSTSCRIPT

I am delighted to report that Professor James L. Rice of the Department of Russian at the University of Oregon has recently completed the most extensive study ever made of the accounts of epilepsy in Dostoievsky's personal papers and in his fiction. He has not only brought to his work a knowledge of the original Russian texts, but has also explored with great care the contemporary medical writings of the period. His work will stand as a landmark contribution to the literature on Dostoievsky, and should be read not only by students of literature but also by neurologists and psychiatrists.

REFERENCES

1. Alajouanine T: Dostoewski's epilepsy. *Brain* 86:209–218, 1963

2. Freud S: Dostoevsky and parricide, in *Standard Edition of Complete Psychological Works, Vol 21*. Edited by Strachey J. London, Hogarth Press, 1961, pp 177–194

Index

(Page numbers in **bold** type refer to tables in the text.)